Baroness Susan G Fellow at Lincoln Colleg ntist, writer, broadcaster and cr er in the House of Lords, she specialises in applying neuroscience to fundamental issues such as the impact of twenty-first-century technologies on the mind, how the brain generates consciousness, and the development of innovative approaches to neurodegenerative diseases such as Alzheimer's and Parkinson's.

She is the recipient of 31 honorary degrees from both British and foreign universities, and of many awards including Chevalier Legion d'Honneur from the French Government, and an Honorary Fellowship from the Royal College of Physicians, as well as being selected as Honorary Australian of the Year in 2006. She appears frequently on radio and television and frequently gives talks to both the public and private sectors.

By the same author

2121: A Tale from the Next Century

You and Me: The Neuroscience of Identity

ID: The Quest for Meaning in the 21st Century

Tomorrow's People: How 21st-Century Technology is Changing the Way We Think and Feel

The Private Life of the Brain

Brain Story: Unlocking Our Inner World of Emotions, Memories, Ideas and Desires

The Human Brain: a Guided Tour

Journey to the Centers of the Mind: Toward a Science of Consciousness

MIND CHANGE

How digital technologies are leaving their mark on our brains

SUSAN GREENFIELD

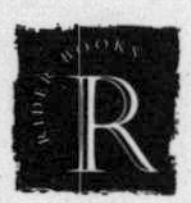

LONDON • SYDNEY • AUCKLAND • JOHANNESBURG

1 3 5 7 9 10 8 6 4 2

Rider, an imprint of Ebury Publishing,
20 Vauxhall Bridge Road,
London SW1V 2SA

Rider is part of the Penguin Random House group of companies
whose addresses can be found at global.penguinrandomhouse.com

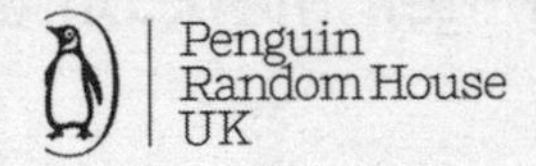

First published in Great Britain by Rider in 2014
This paperback edition first published in 2015

www.eburypublishing.co.uk

A CIP catalogue record for this book is
available from the British Library

ISBN 9781846044311

Printed and bound by CPI Group (UK) Ltd, Croydon CR0 4YY

Penguin Random House is committed to a sustainable future for our business, our readers and our planet. This book is made from Forest Stewardship Council® certified paper.

Copies are available at special rates for bulk orders. Contact the sales
development team on 020 7840 8487 for more information.

For John – invaluable friend,
mentor and colleague.

CONTENTS

PREFACE

The events leading up to the writing of *Mind Change* have been unfolding for the past five years, and arguably for much longer than that – perhaps unknowingly ever since I started neuroscience research and began to realise the power and vulnerability of the human brain. True, my main focus over several decades has been trying to uncover the basic neuronal mechanisms accountable for dementia, literally a loss of the mind; but even before I ever put on a white coat, it was the still broader and more general question of what might be the physical basis for the mind itself that held an utter fascination. Having made the rather unconventional journey to brain research from classics via philosophy, I was always interested in the big questions of whether we truly have free will, how the physical brain might generate the subjective experience of consciousness, and what makes every human being so unique.

Once in the lab, some aspects of these tantalising issues could be translated into specific questions that might be tested experimentally. Accordingly, over the years, we've researched the impact of a stimulating, interactive 'enriched' environment on brain processes, as well as the release and action of the versatile and hard-working chemical messenger dopamine, in turn linked to the subjective experiences of reward, pleasure and addiction. At a more applied level, we've investigated how the anti-ADHD (attention deficit hyperactivity disorder) drug Ritalin might have its effects, and how insights from neuroscience can contribute to improved performance in the classroom. Yet there has always been an underlying theme common to all these diverse areas of enquiry, including our research on neurodegenerative disorders: the theme has been novel brain mechanisms, how they might be inappropriate when activated in disease and, more generally, how these as yet under-appreciated neuronal processes enable each of us to adapt to our individual environment – to become individuals.

This wonderful *plasticity* of the human brain served as a natural segue into thinking about the future, and how upcoming generations might adapt to the very different, highly technological landscape of the decades to come. Accordingly, in 2003 I wrote *Tomorrow's People*, exploring the possible new kinds of environment and lifestyle that information technology, biotechnology and nanotechnology would in combination deliver. In turn, this very different, potential world led me to reflect more on the implications for identity. In 2007, these ideas were set out in *ID: The Quest for Meaning in the 21st Century*, which subsequently was to inspire a dystopic novel of the future (*2121*). In *ID*, I suggested that three broad options had historically presented themselves for self-expression. The *somebody* scenario of defining oneself via consumerism offered an individual identity without true fulfilment, while the *anyone* alternative of a collective identity resulted in the opposite: fulfilment which was subsumed into a wider impersonal narrative. Finally, there was the *nobody* possibility traditionally achieved with wine, women and song, where the sense of self is abnegated in favour of being a passive recipient of the incoming senses. When you have a 'sensational' time, I argued, you were no longer 'self'-conscious.

But might the supra-sensational digital technologies of the twenty-first century be shifting the balance, away from an occasional and contrived situation (drinking, fast-paced sports, dancing), in favour of the 'mind-blowing' scenario becoming more the default cognitive mode? These thoughts were in the background of my mind when, in February 2009, I had the chance to articulate them more clearly.

There was a debate in the House of Lords on the regulation of websites, particularly with regard to children's well-being and safety. If you sign up to speak at such an event, the convention is that you present an argument based on your own specific area of expertise. Since I knew nothing whatsoever about legislation and regulatory practice, I decided to present a perspective through the prism of neuroscience. The syllogism was quite straightforward and not particularly original. Any neuroscientist might well have said the same thing: firstly, the human brain adapts to the environment; secondly, the environment is changing in an unprecedented way; so thirdly, the brain may also be changing in an unprecedented way.

The reaction by the international print and broadcast media to this seemingly bland and logical argument was out of all proportion to its content. Needless to say, I had to endure the inevitable press misrepresentation resulting from a priority of selling copy over the actual truth: 'Baroness says computers rot the brain' was just one of the more lurid headline-grabbing efforts of one sub-editor. Meanwhile I was also told by journalists interviewing me, with the glee that people have for imparting bad news, how reviled I was by some quarters of the blogosphere, and asked how I felt about it.

My reaction was, and has been, that I'm happy to discuss the science prompting my ideas and, if trumped by hard facts, then wave the white flag. That is what scientists do: it's how we publish our peer-reviewed papers and it's how we develop theories. Most of us take professional criticism as the warp and weft of the research process. However, what was really interesting here was, in some cases, the apparent ferocity of the personalised animosity. Had I said the earth was flat, I doubt if anyone would have cared. Clearly I was touching a very raw nerve whereby some people felt threatened or in some way undermined. Until then, I hadn't realised just how important an issue this was for our society. I therefore continued to read more, to think and to speak in a wide range of forums about the brain of the future, indeed the future of the brain.

Then, on 5 December 2011, the House of Lords presented a further opportunity for more formal open discussion. I had the chance to introduce a debate to 'ask Her Majesty's Government what assessment they have made of the impact of digital technologies on the mind'. As you can imagine, securing parliamentary time in the historic red and gold chamber is not easy, and I felt very fortunate even to have been given the brief slot that is known as a 'Question for Short Debate'. Present at this debate was a range of representatives from diverse sectors such as business through to education and medicine.

Interestingly enough, most of the noble Lords seemed keen to emphasise the benefits of technology, and the general tone from the majority of those speaking gave the impression, on the whole, that there was no need for immediate concern. In his summing up, the Parliamentary Under Secretary of State for Schools, Lord Hill of Oareford, concluded that he was 'not aware of an extensive evidence base on negative impact from the sensible and proportionate use of technology', although, 'just as any technological revolution can lead to great progress, so it always also leads to unexpected problems, to which we must indeed always be alert'.

One of the drawbacks of the format of Questions for Short Debate is just that: time is short and, unlike lengthier slots of different types, the peer who has instigated the particular topic, as I had done on this occasion, is unable to reply to the ideas and conclusions that have been aired. Needless to say, if I had had the chance, I would have questioned the Minister on four basic points.

First, very little is currently being done by the UK government to promote research into the effects of screen culture on the young mind, or indeed the mind of any age. And if such an initiative were possible, it would be vital to know what kind of research, in what kind of areas, funded by just how much money, and over what period of time they were anticipating.

My second point would have been that, by definition, if technology is being used 'sensibly', in itself a subjective judgement, then it would be a paradox in terms if such 'sensible' practices had a significantly 'negative' impact. The whole point I had been trying to make was that technology is not necessarily being used in moderation and, as apparent from various surveys, has been estimated to be used for up to eleven hours a day: would this really qualify as 'proportionate'?

Moreover, my third point would have been that when we come to look at the various aspects of cyberculture, we'll see that there is indeed evidence for 'concern'. Yet this ministerial speech serves as a good example of a strategy popular not just with politicians and civil servants, but with anyone wanting a quiet life: prevarication while more evidence comes in, without any indication of just how much and what type of evidence would be convincing enough to launch wide consultation with policymakers, parents, teachers and indeed the taxpayer. So my fourth and final point would have been that the unspecified 'problems' mentioned by the Minister will be 'unexpected' only if we neither anticipate nor discuss them.

And just at that very moment, with the uncanny coincidences that can sometimes occur in life, I was approached by Random House to write this book. *Mind Change* could therefore be viewed in one sense as an answer to the Minister, but its main purpose is to meet the needs of a society that should be squaring up to take some active decisions and directions. In order to do so, it requires a balanced and comprehensive overview of the scientific research which, while it can never be exhaustive, covers the most significant findings – and that is what you will find in this book. It's worth noting, however, that one deliberate omission is the field of Internet pornography, where the controversy and debate are obviously not so much about whether it is 'good' or 'bad', or about how it impacts on types of thinking, but more about legislation and regulation, which are outside the scope of the journey here.

The main goal of *Mind Change* is to explore the different ways in which the digital technologies could be affecting not just thinking patterns and other cognitive skills, but lifestyle, culture and personal aspirations. Accordingly, in addition to coverage of the peer-reviewed scientific literature, you'll find discussion of the various goods and services that could be revealing a new type of mind-set, as well as commentaries and reports in the popular press that act as a mirror to the society in which we all live.

Discovering and collating such a wide range of diverse types of material would be, indeed *is*, extremely daunting. However, once again fate took a hand, and, at a beach party in Melbourne in December 2012, I was fortunate enough to meet Olivia Metcalf. Olivia had just finished a PhD on video games at the Australian National University in Canberra and was unsure of the path she wished to take. Amazingly, she was available and willing to help ensure that the manuscript, then in first draft, encompassed the wide range of research into digital technologies. Over the subsequent year, Olivia's contribution has been invaluable. Her scrutiny and critique of the work have truly raised the game of what *Mind Change* can offer: a real in-depth perspective of a highly complex and fast-moving field.

Some thirty-five years ago, while working in Paris, a colleague showed me the front page of a newspaper featuring a heavily bearded man in a sweater of dubious taste. 'He's from the green movement', he sneered, laughing at the individual as a weird eccentric. The idea of a 'green' movement certainly seemed strange to me, as did the phrase 'climate change'. Now this concept significantly impinges on much of public policy and influences individual lifestyle. *Mind Change* is so called because I suggest that there are similar parallels with climate change, albeit lagging behind by several decades: both are global, controversial, unprecedented and multifaceted. Yet while the challenges of climate change require exercises in damage limitation, *Mind Change* could open up the most exciting possibilities for twenty-first-century society to realise the full potential of each human mind as never before, if only we can discuss and plan what kind of world we want to live in or, more specifically, what kind of people we actually want to be.

A GLOBAL PHENOMENON 1

Let's enter a world unimaginable even a few decades ago, one like no other in human history. It's a two-dimensional world of only sight and sound, offering instant information, connected identity and the opportunity for here-and-now experiences so vivid and mesmerising that they can out-compete the dreary reality around us. It's a world teaming with so many facts and opinions that there will never be enough time to evaluate and understand even the smallest fraction of them. For an increasing number of its inhabitants, this virtual world can seem more immediate and significant than the smelly, tasty, touchy 3-D counterpart: it's a place of nagging anxiety or triumphant exhilaration as you are swept along in a social networking swirl of collective consciousness. It's a parallel world where you can be on the move in the real world, yet always hooked into an alternative time and place. The subsequent transformation of how we might all be living very soon is a vitally important issue, perhaps even *the* most important issue of our time.[1] Why? Because it may be that a daily existence revolving around the smartphone, iPad, laptop and Xbox is radically changing not just our everyday lifestyles, but also our identities and even our inner thoughts, in unprecedented ways.[2] As a neuroscientist, I'm fascinated by the potential effects of a screen-oriented daily existence on how we think and what we feel, and I want to explore how that exquisitely adaptable organ, the brain, may now be reacting to this novel environment, recently dubbed 'the digital wildfire'.[3]

In the developed world, there is now a one in three chance that children will live to 100 years of age.[4] Thanks to the advances of biomedicine we can anticipate longer and healthier lives and, thanks to technology, an existence increasingly freed from the daily domestic grind that characterised the lives of previous generations. Unlike so much of humanity in the past and still in many nightmare scenarios around the world, we take it as the norm and as our entitlement not to be hungry, cold, in pain or in constant fear for our lives. Unsurprisingly, therefore, there are many in our society who are convinced that we're doing just fine, that these digital technologies are not so much a raging wildfire but more of a welcoming hearth at the heart of our current lifestyles. Accordingly, various reassuring arguments are ready to hand to counter reservations and concerns that might otherwise be viewed as exaggerated, even hysterical.

One starting premise is that surely everyone has enough common sense to ensure that we don't let things get out of hand with a wholesale hijacking of daily life by the new cyberculture. We are sensible and responsible enough to self-regulate how much time we spend online, and to ensure that our children don't become completely obsessed by the screen. But the argument that we are automatically rational beings does not stand the test of history: when has 'common sense' ever automatically prevailed over easy, profitable or enjoyable possibilities? Just look at the persistence of hundreds of millions worldwide who still spend money on a habit which caused 100 million fatalities in the twentieth century and which, if present trends continue, promises up to 1 billion deaths in this century: smoking.[5] Not much common sense at work here.

Then again, the reliability of 'human nature' might work in our favour, if we could only assume that most of us were in some way protected by our innate genetic make-up to do the right thing, impervious to any corrupting external influences. Yet, in itself, this idea immediately runs counter to the superlative adaptability of the human brain which allows us to occupy more ecological niches than any other species on the planet. The Internet was initially created as a way for scientists to contact each other, and this invention spawned phenomena like 4chan,[6] allowing no-holds-barred self-expression as a new niche to which we may adapt, with consequences as extreme as the medium itself. If it is the hallmark of our species to thrive wherever we find ourselves, then the digital technologies could be in danger of bringing out the worst in 'human nature', not be rendered harmless by it.

Another way of dismissing out of hand the concerns that the effects of digital technology may bring is a kind of solipsistic stance, where the screen enthusiast proudly points to his or her own perfectly balanced existence, which combines the pleasures and advantages of cyberculture with life in three dimensions. Yet psychologists have been telling us for many years that such subjective introspection is an unreliable barometer of mental states.[7] In any case, and this should be obvious enough, just because a single individual may be able to achieve an ideal mix between the virtual and the real, it does not automatically mean that others are capable of exercising similar restraint and sound judgement. And even those individuals who think they've got everything just right will often admit in an off-guarded moment that 'It's easy to waste a lot of time on Facebook' or that they are 'addicted' to Twitter or that, yes, they do find it hard to concentrate enough to read a whole newspaper article. In the UK, the advent of *I*, an abbreviated version of the national quality paper *The Independent*, or the introduction on the BBC of the *90 Second News Update*, stands testimony to the demands of an ever larger constituency, not just the younger generation, of viewers and readers with a reduced attention span demanding a print and broadcast media to match.

Another consolation is the conviction that the next generation will work out just fine, thanks to the simple pragmatic default of parents taking control and intervening where necessary. Sadly, this idea has already proved to be a non-starter. For reasons we shall explore shortly, parents often complain that they cannot control what their offspring do online, and many already despair at their inability to prise them away from the screen and back into a world of three dimensions.

Marc Prensky, an American technologist, coined the term 'Digital Native' for someone defined by his or her perceived outlook and abilities, based on an automatic facility and familiarity with digital technologies.[8] By contrast, 'Digital Immigrants' are those of us who, according to Prensky, 'have adopted many aspects of the technology, but just like those who learn another language later in life, retain an "accent" because we still have one foot in the past'. It is unlikely that anyone reading these words will not have strong views, firstly, as to which side of the divide they themselves belong; and, secondly, as to whether in any event the distinction is cause for unalloyed celebration or deep anxiety. Generally speaking, it corresponds to age, although Prensky himself did not pinpoint a specific line of demarcation. The date of birth of the Digital Native seems therefore to be uncertain: we could even go back as far as the 1960s when the term 'computer' entered into common parlance or as late as 1990 when emailing, which started around 1993, would have become the default way of life by the time the young Digital Native could read and write.

The important distinction is that, today, Digital Natives know no way of life other than the culture of Internet, laptop and mobile: they can be freed from the constraints of local mores and hierarchical authority and, as autonomous citizens of the world, they will personalise screen-based activities and services while collaborating with, and contributing to, global social networks and information sources. But then a much gloomier portrait of the Digital Native is being painted by pundits like the British American author Andrew Keen:

> MySpace and Facebook are creating a youth culture of digital narcissism; open-source knowledge sharing sites like Wikipedia are undermining the authority of teachers in the classroom; the YouTube generation are more interested in self-expression than in learning about the world; the cacophony of anonymous blogs and user-generated content is deafening today's youth to the voices of informed experts.[9]

Then again, perhaps the Digital Native doesn't actually exist after all. Neil Selwyn from the Institute of Education in London argues that they are actually no different from preceding generations: they are not 'hard-wired' to have unprecedented brains.[10] Rather, many young people are using technology in a far more sporadic, passive, solitary and, above all, unspectacular way than the hype of the blogosphere and zealous proponents of cyberculture might have us believe.

Irrespective of whether the digital age has spawned a new type of superbeing or just ordinary humans better adapted to screen life, suffice it to say that, for the moment, parents are most likely to be Digital Immigrants and their children Digital Natives: the former are still learning the enormous potential of these technologies in adulthood, while the latter have known nothing else. This cultural divide often makes it hard for parents to know how best to approach situations that they intuitively perceive to be a problem, such as seemingly excessive time spent on computer-based activities; meanwhile children may feel misunderstood and impatient with views they regard as inappropriate and outdated for present-day life.

Although reports and surveys have focused largely on the next generation, the concerns I want to flag are not limited to the Digital Native alone. Far from it. But a generational divide has undoubtedly arisen from the vertiginous increase in the pace of ever smarter digital devices and applications. What will be the effects on each generation, and on the relationship between them?

In a 2011 report *Virtual Lives*, researchers for the UK children's charity Kidscape assessed the online activities of over 2,000 11- to 18-year-olds: just under half of the children questioned said they behaved differently online compared to their normal lives, with many claiming it made them feel more powerful and confident. One explained: 'It's easier to be who you want to be, because nobody knows you and if you don't like the situation you can just exit and it is over.' Another echoed this sentiment: 'You can say anything online. You can talk to people that you don't normally speak to and you can edit your pictures so you look better. It is as if you are a completely different person.' These findings, the report argues, 'suggest that children see cyberspace as detachable from the real world and as a place where they can explore parts of their behaviour and personality that they possibly would not show in real life. They seem unable to understand that actions online can have repercussions in the real world'.[11] The easy opportunity of alternative identity and the notion that actions don't have consequences have never previously featured in a child's development, and as such are posing unprecedented questions as to what might be for the best. While the brain is indeed not 'hard-wired' to interface effectively with screen technologies, it has evolved to respond with exquisite sensitivity to external influences – to the environment it inhabits. And the digital environment is getting ever more pervasive at an ever younger age. Recently Fisher-Price introduced a potty-training seat complete with iPad stand,[12] presumably to complement an infant lifestyle where the recliner in which the baby may spend many hours is also dominated by a screen.[13]

This is why the question of the impact of digital technologies is so very important. Hardened captains of industry or slick entrepreneurs will often sidle up in the coffee break at corporate events and let their professional mask slip as they recount in despair the obsessional fixation of their teenage son or daughter with the computer. But these anxieties remain unchannelled and unfocused. Where can these troubled parents share their experiences with others on a wider platform and articulate them in a formal and cogent way? At the moment, nowhere. In the following pages, we'll be looking at many studies on pre-teens as well as teenagers: unfortunately there are far fewer studies on adults, perhaps because they are less cohesive and identifiable as a group than a volunteer student body or a captive classroom. But, in any event, it's important to view the data *not* as a self-help guide for bringing up kids, but rather as a pivotal factor in the bigger picture of society as a whole.

Another argument sometimes used to dismiss any concerns about digital culture is the idea that, as long as appropriate regulation is in place, we'll muddle through. All too often this can be the mood music of professional policymakers and government ministers: there is no conclusive evidence for concern as yet. If and when there is, all the appropriate checks and balances will of course be duly put in place. In the meantime, as long as we are sensible and proportionate, we can enjoy and benefit from all the advantages of cyber life. Technology clearly brings us previously unimagined opportunities, and such advances will of course be balanced out by always being alert to potential negative impacts.[14] Yet, while moderation may well be the key, technology is *not* necessarily being used in moderation. Entertainment media use in the United States among the young is, on average, more than 53 hours per week.[15] When media multi-tasking, or using more than one medium at once, is taken into account, young people average nearly 11 hours' worth of entertainment media use per day: hardly moderate.

The deeper problem with regulation as the 'solution' is that it is always reactive, it has to be: otherwise how could rules and policies control something that hasn't yet happened? Regulatory procedures can only respond to, and then sweep up behind, some new event, discovery or phenomenon in order to eliminate clear harm, as with junk food or air pollution or, in the case of the Internet for example, the sexual grooming of children or their access to extreme violence. But regulation always has to play catch-up: the politicians and civil servants will always be leery about predictions because they are rightly aware they are spending taxpayers' or donors' money on what could be regarded as speculation. However much guidelines and laws may be needed for the obvious and immediate dangers of the cyber world, they are inadequate to the task of looking forward, of imagining the best uses to which new technologies can be put. For that you need long-term imagination and bold thinking, qualities not necessarily associated nowadays with cash-strapped civil servants or politicians with an eye to imminent re-election and easy wins in the short term. And so it is up to the rest of us. Technology can be empowering, and can help us shape more fulfilling lives, but only if we ourselves step up to the plate and help take on the task.

Digital technologies are eroding the age-old constraints of space and time. I'll always remember a speech by Bill Clinton that I attended in Aspen back in 2004, where he described how the history of civilisation could be marked by three stages: isolation, interaction and integration. 'Isolation' characterised the segregation of the remote empires of the past, access to which even until the last century was intermittent, time-consuming and hazardous. 'Interaction', as Clinton pointed out, proved then to be subsequently both positive in the form of trade, exchanges of ideas and so on, but also negative, with the increased facility and scale of warfare. But this century is perhaps exemplifying for the first time the realisation of a massive 'integration'.

And yet this idea, at least as a hypothetical scenario, is not that revolutionary. As long ago as 1950, the French philosopher and Jesuit priest Pierre Teilhard de Chardin developed the idea of globalised thought, an eventual scenario he dubbed the 'noosphere'.[16] According to Chardin, the noosphere would emerge through, and be composed of, the interaction of human minds. As humanity progressed into more complex social networks, so the noosphere would be elevated in awareness. Chardin saw the ultimate apotheosis of the noosphere as the Omega Point, the maximum level of complexity and consciousness towards which he believed the universe was evolving, with individuals still as distinct entities. Tempting as it is to believe that the digitally induced globalisation in instant thought sharing and worldwide communication is realising Chardin's vision, we cannot assume that this erstwhile hypothetical idea is now becoming our reality. What if one immediate outcome of global outreach and a correspondingly homogenised culture might be that we all start to react and behave in a more homogeneous style, one that eventually blurs cultural diversity and identity? Obviously, while there are huge advantages to understanding previously alien lifestyles and agendas, there is a big difference between a world enriched by other, contrasting ways of living and one that shares one standardised cookie-cutter existence. While diversity in societies brings great insights into the human condition, such comparisons mandate a clear and confident identity and lifestyle on which to base those comparisons. A mere global homogenisation of mind-set might in the long run have serious consequences for how we see ourselves and the societies in which we live.

While speed, efficiency and ubiquity must surely be good things, this new life of integration may have other, less beneficial effects that we need to think about. In days gone by we waited for the delivery of the post, at fixed times only two or three times a day. An international phone call was, for everyone other than the very rich, generally an option only for special or emergency circumstances. But we now take for granted the constant availability of international communication as readily as with the person in the neighbouring office or apartment. We tend to expect instant responses, and in turn assume we ourselves will reply immediately, oscillating incessantly between transmit and receive modes.

At a formal breakfast I attended recently where the main speaker was the British deputy prime minister, Nick Clegg, the woman sitting next to me was so busy tweeting that she was at a breakfast with Clegg that she wasn't actually listening to what he was saying. Twenty-four per cent of users of US adult social networking sites reported a curious phenomenon in 2012 – that they missed out on a key event or moment in their lives because they were so absorbed in updating their social networking site about that event or moment.[17] Alternatively, you can monitor the flood of consciousness of others, almost as a way of life. When I asked a colleague how often she used Twitter, she showed me an email from a friend that is not uncommon in what it describes: 'I have Twitter open on my PC all day so I look at it between calls, when on hold on the phone etc. I'd say pretty much our whole office does.'

We no longer need to wait, to acknowledge the passing of time between cause and effect, action and reaction. For most people who, a few decades ago, would never have contemplated foreign travel, or having a network of friends beyond the local community into which they were born, there are now non-stop thrilling opportunities for encompassing the entire planet. The advantages of this effortless communication are many. No one could make a convincing case for turning back the clock to when postal deliveries took days. But perhaps there is some merit in having time to reflect before responding to views or information. Perhaps there are benefits in pacing your day according to your own choice, at your own speed.

The crucial issue here is how we digest, internally, what is happening around us as we travel through each day: how we think, and the time required for thinking. Back in the 1960s, someone once said, 'Thinking is movement confined to the brain.' A movement is characterised by a chain of linked actions that take place in a particular order. The simplest example, walking, is a series of steps where placing one foot forward leads to the other foot overtaking, where one step thus leads to the next in a cause-effect chain that is not random. It is a fixed linear sequence. So it is with thought: there is a beginning, a middle and an end in a specified linear sequence in a cause-effect chain. Any thought, be it a fantasy, a memory, a logical argument, a business plan, a hope or a grievance all share this basic common characteristic of a fixed sequence. And since there is clearly a defined beginning, middle and end, there has to be a time-frame. As I see it, it is this idea of sequence that is the very quintessence of a thought, and it is the mental steps that are needed that will distinguish a *line* or *train* of thought from a one-off instantaneous emotion captured in a shriek of laughter or a scream. Unlike a raw feeling that occurs as a momentary reaction, the thought process transcends the here and now and links a past with a future.

Human beings are not alone in possessing sufficient memory to link a previous event, a cause, with a subsequent one, an event, and even to see a likely result in the future. A rat that receives a food pellet for pressing a bar, can soon 'think' about its next best move and learn to press the bar again. The link between stimulus and response has been forged. But we humans are unique in being able to link events, people and objects that are *not* physically present in front of us into a stream of thought. We have the ability to see one thing, including an abstract word, in terms of another. Unlike all other animals, and indeed infants, we have spoken and written language. We are liberated from the press of the moment around us because we can turn towards the past and then to the future by using symbols, words, to stand for things that are not in front of us: we can remember and plan and imagine. But it takes time to do so, and the more complex the thought, the more time we need to take the necessary mental steps.

But if you place a human brain, with its evolutionary mandate to adapt to its environment, in an environment where there is no obvious linear sequence, where facts can be accessed at random, where everything is reversible, where the gap between stimulus and response is minimal, and above all where time is short, then your train of thought could be derailed. Add in the sensory distractions of an all-encompassing and vivid audio-visual universe encouraging shorter spans for sustained attention, and you might become, as it were, a computer yourself: a system responding efficiently and processing information very well, but devoid of deeper thought.

Thirty or so years ago, the term 'climate change' meant little to most people; now it is understood by virtually everyone as an umbrella concept encompassing a wide variety of topics, be it carbon sequestration, alternative energy sources or water use, to cite just a few examples. Some feel that we're doomed, others that the different problems are exaggerated, and still others that science can help. Climate change is therefore not only global and unprecedented, but also multifaceted and controversial. When we turn to the question of how future generations will think and feel, 'Mind Change' can be an equally useful umbrella concept.

The argument underlying Mind Change therefore goes like this: the human brain will adapt to whatever environment in which it is placed; the cyber world of the twenty-first century is offering a new type of environment; the brain could therefore be changing in parallel, in correspondingly new ways. To the extent that we can begin to understand and anticipate these changes, positive or negative, we will be better able to navigate this new world. So let's probe further into how Mind Change, just like climate change, is not only *global*, as we've just seen, but also *unprecedented, controversial* and *multifaceted.*

2 UNPRECEDENTED TIMES

Humans adapt: it is what we do better than any other species. Accordingly, our predecessors have always had to embrace a changing world where new inventions and technologies have, in turn, driven lifestyles, insights, tastes and priorities. So why should this digital age be any different?

The automobile, for example, had vast, life-transforming effects. Using this kind of analogy, you could view digital devices as just the latest in a long line of innovation, exciting and disturbing at first, then ultimately incorporated into our lives as the driver of some newest development that will always have been hard for some traditionalists to accept. Take the printing press, whose introduction into Europe by Johannes Gutenberg around 1439 was undeniably a milestone in the progress of civilisation. It democratised knowledge and the reactionary forces of the *status quo* just didn't like it, just like, you might argue, those who seem to be techno Luddites nowadays. Books began to disseminate insight to ever greater numbers of individuals who then could, and did, foment social change, which led to personal advancement and universal education. Even fiction invariably raised issues about the human condition that enabled the reader to see the world through the eyes of others in other eras and locations, all the better to appreciate and shape one's own perspective and self-understanding: how could anything ever be more transformational?

Then there was electricity. Up to the end of the nineteenth century, night-time would have brought uncontrollable darkness: the only redress for our ancestors would have been candlelight to fend off whatever unknown perils, real or supernatural, might be lurking just beyond that feeble pool of light. The light itself would be flickering and casting shadows on the wall and that would have been the only reality. Our ancestors' experience of daily life would, for much of the time, be one of half-formed shapes, half-light and a helpless inability to control their surroundings. Imagine the cataclysmic difference when eventually that dark and sinister world was flooded with electric light: what kind of new thinking and mind-set might have occurred? Whatever it was, it was clearly a dramatic revision of reality, to which our species adapted, and which thereby changed us.

Let's move to a more recent development: television. From the time of its invention around the middle of the twentieth century, the concern was that television would be bad for children's brains, that they would get 'square eyes' and stop reading and playing outside. However, since television was broadcast only at limited times in the evening, and since there was at the time a dominant culture of outdoor games, reading and collective family meals, the TV, in fact, complemented an existing lifestyle rather than disrupting it. In one sense, rather than being an early forerunner to the home computer, the TV was more like the Victorian piano in being a means of cohesive family activity and interaction.

This is no nostalgia for the golden days gone by. The middle years of the twentieth century were physically uncomfortable and tough, and turning back the clock, even if it were in some way possible, is not an attractive proposition: who in their right mind would ever opt for an unheated bedroom with uncooperative layers of thin scratchy blankets. But they *were* different times. There was only one TV set to a household if you were lucky; at first, usually only one home in a street might boast of such a marvel, attracting endless visitors to share in the wonderment. And even into the 1960s, watching TV had a communal feel.

Nothing could have been further from the twenty-first-century scenario of a family member rushing in from work or school to sit for hours in voluntary solitary confinement in front of the screen. One of the big differences between the earlier technologies and the current digital counterparts is quantitative; the *amount* of time the screen monopolises our active and exclusive attention in a way that the book, the cinema, the radio and even the TV never have. The futurologist Richard Watson certainly thinks that the *degree* to which digital technologies are dominating our lives makes the crucial difference: 'We've always invented new things. We've always worried about new things and we've always moaned about younger generations. Surely most of (this) is conjecture mashed up with middle-aged technology angst? I think the answer to this is that it's a little different this time. (Screens) are becoming ubiquitous. They are becoming addictive. They are becoming prescribed.'[1]

It's not so much the physical ubiquity of screens that might now differentiate the appearance of the average home from its predecessors, but an invisible feature, inconceivable a decade ago, whereby family members can be constantly connected beyond the household more intimately than with the immediate family members with whom they live in close proximity. Each individual adult and child now owns multiple digital devices that they use for entertainment, socialisation and information.[2]

There is a push and pull, respectively, *towards* the cyberspace offered by, say, the isolation of the mobile device and/or the multifunctional bedroom and *away* from the erstwhile epicentre of the family. In the past, bedrooms were places of punishment to which you would be exiled for bad behaviour, and a far cry from the havens they are regarded by many young people today. The warm drawing room where the nuclear family sat together was the primary forum for interaction and information which provided a framework and a timetable for daily existence. Now the world of the screen in the bedroom, or anywhere, has in many cases offered an alternative context for setting the pace, setting standards and values, offering conversations and providing entertainment, while the nuclear familiar eating a meal together is becoming less central in the midst of more complex societal trends of divorce and remarriage, as well as more variable and demanding work patterns.

Beyond the all-pervasiveness of digital technologies compared to inventions from previous eras, another difference is the shift from technology as a means to its being an end in and of itself. A car gets you from place to place; a fridge keeps your food fresh; a book can help you learn about the real world and the people in it. But digital technology has the potential to become the end rather than the means: a lifestyle all on its own. Even though many will use the Internet to read, play music and learn as part of their lives in three dimensions, the digital world offers the possibility, even the temptation, of becoming a world unto itself. From socialising to shopping to working to learning and having fun, everything we do every day can now be done very differently in an indefinable parallel space. For the first time ever, life in front of a computer screen is threatening to out-compete real life.[3]

You wake. The first thing you do is check your smartphone (62% of us), and in all probability (79%), you'll be checking your phone within the first fifteen minutes of consciousness.[4] In 2013, 25 per cent of US smartphone users aged 18–44 could not recall a *single* occasion during which their smartphone was not within reach of them or in the same room. After waking, you grab a cup of coffee and a Danish while checking out emails that may have come in overnight as well as sending some yourself. Let's say your job enables you to work from home, as some 20 per cent of American professionals do:[5] you'll then get down to business. While you have your tasks up in front of you, you will also have Twitter open to follow your favourite celebrity and your Facebook page to ensure that you don't miss out on any news. You'd also need to keep checking your social network sites, such as Instagram updates or Snapchat, and taking quick photos of what you're having for lunch (time has flown), all at the same time as being on the alert for good old-fashioned text messages. Exhausted by all this multi-tasking while working, you then relax by watching a YouTube video that was rated with high views, or download the latest episode of a TV show. Next it's time to place your grocery order and have more serious retail therapy with some online shopping. In 2011, 71 per cent of adult US Internet users bought goods online[6] and the following year a comparable number, 87 per cent, of UK adults aged 25–44 were shopping online.[7] By 2017, online sales are projected to account for 10 per cent of all retail sales in the United States. Needing stimulation, excitement and escapism after it hits home how much money you've just spent, you'll then immerse yourself in a thrilling video game, just like some 58 per cent of all Americans.[8] But now you feel a bit isolated and in need of some company. So you check out social networking, but this time looking more closely at online dating sites. US Internet users spend 22.5 per cent of their online time on social networking sites or blogs.[9] More than a third of couples who married between 2005 and 2012 in the United States reported meeting their spouse online, with about half of these meeting in online dating sites, and the rest through other online sites such as social networking sites (SNS) and virtual worlds.[10] The real, physical world and what we do in it may be becoming less and less relevant, as traditional constraints of time and space are fading. And as each of us adapts to an unprecedented new dimension, what sort of individual might eventually emerge?

For certain, someone who is less attuned to the outdoors. Since 1970, the radius of activity for a child, namely the amount of space in which they freely wander around the area surrounding the home, has shrunk by an astonishing 90 per cent.[11] And this restriction on play is unprecedented. In his book *A History of Children's Play and Play Environments,* Dr Joe Frost traces the history of children's play from their early records in ancient Greece and Rome to the present time and concludes that 'Children in America have become less and less active, abandoning traditional outdoor play, work and other physical activity for sedentary, indoor virtual play, technology play or cyber playgrounds, coupled with diets of junk food. . . '.[12] The consequences of play deprivation and the abandonment of outdoor play may well become fundamental issues in the welfare of children. For example, they may no longer develop a realistic sense of risk, nor an imagination that allows them to suggest to their friends, as all previous generations have done, 'Let's make up a game . . .'

The content of a screen-based lifestyle is unprecedented in how it shapes thoughts and feelings, and also because of the corollary effects of *not* exercising and *not* playing and learning outside. While an increasing number of digital aficionados may eventually opt for mobile technologies exclusively, for the time being an appreciable amount of time is still spent sitting down in front of a computer screen. In any case, if we're busy texting on our mobile phones, or tweeting, even if we're out walking, we're still less likely to be taking more strenuous physical exercise than we may otherwise do. A clear corollary of a sedentary disposition is that we put on weight. Obesity stems from many factors, including the wrong kind and quantity of food, but also from reduced energy expenditure. It is hard to clarify a specific order of events: whether a child who doesn't much like sport will be more attracted to the screen, or a screen lifestyle has an allure that trumps climbing a tree, is a chicken-and-egg scenario that is impossible to resolve here. Rather, we need to look in the round at the whole digital lifestyle, both the increase in time spent in two dimensions and the simultaneous decrease in time spent in three.

For example, I recently received an email from a father of two young children in Australia which sums things up in a really arresting way:

> Last weekend I had an eye opening moment where the children had been lazing around the house, using and fighting over technology. When finally I was able to coerce them out for a short walk, we took bikes and I watched with delight the laughter and fun the kids had purely riding up and down this one particular steep-ish dog leg's bend on this quiet country road. The enjoyment, laughter and giggles from one's children is truly music to the ears of a parent. I do not ever hear that laughter when they are using technology.

A former teacher, Sue Palmer, flagged this issue back in 2007. Her book *Toxic Childhood* contained a list of simple activities that a child should have experienced before they reached adolescence, such as climb a tree, roll down a really big hill, skim a stone and run around in the rain.[13] How sad it is that these childhood activities, which would have been taken for granted a generation or so ago, should now be listed as identifiable goals that might otherwise not be achieved. Meanwhile, in a recent National Trust report, the term 'nature deficit disorder' was coined to articulate, not a genuine medical condition, but as a vivid expression of another endemic pattern of behaviour, indicating for the first time ever that we have become dissociated from the natural world with all its beauty, complexity and constant surprise.[14] Even the most diehard digital zealot cannot escape the simple fact that every hour spent in front of a screen, however wonderful, or even beneficial, is an hour spent *not* holding someone's hand or breathing in sea air. Perhaps even simply being at ease and happy in total silence could become a rarefied commodity that, instead of being a normal part of the human repertoire, will find itself on a wistful wish list of the future.

Professor Tanya Byron, a British psychologist best known for her work as a child therapist on television, was initially concerned specifically with regulation of the Internet: however, only two years later she recognised that the issue wasn't merely one of doing no harm, but of identifying the best possible environment beyond screen experiences: 'The less children play outdoors, the less they learn to cope with the risks and challenges they will go on to face as adults . . . Nothing can replace what children gain from the freedom and independence of thought they have when trying new things out in the open.'[15] In the past, play was most usually outside in fields and woods or in urban backstreets. Just look at the many books from the children's author Enid Blyton, written around the mid-twentieth century, where the young heroes and heroines were so busy catching smugglers and other shady villains that they only ever went indoors at mealtimes and to sleep.

At that time, in both fiction and fact, the environment in which you happened to be growing up provided a backdrop and props, not the actual narrative. The story came from inside your head – it had to – and arose from interaction with your friends as you became a cowboy or an Indian; and it was the same inside the home as plots were devised and story-lines emerged from playing with dolls or soldiers or dressing up. A tree never called out to be climbed, or a blank drawing pad demand that you paint in it. Dolls and soldiers, typically along with the cardboard boxes they may have come in, were the mere inanimate tools and prompts for *your* game, *your* story, *your* internally driven scenario above all for *your* imagination. Sometimes, even quite regularly, you might be bored. But it was that very state of under-stimulation that impelled you outside to play, or to stay inside to draw a picture or make up a game. The point I want to stress is that *you* were the driver and *you* would be in control of your own inner private world, your own inner reality.

But now the screen can be the driver. Admittedly you have to be mildly proactive in turning the device on and navigating your options, but, once you have selected an activity, spectacular cyber experiences contrived by someone else engulf you. You are now a passive recipient, and even though games like *Sims*, for example, allow you to modify and create worlds, it is always within the second-hand parameters of the game world designer's thinking. I wonder how much of the time that would previously have been spent walking in the fresh air, playing the piano or having a face-to-face conversation has now been forfeited in favour of a cyber activity, a completely new type of environment where taste, smell and touch are not stimulated, where we can be completely sedentary for long periods of time, yet where the ensuing experience trumps more traditional ways of life for appeal and excitement.

It would be simplistic in the extreme to think of the powerful and pervasive new digital lifestyle as either the apotheosis of human existence or the most toxic culture ever. We are being offered an unprecedented and complex cocktail of opportunity and threat, but then not everyone is likely to agree on exactly what constitutes which.

A CONTROVERSIAL ISSUE 3

The American journalist H. L. Mencken once quipped, 'There is always a well-known solution to every human problem - neat, plausible, and wrong.'[1] Agonising over whether digital technology is 'good' or 'bad' for the human mind is about as meaningless as arguing over whether a car is 'good' or 'bad'. But, nonetheless, debates on the complex issue of Mind Change are inevitable as they will question the way we live our lives and the kind of people we might end up being. Rather than adopt simplistic and entrenched stances of 'good' or 'bad', 'right' or 'wrong', we need first to see where the various battle lines are actually being drawn, and then how we might resolve any resultant conflict in understanding and expectation.

Inevitably the biggest controversy revolves around the basic question of evidence: how strong it is and what it's actually demonstrating. Two reports in particular, surveying the evidence over the last few years, have suggested a 'glass half-full' state of affairs. One was authored by psychologist Professor Tanya Byron in 2008 on the risks that children face from the Internet and video games.[2] Her report came to the unsurprising conclusion that 'the internet and video games are very popular with children and young people and offer a range of opportunities for fun, learning and development'. However, Byron had concerns over potentially inappropriate material, ranging for example from violent content, through to the behaviour of children in the digital world. She also drew attention to the notion that we shouldn't just be thinking about a child with a digital device in isolation, but should realise that the wider lifestyle picture is highly relevant, not least the child's relation to the parents.

The generational digital divide means that parents do not necessarily feel equipped to help their children in this unfamiliar space, which can lead to fear and a sense of helplessness. This sad state of affairs can be compounded by a wider risk-averse culture that is increasingly disposed to keep children indoors despite their developmental needs to socialise and take risks. While a risk-averse culture cannot by any means be the result exclusively of screen living, it obviously provides an attractive incentive and alternative for a child to be readily persuaded not to venture outside. Another uncontroversial point made by the Byron Report was that, while children are confident with the technology, they are still developing critical evaluation skills and need adult help to make wise decisions. In relation to the Internet we need 'a shared culture of responsibility'.

Byron's real emphasis has been on protection, but her report also touched on the wider issue of the empowerment of children: 'Children will be children pushing boundaries and taking risks. At a public swimming pool we have gates, put up signs, have lifeguards and shallow ends, but we also teach children how to swim.' All that said, for the time being, anyone reading the Byron Report would feel that there was no immediate need just now for any revolutionary, or even merely interceptive, action.

It was a similar story a little later in 2011, when neuroscientist Dr Paul Howard-Jones of Bristol University was commissioned to produce a 'state of the art review' on the impact of digital technologies on human well-being. Howard-Jones accordingly set about discussing what the field of neuroscience has established regarding the implications of using interactive technologies for impacting the brain, behaviours and attitudes of everyone, but emphasising the effects on children and adolescents specifically. After all, 'The vanguard of our advance into this new world is our children, and especially our teenagers. We know that the developing brain of a child is more plastic, and responds more malleably to experience than an adult's brain.'[3]

Commendably, Howard-Jones highlighted the need to understand the uses of technologies in a specific context rather than to label particular technologies, or technology, with a blanket description of 'good' or 'bad'. He also highlighted the findings that some technology-based training, such as computerised working memory tasks, can improve the working memory and that others can provide mental stimulation that slows cognitive decline, while some types of gaming can improve visual processing and motor response skills. However, his review also identified three potential risks for children, namely violent video games, the use of games and other technology leading to sleep problems, and excessive use of technology having a negative physical or mental impact or interfering with daily life. He went on to point out that any changes in the mind-set of the upcoming generations are, most crucially, anticipating changes in society as a whole - so the issues are relevant to all of us, whatever our age.

These snapshots from Byron and Howard-Jones depict an image of the Digital Native that is still currently blurred and uncertain, yet cautiously sanguine. Both reports leave at best an overall feeling of reserved optimism and at worst the usual academic-type conclusion that the jury is still out because 'more research is needed'. Both Byron and Howard-Jones paint an equivocal but generally positive picture of work in progress, so long as we are constantly alert to ever present dangers such as bullying, sexual grooming and violent gaming. Any concerns either author has are more to do with regulation. On the whole, the conclusions in both cases err on the side of the mildly positive with regard to learning, socialising and harnessing games to the benefit of mental functions. The glass is half-full, so long as everyone acts sensibly.

But such comforting assessments seem significantly outnumbered by voices from various professionals around the world who were not commissioned to provide a generalised snapshot of the current moment, but who deal with what happens when the use of digital technologies is *not* sensible. The glass then appears half-empty.

First, there's the perspective of experts from different relevant sectors, for instance those articulated in books such as *iDisorder* by clinician Larry Rosen[4] or *Alone Together* by the MIT psychologist Sherry Turkle,[5] who suggest that the more people are connected online, the more isolated they feel. In both cases, the concern is for when Internet use becomes obsessive. Perhaps surprisingly, captains of the digital industries themselves are also worried. Biz Stone, the co-founder of Twitter made headline news by stating at a conference: 'I like the kind of engagement where you go to the website and you leave because you've found what you are looking for or you found something very interesting and you learned something.'[6] The idea would be that you use Twitter to enhance the quality of your real life: but even he believes that using Twitter for hours at a time 'sounds unhealthy', presumably because his invention had become a lifestyle in itself. Then there's Eric Schmidt, the erstwhile CEO, now chair, of Google: 'I worry that the level of interrupt, the sort of overwhelming rapidity of information . . . is in fact affecting cognition. It is affecting deeper thinking. I still believe that sitting down and reading a book is the best way to really learn something. And I worry that we're losing that.'[7]

This worry is prescient in the light of what many neuroscientific and medical experts are voicing.[8] For example, neuroscientist Michael Mezernich, one of the pioneers in demonstrating the incredible adaptability of the nervous system, has concluded, in the typically restrained language required of his profession: 'There is thus a massive and unprecedented difference in how their [Digital Natives'] brains are plastically engaged in life compared with those of average individuals from earlier generations, and there is little question that the operational characteristics of the average modern brain substantially differ.'[9]

Educators are also voicing worries. In a 2012 report from 400 British teachers, three-quarters reported a significant decline in attention spans.[10] In the same year, a survey of over 2,000 US secondary school teachers showed that 87 per cent of teachers believed that digital technologies are creating an 'easily distracted generation with short attention spans', whereas 64 per cent agreed that they have more of a distracting than a beneficial effect on students academically.[11] The diversity of different professions expressing the drawbacks of digital devices was well illustrated in an open letter written in September 2011 to the respected British newspaper the *Daily Telegraph* and signed by 200 teachers, psychiatrists, neuroscientists and other related sectors expressing alarm over the 'erosion of childhood'.[12]

However, perhaps one of the most telling surveys has been to target cyber aficionados themselves: the Pew Research Center in the United States, along with Elon University, asked over 1,000 technology experts how the brains of 'millennials' (a term pretty much interchangeable with 'Digital Natives') will change by 2020 as a result of being so connected to online digital technologies.[13] These professionals were asked which of two predictions was the more likely for the immediate future, as articulated in two contrasting statements. One was extremely positive:

> Millennials in 2020 do not suffer notable cognitive shortcomings as they multitask and cycle quickly through personal- and work-related tasks. They learn more and are adept at finding answers to deep questions, in part because they can search effectively and access collective intelligence via the Internet. Changes in learning behaviour and cognition generally produce positive outcomes.

However, the more negative statement warned:

> Millennials in 2020 do not retain information; they spend most of their energy sharing short social messages, being entertained, and being distracted away from deep engagement with people and knowledge. They lack deep-thinking capabilities; they lack face-to-face social skills; they depend in unhealthy ways on the Internet and mobile devices to function.

The group of digital experts was actually split evenly on what they predicted for the future: but perhaps most tellingly, for those who went along with the positive prediction, many noted it was *more their hope than their best guess*. So even the 50 per cent or so of professionals who regard the screen culture in a favourable light overall do so, in many cases, from a stance of wishful thinking rather than of certainty or rational argument.

Further 'evidence' indicating that something might be going awry is perhaps every bit as compelling as expert opinion or epidemiological and experimental research: the very apps and websites that indicate clear trends in the tastes and proclivities of current society. One app, paradoxically called *Freedom*, will block your Internet access for an agreed amount of time each hour, while *SelfControl* will enable you to blacklist and be barred from websites that you feel you are following too slavishly but are helpless to resist. Zadie Smith, author of the acclaimed bestseller *White Teeth*, for instance, credits these two Internet applications in the acknowledgements section of her latest work.[14] Apparently she was struggling to maintain her concentration while writing her new book because of the diversions available just a click away on the Internet. So she was grateful to the apps for 'creating the time' in which she could write.

And Zadie Smith is not alone. The success of these flourishing enterprises obviously begs the question as to why they are doing so well: why should increasing numbers of people require some external service to stop them using the Internet, rather than just switching it off for themselves? As with junk food or cigarettes, we become addicted to the distraction of an external input which determines and shapes our actions, choices and thoughts. The existence of these apps in themselves does not mean that there's an epidemic of screen addiction, but it *does* imply that there are enough customers who experience these problems for the apps to be profit-making enterprises. We cannot ignore that even the platforms and users themselves implicitly acknowledge the clear effect that screen technologies are having on the mind-set of our society, namely, that they can become compulsive.

Another unprecedented feature of our current society is the lightning-speed dissemination of information. The hyper-connected blogosphere, unlike the equally swift satellite radio and television, reaches more people more quickly: the Pakistani citizen who unwittingly tweeted live updates of the raid on Osama bin Laden's house was able to access a large audience more quickly than any other form of media could get to the information. Yet, for precisely that reason, the blogosphere is the perfect medium for spreading misinformation relating to complex issues, or even for just oversimplifying them. Such is the concern of the World Economic Forum's Risk Response Network, which provides leaders from the private and public sectors with an independent platform to map, monitor and mitigate global risks. Its 2013 annual *Global Risks Report* analysed the perceived impact and likelihood of fifty prevalent global risks over a ten-year time horizon: among those listed are 'digital wildfires in a hyperconnected world'.[15]

I first joined the fray over the impact of digital technologies back in February 2009 with a speech in the House of Lords on the possible, unexpected effects on the human mind of social networking.[16] All I did was make the neuroscientific case for the well-accepted plasticity of the brain and point out that new types of screen experience would thus have a new type of impact on mental processes. The reaction, worldwide, was disproportionate to the tentative syllogism I was putting forward. While some seemed to agree with me, others were emphatic in insisting that there was 'no evidence' for what I was saying. Surely this would be an easy issue to resolve one way or the other? Not quite . . .

The problem with a simple negative argument is that *even if* there were no scientific findings at all to back up the argument, absence of evidence is not evidence of absence. In science, you can only conclusively establish with experiments that a finding is positively the case, never the reverse. After all, it might simply be that the test you are using isn't the most appropriate, or that the measuring instruments are not sensitive enough, or that the effects will be delayed or too immediate to fit the time window of your particular observation period. The point is that you cannot be conclusive, and you must therefore leave open the possibility that there is indeed an effect, albeit one that you haven't been able to detect. Thus it is impossible to demonstrate definitively that screen-based activities have no effect at all on the brain or behaviour, any more than I or anyone could prove definitively, to use an age-old example, that there is *not* a teapot in orbit around Mars.

This constraint poses a problem for both sides, since it is impossible to demonstrate just as conclusively that screen-based activities *are* having an unequivocal effect on the brain and consequent behaviour.[17] Let's assume a finding *is* reported of some definite effect, good or bad. Even then, in the evaluation of 'scientific' findings, a flock of swallows rarely make a summer and few single peer-reviewed papers, that gold-standard of professional probity, are viewed unanimously by all scientists as conclusive; it is normal practice for research to continue, and for interpretations to be revised as results accumulate. Interpretations of the evidence are inevitably subjective, with different scientists placing different emphases on different aspects or priorities within the experimental protocol. There is very rarely a Rubicon that, once crossed, means that a finding is universally accepted as 'the Truth'. Truth is always provisional in science, waiting for the next discovery to come along that could displace the current view or, as it would by then be disparagingly called, 'the current dogma'. When enough doubt accumulates to challenge this dogma, when accepted patterns of thought are straining to account for just too many anomalies or red herrings, the reappraisal of what is true amounts to a 'paradigm shift' - a concept Thomas Kuhn first introduced in 1962 in his now classic work, *The Structure of Scientific Revolutions*.[18]

A wonderful example of how scientists can stick rigidly to dogma and have closed minds to highly novel ideas is the revolution in the treatment of ulcers that developed in the 1990s. The hero of the story is an Australian physician, Barry Marshall. As part of his training, Marshall was working in a lab with another scientist, Robin Warren, studying bacteria. Contrary to accepted dogma, they found that a certain bacteria, *Helicobacter pylori*, could survive in a highly acidic environment, such as the stomach. Marshall and Warren started to doubt the well-accepted and established body of knowledge that ulcers were caused by excess acid, and thus were primarily the result of stress. What if ulcers were the result of bacterial infection instead? What would happen to the blockbuster drugs currently on the market for ulcers, but perhaps designed for the wrong biological target after all? The implications for the pharmaceutical industry, as well as for the medical establishment, were huge. 'Everyone was against me,' Marshall recalls.[19] For many years, good old unscientific prejudice delayed significantly the final acceptance of Marshall and Warren's theory. Starved of funding, but convinced of the merits of their theory, Marshall actually drank a glass of the medium containing the bacteria and duly gave himself an ulcer, which was cured by antibiotics. Vindicated at last, he and Warren won the Nobel Prize.

Even without the need to wait for a seismic paradigm shift, disagreement is fundamental to science: what one individual researcher will see as an exciting discovery, another may view as an epiphenomenon, while a cynic might regard it as unproven. It is not in the act of empirical observation, but in the consequent subjective evaluation, that there is most room for controversy and doubt. In all branches of science, the explanation that is formulated as scientists pore over the latest data is never ever conclusive. Any scientist writing the final 'Discussion' section of a paper for a peer-reviewed journal will invariably be tentative and provisional, always acting in the knowledge that not all potentially salient facts and factors are known. Scientists inhabit a hesitant world that is far from absolute but instead is conditional, and where doubt is as natural as breathing. So disagreement in science is normal and unavoidable if not necessarily understandable at first; but the flat refusal even to debate and to think about possibilities, as can happen with the question of screen technologies, is not.[20] The only realistic way forward is to plough through as many individual papers as possible that each tackle a specific issue and that collectively form a general overall picture.

In the case of cyber-induced long-term changes in the brain and resultant behaviour, we are faced with a complex situation, which is not readily disposed to a definitive litmus test or a single one-off smoking-gun experiment. What kind of evidence might one hope for, in a realistic and therefore constrained window of time, that could demonstrate to everyone's satisfaction that screen culture is inducing long-term transformations in wide-ranging phenomena as diverse as empathy, insight, understanding, identity and risk-taking? What single, one-off finding would it take for those who resist the possibility that there's any issue to accept that there just might be something amiss after all, or at least that we are missing opportunities?

Concepts such as Mind Change are, in Kuhn's terminology, 'paradigms', not specific single hypotheses that can be empirically tested in highly constrained and specific experiments. It is important not to confuse a hypothesis, which is always a statement that can be tested, with a generalised idea. An umbrella concept like Mind Change, as we're about to see, draws together threads from apparent societal trends and expert professional views, as well as a wide range of direct and indirect scientific findings from different disciplines in diverse scientific research papers. The majority of the scientific studies reported in the chapters to come will have been peer reviewed: this process ensures that they have demonstrated 'statistically significant' findings, which means that any differences reported are not subjective judgements but the results of a standardised and well-established system of testing.[21]

Irrespective of the different types of evidence that supports it, inevitably the notion of Mind Change as a new paradigm has set the hares running with allegations of scaremongering and inciting moral panic. But bear in mind that scaremongering is predicated on the notion that there is really nothing to be scared of in the first place. Do we in fact know that this is the case? However, if and when the validity of the scare is irrefutably demonstrated, then the scare is no longer a scare at all but turns into an established danger. So now the original prediction would actually have been something very different, a wake-up call. Dismissal on the grounds of scaremongering should be, if anything, a final conclusion and not an opening gambit.

As for moral panic, perhaps any criticism of the digital world could be interpreted mistakenly by cyber aficionados as an attack on their personal lifestyle, and therefore ultimately on them as individuals. But there is no need to panic at the moment: quite the reverse. If we allow ourselves the opportunity, we have the chance to examine and take stock of where we are and where we wish to go, and to work out how to get there in terms of what we want the twenty-first-century lifestyle and society to look like. But in order to do that we need to first unpack the various very different issues that Mind Change embraces.

A MULTIFACETED PHENOMENON 4

Climate change, according to the Intergovernmental Panel on Climate Change (IPCC), 'may be due to natural internal processes or external forcings, and/or to persistent anthropogenic changes in the composition of the atmosphere or in land use.'[1] Nobody could dispute that there's a multitude of issues here: so it is with Mind Change, which I'm suggesting is comparably multifaceted, throwing up a range of different questions that need to be explored independently. These different questions fall into three main and yet very different areas, worth previewing here: social networking and the implications for identity and relationships; video gaming and the implications for attention, addiction and aggression; and, finally, search engines and the implications for learning and memory.

In no particular order of priority, let's start with social networking. A recent radio programme on the BBC featured 'Kaylan', an 18-year-old young man who had decided to take advantage of the opportunity offered by Facebook as of September 2011 to remove all privacy settings on his page so that any number of followers could track his daily life in the public domain: he boasted at the time of broadcasting to some 100,000 followers. Kaylan also admitted he had done nothing at all to deserve fame. His posts were often mundane photos of himself throughout the day leading a 'crazy life'.

So what was it that was so attractive to his followers? Well, there were a whole bunch of similar folk like him who could create arguments with each other, have bust-ups and leak photos. Then the followers could take sides. Yes, Kaylan had his fair share of 'haters'. After all, he added, 'You can't be nice on Facebook.' By saying unpleasant things, these haters would then garner maximum praise and 'fame' themselves. What kind of things might they say which met with such approval? The majority would say, 'Kill yourself'. While Kaylan is obviously very far from being a typical Facebook user, both he and his 100,000 followers serve as an example of the unprecedented extremes to which the facility can be used. Your importance as revealed by social networking activity can even now be quantified.[2]

Even in the far less dramatic cases of the majority of Facebook users, if you haven't rehearsed the basic non-verbal communication skills of eye contact, voice modulation, body language perception and, above all, physical contact, you'll not be particularly good at them. And if so, it will be harder for you to empathise with others. In a Pew Research Center survey of US social networking among an adolescent cohort aged 12–19, data indicated that they overwhelmingly chose negative rather than positive adjectives to describe how people act on social networking sites, including 'rude, fake, crude, over-dramatic and disrespectful'.[3] For example, one middle school girl respondent commented: 'I think people get, like when they get on Facebook, they get ruthless, stuff like that . . . They act different in school and stuff like that, but when they get online they're like a totally different person, you get a lot of confidence.' Another girl said: 'That's what a lot of people do. Like they won't say it to your face, but they will write it online.'

A recent meta-analysis looking at data collected over thirty years from 14,000 US college students indicates that overall levels of empathy may be declining, with an especially steep drop in the last ten years – a time-frame that corresponds well with the advent of social networking among Digital Natives.[4] Of course a correlation is not a causal link, as the tobacco companies back in the 1950s were keen to point out: but this is just the type of close correspondence that should serve as a starting point for rigorous epidemiology to establish whether there might be a direct causal link between screen time and a reduction in empathy. We should also be asking why those who already have problems empathising - individuals with autistic spectrum disorder for example - are particularly comfortable in the cyber world. And, more generally, could this sanitised and limited type of interaction account for the ease with which bullying, always a dark part of human nature, has now found unconstrained expression in the cyber world?

Over a billion people in the world use Facebook to keep in touch with friends, share pictures and film clips, and post regular updates of their movements and thoughts.[5] Another estimate is 12 per cent of the entire global population, with 50 per cent of North Americans, 38 per cent of Antipodeans, 29 per cent of Europeans and 28 per cent of Latin Americans all signed up.[6] Remember that these numbers are percentages of total societies and therefore do not exclude newborn babies, the severely infirm or older people with a prohibitive lifestyle resulting in no computer access: so the proportion of potential users is probably far higher still. A further 200 million actively use Twitter, the 'micro-blogging' service that lets users circulate short messages about themselves, post pictures and follow in momentary minutiae the stream of consciousness or daily routines of others.[7]

Nowadays, all generations are represented on the sites, with octogenarians who may now live on their own able to stay in touch with their grandchildren, but it is the Digital Natives that are the most avid users. In the United Kingdom, 64 per cent of adult Internet users aged 16 and over are social network site users, whereas 92 per cent of those aged 16–24 who use the Internet have profiled themselves on a social networking site.[8] In the United States, 80 per cent of online teens aged 12–17 use social networking sites, mostly Facebook and Myspace.[9] US users have on average 262 friends,[10] a figure higher than the world average of roughly 140 friends.[11] Twelve- to 24-year-old Facebook users have, on average, over 500 Facebook friends.[12] Roughly 22 per cent are from high school, 12 per cent are immediate family, 10 per cent are co-workers, 9 per cent are from college and 10 per cent of friends have never been met in person or only been met once.[13]

On an average day, 26 per cent of users 'like' a friend's status, 22 per cent comment on a friend's status whilst only 15 per cent update their own status.[14] So more people spend the time interacting with other users' content rather than posting their own. All of which points to a blindingly obvious truth: social networking has become a central factor in the culture of all but the very poorest and most deprived regions in the world, or the most ideologically repressed. A critical question then is, quite simply, what is so special about social networking? What is the basic need that this new culture is meeting in an apparently unprecedented and yet effective way? If we are to understand and appreciate the changing mind of the mid-twenty-first century, this is one of the most important questions to ask.

The benefits of social networking seem irrefutable: direct marketing to the consumer, dating sites, career building, contact with old friends. Being 'connected' is often pronounced with an enthusiasm that automatically assumes it is a desirable scenario. But what worries me is whether this almost incessant communication through the screen might have a downside as well. As always, there's the key issue of being 'sensible':

while social networking sites could provide harmless fun and complement real friendships, if used excessively or to the exclusion of real relationships, they might perhaps impact in a very fundamental and unforeseen way on how you view your friends, friendship and, ultimately, yourself.

If you're increasingly anchored in the present and consequently devoting all your time to the demands of the outside world, a robust sense of inner identity might be harder to sustain. Perhaps the constant accessing of social networking sites will mean living a life where the mere thrill of reporting and of receiving information completely trumps the ongoing experience itself – a life where checking in at a restaurant, posting pictures of a meal and yearning for 'likes' and 'comments' generates more excitement than the occasion of dining out itself. The momentary exhilaration you'd be feeling would shift from being generated by a first-hand life experience itself towards the slightly delayed indirect experience of the continuing reaction and approval of everyone else. If we're going to be living in a world where face-to-face interaction, unpractised as it might become, is thereby uncomfortable, then the 'push' of such an aversion to messy real-life, three-dimensional communication, combined with the 'pull' of the appeal of a more collective identity of external reassurance and approval, may be transforming the very nature of personal relationships themselves. The knee-jerk speed required for reaction and the reduced time for reflection might mean that those reactions and evaluations themselves are becoming increasingly superficial: already, people are using phrases like 'kill yourself' and 'hater' on Facebook in a context that conveys far less depth of real feeling and of individual background history than these terms would previously have implied.

Already privacy appears to be a less prized commodity: among 13–17-year-old US youths, more than half have given out personal information to someone they don't know, including photos and physical descriptions.[15] Meanwhile, Digital Natives post personal information on their Facebook page that is typically shared with over 500 'friends' at a time, fully aware that each of these friends could then pass on that information to further hundreds in *their* networks.

It has become more important to have attention, to be 'famous'. The trade-off for such disclosure and indeed fame is, and always has been, as the mid-twentieth-century film star Greta Garbo famously exemplified, loss of privacy. So why is it that the privacy we so treasured previously we now hold in increasingly casual disregard? Until now, privacy has been the other side of the coin to our identity. We have seen ourselves as individual entities, in contact with the outside world, yet distinct from it. We interact with that outside world, but only in a way and at the times we choose. We have secrets, memories and hopes to which no one else has automatic access, a *secret* life, distinct from a *professional* one, and even more intimate than a *private* life of individual friendships where we vary what and how much we confide to others. This 'secret' life is a kind of inner narrative that, until now, has provided each individual with their own way of linking past, present and future so that they have an ongoing subjective, internal commentary that meshes past memories and future hopes with the happenstance of each day. Now, for the first time, this secret story-line is being opened up to the outside world, to an external audience that can be uncaringly capricious and judgemental in its reaction. A particular identity is therefore no longer an internal, subjective experience, but is constructed externally and therefore is much less robust and more volatile, as has already been suggested in a recent report to the British government on 'future identities'.[16]

A second cornerstone of the digital lifestyle is video gaming. In the mid-1980s, children might have spent about four hours a week on average playing video games at home and in arcades.[17] But spool on a decade or so and the video game has become an integral part of the home scene and beyond.[18]

A 2012 study of adolescents from a US high school reported that 10–13-year-old boys were playing video games on average a staggering *43 hours a week* although, admittedly, the number of subjects was fairly small, 184.[19] Yet, even conservative estimates (from 2009) indicate that the average US 8–18-year-old is spending 73 minutes a day recreationally in this one screen-based activity, up from 23 minutes in 1999.[20] That means at least an hour a day spent not interacting with the real world, and in particular not studying. In a survey of US youth aged between 10 and 19, gamers spent 30 per cent less time reading and 34 per cent less time doing homework.[21] Granted, it is hard to separate the chicken from the egg: perhaps children who perform more poorly at school are likely to spend more time playing games, which may give them a sense of mastery that eludes them in the classroom. We need to go beyond correlation to cause: but what we can't do is just ignore the issue altogether.

Video games open up fertile territory for controversy. On the one hand, there are clear positives, as we'll explore in detail later: for example, improved sensorimotor coordination and perceptual learning. On the other hand, various and many stories around the world can paint a terrible picture of a modern lifestyle of overindulgence in the unfettered fun of playing video games. For example in Taiwan in February 2012 Chen, a 23-year-old man, was found dead in an Internet cafe after 23 hours of continuous gaming.[22] Another young man aged 18 in Taiwan died in July 2012 after 40 hours of continuous gaming.[23] Then there was the report of two parents neglecting their own real baby, who subsequently died, in order to raise an online virtual baby.[24]

In December 2010 a man in the north of England received a life sentence after killing a toddler immediately after losing in a violent video game.[25] Then there was the case of a gamer who hunted down his virtual opponent in real life and stabbed him as revenge for being stabbed in a game,[26] not to mention the list of high-profile suicides of gamers.

The immediate defence of a gaming fan would probably be that (1) this is all scaremongering and unlikely to be true; (2) it is unlikely to be the whole story, with other more important factors really to blame or to mitigate the circumstances; or (3) these examples, horrendous though they may be, are isolated cases that are actually extremely rare. All of these possibilities are not mutually exclusive and may indeed be the case, but they should be conclusions, not starting premises. Moreover, even if such stories are exaggerated and uncommon, they may still be important as caricature scenarios of certain prevailing trends now emanating from society, albeit in a much milder form: a profile of addiction, aggression, impulsivity and recklessness.

In modern video games, the gamer enters a visually rich world where they can assume a character completely unlike themselves, or in some games create a character (avatar) in whatever way they desire. They navigate these fictional beings through situations involving moral choices, violence/aggression and role-playing, with intricate reward systems built into the games that provide the incentive to carry on living out the fantasy. Some individuals can become so immersed that they lose track of the real world and time; they report that they turn into their avatars when they load the game, and become their characters. Alternatively, gamers may develop an emotional attachment to their character. So how are these highly stimulating, often violent games with possible addictive qualities, actually affecting us?

One outcome could be enhanced aggression. Experimental studies are revealing that violent video games lead to increases in aggressive behaviour and aggressive thinking accompanied by decreases in prosocial behaviour.[27] It seems that video-game-induced aggression is directly caused not only by immediate provocation, but also by more indirect biological predispositions and environmental influences, as an individual gradually develops a more adversarial world view. Although violent games have not been proven to be directly the reason for immediate criminally violent behaviour, there is strong evidence that playing them may increase the type of low-grade hostility that happens every day in school or office corridors.

It may also be that video games lead to excessive recklessness. In one recent investigation using brain imaging, the key finding was of an enlargement of a specific area of the brain typically seen in the brains of compulsive gamblers.[28] Most intriguing of all is that a substance (dopamine) is released from this particular brain region (the nucleus accumbens) that is a key chemical messenger enhanced by all addictive psychoactive drugs. These chemical similarities between the brains of gamers and gamblers do not prove that gaming is technically addictive, but nonetheless both may well share a further feature: recklessness. After all, it is a dangerous lesson to learn that death lasts only until the next round, that actions don't have consequences, even when they subsequently occur in the real world.

The crucial factor once again will be whether an individual is being, in the minister's words in our House of Lords debate back in 2011, 'sensible and proportionate', and how much they indulge in playing games. It's a bit like eating chocolate: the occasional treat in an otherwise balanced diet is relatively harmless and enjoyable, whereas an unremitting daily diet exclusively of chocolate would have dire consequences. The problem is not with those who might play games occasionally as a pastime in a portfolio of other interests and activities in the real world, but the number of frequent gamers who, from the number of hours they spend on gaming to the exclusion of all else, end up being obsessional or compulsively hooked.

Finally, in addition to social networking and video gaming, there's a third aspect to Mind Change: surfing the Internet, particularly with search engines. If you are not using digital technologies interactively to engage in a relationship or to play a game, then the screen can still have intoxicating appeal as a one-way street, simply in what it can tell and show you – some might go so far as to say teach you. It's almost unbelievable that this essential facility started less than 20 years ago, in 1994, when Yahoo! was created by Stanford University students Jerry Wang and David Filo in a campus trailer, originally as an Internet bookmark list and directory of interesting sites. Then, in 1996, Sergey Brin and Larry Page, also two Stanford University students, tested Backrub, a new search engine which ranked sites according to relevance and popularity. Backrub was destined to become Google, which currently has around 80 per cent of the global market share in search while their nearest competitors are in single figures.[29] The brand name has become a verb: almost everyone 'googles'.

Sometimes, for no obvious reason in particular, seemingly pointless activities draw crowds, such as striking a funny pose, 'planking' or performing a little dance like the Harlem Shake. I have my own direct experience of how powerful such viral phenomena can be. Back in April 2010 I was being interviewed by Alice Thomson of *The Times* about the impact of digital technology on how we feel and think. We had progressed to discussing how the fast-paced technology might mandate correspondingly fast, knee-jerk views and reactions. Summarising in the (as ever) much sought-after journalistic sound bite, I suggested the prospect of humans reduced to simple positive or negative gut reactions 'Yuck' or 'Wow' to whatever flashed up on the screen. Because I tend to talk quickly, Alice misheard and transcribed what I'd said as 'Yaka-Wow'. This may be amusing enough in itself, but the point is that, in just twenty-four hours, this simple nonsense term captured the imagination of some 75,000 people on Google. Moreover, someone took out the domain name and soon I was astonished to see mugs and T-shirts sporting YAKA-WOW. On one website, the First Church of the Yaka-Wow welcomed 'breezy people to a world of no consequences'. The term had gone viral with an outreach and repercussions within a time-frame that would have been unthinkable only a decade or so earlier.

So what is the potential of digital technologies to help everyone, of any age, to learn things, anything, in the broadest sense of the term? Presumably, when people surf they are feeding in, if not formal questions, then at least specific terms or names, and receiving relevant information in response. They are 'learning'. The dictionary defines learning as 'the act or process of acquiring knowledge or skill'. The current digital technology may well enhance, or then again jeopardise, this ancient, superlative human talent, but we need to unpack the various different issues at stake. The appeal of the surfing experience, the differences between silicon and paper, the educational value of digital technologies and, above all, access to an infinite amount of information, all impact as different and unprecedented factors to shape our thought processes.

Search engines are now part of our lives, and for many they are the immediate and obvious first stop for finding out a fact or learning more about a subject. So screens could shape our cognitive skills in a fundamentally new way. Surely one of the most important issues to explore, for the next generation, is whether they might be learning very differently compared to their predecessors who used books. The most obvious difference is a tactile one, for paper can be thin, light, porous and opaque, and as such allow activities such as grasping, carrying, folding, writing and so on. That being so, how might the pleasures of reading on a screen match up to those of paper? Flicking pages back and forth, highlighting sentences and scribbling in the margin may all be positive features that contribute to the absorption of what you are reading, so the potential for personal interaction with a paper book may be greater than with a screen.

Anne Mangen at the University of Oslo explored the importance of actually touching paper, by comparing the performance of readers of paper to that of readers of the screen. Her investigation indicated that reading on a computer screen entails various different strategies, from browsing to simple word detection, that together lead to poorer reading comprehension in contrast to reading the same texts on paper.[30] Moreover, apart from the physical features of the printed page compared to the pixelated one, there is the additional feature of the screen that the book can never have: hypertext. Above all, a hypertext connection is not one that you have made yourself and it will not necessarily have a place in your own unique conceptual framework. Therefore it may not help you understand and digest what you're reading at your own appropriate pace, and it may even distract you.

But the whole point of screens is not that they can simply serve as substitute books. A still deeper issue is how computers and iPads can also provide information in an utterly different, non-verbal way, and thereby perhaps actually transform how we think. If inputs arrive in the brain as images and pictures rather than as words, might it, by default, predispose the recipient to view things more literally rather than in abstract terms?

These, then, are the ever more invasive and pervasive technologies that have the power to transform not just what, but how, we think. Yet Mind Change involves more than innovative gadgetry: just as critical is the mind that is to be changed. It is the growth and connections between the brain cells we are born with that will turn us into the unique beings we are, with brains capable of individual and original thought. There are many talents we as a species lack: we don't run particularly fast or see particularly well, nor are we particularly strong compared to others in the animal kingdom. But our brains have the superlative talent to adapt to any environment into which we are placed, a process known as 'plasticity'. As we make our personal, idiosyncratic way through life, so we develop our own particular perspective as a consequence of these personalised connections in our brains and it's this unique pattern of connectivity that I'd like to suggest amounts to an individual 'mind'. So, in order to appreciate the impact of these global, unprecedented, controversial and multifaceted technologies on the twenty-first-century human mind, we need next to look through the prism of neuroscience.

5 HOW THE BRAIN WORKS

How could an experience, screen-based or otherwise, literally leave its mark on a sludgy brain? If we neuroscientists are to contribute anything significant at all to appreciating the effects of the digital lifestyle on our mental processing, then it's by pointing out the actual physical neuronal mechanisms at work: we should be able to demonstrate the causal link between exposure to certain environments and experiences, and ensuing thoughts and behaviour. By understanding as much as possible about how the brain works, we'll be able to get a much more accurate picture as to how, and to what extent, screen technologies could be transformational.

The big challenge for neuroscience has always been to make the intellectual leap between a bit of brain tissue and a thought, an emotion, indeed even a dream, in both senses of the word: the literal phenomenon of that bizarre inner world that unfolds during sleep, as well as the metaphor for planning wonderful outcomes for our lives. It's a journey we'll need to make in three steps: firstly, to find out how the brain itself works; secondly, to discover how it changes throughout life; and, thirdly, to see how these changes in the brain could amount to the 'mind'. Yet it's far from obvious even where to start.

'So how *does* the brain work then?' The little girl in front of me, probably about 11 years old, was insistent. Surely it was simply because I had run out of time in my one-hour talk to her group of school children that I had omitted to clear up this final, trivial question. We had looked at the brain from all angles by taking apart a plastic model. I had told my young audience about the time when I had been a student myself and had held a real human brain in my hands and, because brain tissue is nothing like the hard, bright pink plastic model, but is creamy white, soft and fragile, I had pondered on what would have happened if some of it got caught under my fingernail. Can a memory or an emotion dislodge under a fingernail? Could a bit of brain tissue that somehow related to a particular habit, say, biting your fingernails, actually end up adrift *under* a fingernail? How is the experience of being you, of seeing the world in a way no one else can share first-hand, generated by this unappealing and uncooperative mass that you can cup in one hand?

No model brain, nor indeed its real-life counterpart, offers any obvious starting point. There are no conspicuous moving parts, as there are for the heart or the lungs, that indicate what is going on. All you can do by looking at the brain is appreciate how, on the macro-scale, it is put together. You'll see that there are ever enveloping layers around the top of the spinal cord as it swells out into the most basic part.[1] From there evolution has added further compartments and easily discernible structures, brain 'regions' that vary in size and importance according to the species. But the theme is the same for all mammals: whether you're looking at the brain of a rat or of a human, you'll always see, for example, a small cauliflower-like growth coming out from the back of the brain just above the spinal cord.[2] You'll also always see the two hemispheres that jam against each other like two fists with their outer covering wrapping round like bark wraps around a tree, the cortex (Latin for bark).[3]

The surface area of the cortex has expanded in humans to such an extent that accommodating such vast amounts of brain in the confines of the skull would be like accommodating a sheet of paper in a tight fist: you would have to crumple the paper up. In a sense, and so long as we don't stretch the analogy too far, this is what evolution has done: the surface of the human brain is as wrinkled as a walnut, that of the other primates less so, that of cats and dogs even less still, and the cortex of rodents not at all. This all-enveloping thin outer layer is perhaps the most fascinating and enigmatic. In evolutionary terms, it is the newest part of the brain and, perhaps not surprisingly, the most prominent in humans - the species with the greatest intellectual capacity - so the cortex will feature more than any other brain area as we explore the impact on thinking of the digital technologies.

To get an idea of how the brain is put together, think of a busy metropolis like New York City: the anatomically distinct brain regions would correspond to boroughs, within which would be districts and then neighbourhoods - in brain terms, smaller and smaller groups of cells. By the time we arrive at a block, a street or a line of houses, we are at the basic unit of neuronal communication: the individual gap (the synapse) between any one brain cell and another. And the house on the street? That would be the neuron itself, the rooms within it the organelles, literally the little organs that keep a single brain cell alive, just like any generic cell in the body. While this metaphor may convey the nested hierarchy of the anatomy of the brain areas, the extrapolation can go no further: it is simply a static snapshot of how the physical brain is built up.

In my talk to the young students, I had prised the plastic model apart and shown them all the different and easily discernible regions beneath, how they intertwined around each other, just as I had first seen in the real post-mortem brain so long ago in the dissecting room of the Oxford University Anatomy Department. But would that answer satisfy the little girl standing in front of me, eyes like saucers, impatient for me to tell her in a sentence how the brain 'worked'? The problem is that brain cells are less analogous to fixed structures like bricks and houses, which don't actually do anything, and more comparable to people, their highly dynamic inhabitants. What we really need, therefore, is an image, some kind of scenario that not only describes how the brain is constructed anatomically from the building blocks, the brain cells, but how they then actually function.

Neurons are the basic units of the brain, just as a person is the basic unit of an organisation or a society. Like a person, a neuron is generic, and yet at the same time an individual entity. A person changes gradually over time, and a neuron will also adapt, show plasticity. A neuron gradually makes connections via a small gap (a synapse) using an intermediary, a chemical messenger (a transmitter); actual direct physical contact is possible but features less. Similarly, a person gradually builds relations with others by indirect contact via a language; touching is rarer. With both chemical messengers and languages there's enormous diversity but an adherence to the same common principle: communication between two independent entities without any direct physical connection. Both languages and transmitters come in a wide range of varieties, but they can be categorised into families, defined by geographical provenance (for language) or chemical structure (for a transmitter) respectively. The actual mode of communication in both cases has parallels in that all languages and transmitters can use simple signals through to complex and sophisticated ones. In the most basic scenario, a neuron can signal via its transmitter a simple 'yes' or 'no', which translates into a momentary inhibition or excitation of the activity of the target brain cell.

When a brain cell 'speaks', or more technically, is 'active', it generates a small electrical blip[4] lasting a thousandth of a second (a millisecond) which then zooms down to the end of the cell[5] to communicate with the next neuron. But then there's a problem: there's a gap between one cell and the next, the synapse. Once there, the electrical message can go no further. But all is not lost: the arrival of the blip then acts as a trigger for the tip of the cell to release its chemical messenger, which is then able to travel across the synapse as readily as words travel through air. Once it reaches its destination, on the next cell, it's a little like sound waves hitting an ear, but here the transmitter enters into a molecular handshake with its special target.[6] This interlocking is so tight and tailor-made that a better analogy might be a key fitting into a lock. The complexing of a transmitter with its custom-made target then triggers a brief change in voltage in the target cell, effectively a conversion back from a chemical signal to one that is now again more appropriate, an electrical one. The 'yes' in neuronal communication is when there is a momentary increase in electrical activity (excitation); the 'no' is when activity is suppressed (inhibition).

However, most of the time, verbal communication is more than a simple monosyllable: conversation occurs over time, and the arrangement of words into ordered sentences, then the ordering of sentences into a statement, are crucial. So it is with transmitters: their final effect will depend on the sequencing of different transmitters converging over a particular time window onto any given cell. In both cases the impact of each word, or transmitter signal, will depend on the wider context over the period within which it occurs.[7] Then, as milliseconds turn to seconds, to minutes, to hours and eventually to days, these connections between either neurons or people change too. It's quite fun, and indeed insightful, to explore the various parallels between synapses and personal relations: both strengthen through repeated use, becoming stronger and more intense. For both neurons and people, relationships are most flexible when young. Neurons then become increasingly specialised and more 'individual' as their network grows, as do people. Over time, neurons become more resistant to change in general function, just as people mature and develop particular personality traits. And just as friendships wither if they are not actively maintained, so do supernumerary neuronal connections atrophy through underuse.

As an individual grows, they establish more and more complex relationships, some close and frequent, others less activated and more distant: larger and larger groups eventually interconnect and form a still wider society. So it is with the brain, where a nested hierarchy of ever more complex layers of networks of neurons eventually make up a particular macro brain structure. All brain regions eventually interconnect with each other, even over long brain distances, via fibre tracts like telephone lines which enable incessant dialogues all over the brain. It is a holistic organisation.

Exploring just how this happens is referred to as the 'bottom-up' approach. If you're a neuroscientist specialising in understanding transmitters, receptors and the operations of the synapse, it's a bit like being an expert in interpersonal communication. For example, the transmitter dopamine is linked to many different brain processes, such as arousal, addiction, reward and initiation of movement. But to understand bottom-up how chemicals like dopamine function, we also need a top-down approach, which starts with the macro brain areas and attempts to map out how they work together to give rise to different behaviours and eventual ways of thinking.[8] This time an appropriate analogy might be sociology or anthropology, either of which focuses on collective trends and outcomes rather than on the behaviour of individuals.

Scientists are now using brain scans to image the wholesale activity of different brain areas as a result of different types of inputs, environments and behaviours. When confronted with impressive and often beautiful brain scans, you might see bright blobs pinpointing certain areas in a sea of grey brain, or perhaps multicoloured arrays where white is a hotspot, shading through to yellow to orange to red to a low-activity purple-coloured perimeter. But in the enigmatic cohesion of the brain, all the ongoing chatter between the various brain regions will actually *not* be visible to you. These pictures reveal the brain at work over a protracted window in time. Such scans usually have a resolution of seconds (in the very latest developments, tens of milliseconds), but the universal electrical signature of brain cells at work, the 'action potential' blip, is a hundred or so times faster than that. Brain scans are like old Victorian photographs that show static buildings but exclude any people or animals, which would have been moving too fast for the exposure time. The buildings are perfectly real but they don't constitute the whole picture.

When looking at brain scans, it is also tempting to think that if a certain area of the brain lights up it must be the centre *for* whatever behaviour or response is being studied. This notion of 'centres' of the brain *for* this or that is attractive. If it were true, the brain would be so much easier to understand. Back on the cusp of the nineteenth century Franz Gall introduced the 'science' of phrenology (literally 'study of the mind'). The white china heads covered with black lined rectangles, labelled with, for example, 'love of country' and 'love of children', were intended to provide the template against which the bumps of the individual head being studied could be compared to ascertain the strength of a trait. While these busts remain popular with photographers as a prop to enliven shots of media-worthy brain scientists, the approach inevitably became discredited as systematic examination of the brain itself became possible. But traces of the crazy rationale of phrenology, of there being multiple mini-brains within your head, can still fuel interpretations of real scientific findings.

The idea of 'one brain area, one function' gained traction as medicine blossomed: clinicians became increasingly skilled at keeping patients alive despite dramatic brain damage from, say, a bullet or an injury or stroke that led to a particular deficit. This is where a phrenology-like interpretation was able still to sneak in, by ascribing to the damaged brain area the 'function' that had been lost. Yet, as one psychologist remarked over half a century ago, if you remove a valve from a radio (yes, the analogy is that old), and the device started to howl, you wouldn't claim the function of the valve was to inhibit howling. If the brain area in question malfunctions, like the elderly valve, the holistic system of the radio will be impaired, but the contribution of the valve, or indeed the brain region, cannot be extrapolated backwards from the final net outcome. If a spark plug malfunctions, your car will not start, but you can't deduce how a car works by studying a spark plug. We now know that there is no one function controlled by any one brain area. Vision, for example, involves dividing up different aspects of seeing form, motion and colour between as many as thirty different brain areas. And no one brain area has only one function. Rather, each brain structure contributes to a net final function not as a hierarchy, but more in the way the various instruments in an orchestra produce a symphony.[9]

This internal processing of the brain will determine how you see the world, but whatever external inputs are being fed into your brain at any one time, the experience of that very moment, *will simultaneously change that organisation of brain cells, and hence your thinking*. One leading expert in brain development, Bryan Kolb, sums up: 'Anything that changes your brain, changes who you will be. Your brain is not just produced by your genes; it's sculpted by a lifetime of experiences. Experience alters brain activity, which changes gene expression. Any behavioural changes you see reflect alterations in the brain. The opposite is also true: behaviour can change the brain.'[10] And that is just what we're going to explore next.

6 HOW THE BRAIN CHANGES

London taxi drivers are renowned throughout the world for their detailed knowledge of the streets, traffic configurations and one-way systems of the big city. Unlike most of their counterparts around the world, it's seemingly second nature for them to navigate the streets of the British capital without recourse to a manual. On average it takes a rookie driver two years to absorb the information required to be able to do this, and to eventually pass an ominous oral exam tellingly called 'The Knowledge'. These drivers have chosen a career that places a huge burden on their memory, specifically on their working memory, where rules and facts have to be kept constantly in mind in determining ongoing actions.

In 2000 Eleanor Maguire and her colleagues at University College London were intrigued to find out whether London cab drivers would show any physical changes in their brains as a result of the very unusual daily experience of constantly using their working memory. Amazingly, they saw in brain scans that a particular area of the brain related to working memory (the hippocampus) was actually bigger in the drivers than in non-taxi drivers of the same age.[1] Nor was it the case that having a big hippocampus predisposed these individuals to drive cabs, as the difference in hippocampal size was larger the longer the subjects had been plying their trade. This study captured the attention and fascination of the media, as well as of London taxi drivers, of course, and it remains to this day one of the best and simplest examples of the 'use it or lose it' principle. Neurons, like the muscles of the body, grow stronger and larger with whatever activity is rehearsed. Even though such adaptation is shared not only by mammals but also by far simpler organisms such as the octopus[2] and even the humble sea slug,[3] humans have been able to exploit this talent superlatively, well beyond any other species.

Changes in the brain as a result of experience were actually first shown as long ago as 1783 by the Swiss naturalist Charles Bonnet and the Piedmontese anatomist Michele Vicenzo Malacarne: they discovered that training dogs and birds led to an increase in the number of folds in a part of the brain (the cerebellum), compared to dog littermates or birds from the same clutch of eggs.[4] However, this finding did little to overthrow the dogma of the time, that the brain was unchangeable, until the idea was revisited some time later, in 1872, by the philosopher Alexander Bain: 'For every act of memory, every exercise of bodily aptitude, every habit, recollection, train of ideas, there is a specific grouping or coordination of sensations and movements, by virtue of specific growths in the cell junctions.'

Almost twenty years later, in 1890, the pioneering psychologist William James had a flash of insight: 'When two elementary brain-processes have been active together or in immediate succession, one of them, on recurring, tends to propagate its excitement into the other.' The actual term for this process, *plasticity*, was first introduced a few years later, in 1894 by the great Spanish anatomist Santiago Ramon y Cajal who borrowed the word from the Greek 'to be moulded'[5], well before the advent of the ubiquitous synthetic material.

'Give me a child until he is seven, and I will give you the man,' guaranteed the Jesuits. Just as plasticity had been anticipated by Michele Malacarne and Charles Bonnet long before modern scientists like Eleanor Maguire produced experimental data, so too has it been widely accepted that a young, developing brain is more impressionable and more vulnerable. Of course this sensitivity of the young brain to external influence highlights the importance of shaping the right kind of early environment for the next generation. As Hillary Clinton pointed out in 1997, the experiences of a 0–3-year-old 'can determine whether children will grow up to be peaceful or violent citizens, focused or undisciplined workers, attentive or detached parents themselves'.[6]

In the first years of life the brain has windows of opportunity, characterised by the exuberant growth of connections between neurons which allow for astonishing possibilities. For example, in infants the visual and auditory compartments of the outer layer of the brain (cortex) appear to be functionally interchangeable, equally effectively stimulated by either hearing or vision. Consequently, when there is a loss of vision in early childhood, some form of hearing ends up sharper through a process known as cortical remapping.[7] Because the visual sector is not being used for its normal job, it adapts to whatever inputs are available and takes on an alternative role, helping the brain process hearing with a resulting greater prowess.

This obliging adaptation by the central nervous system is not restricted to the senses. An example of the power of the young brain in compensating for damage was the case of Luke Johnson. Luke made the headlines in a British newspaper in 2001 when he was just a toddler. Soon after he was born, his right arm and leg appeared limp and motionless. Doctors diagnosed severe brain damage due to a stroke in the left side of his brain while in the womb or shortly after birth. But within a few years Luke had recovered the full use of his legs and arms. Over the course of the first two years of his life, his brain had been busy rewiring itself, reorganising nerve pathways to bypass the damaged tissue.[8]

Sadly, these critical periods do not always ensure a positive outcome. Take the case of children who develop cataracts on one or both of their eyes. Visual deprivation through a cataract or another abnormality that impairs sight that occurs between birth and 5 years, leads to permanent damage to vision. But for children who encounter this problem when they are older, vision typically recovers after treatment.[9] Interestingly, different types of vision have different critical periods, meaning that a child with a cataract within a certain time-frame may have impairments in, say, the detection of motion, yet develop normal acuity. As with Luke Johnson, the brain of a young child with a cataract will 'rewire' itself, but this time with the tragic consequences that the territory normally used by the non-operational eye would have been usurped for other purposes.

Critical periods are intuitively easy to grasp, in terms of brain development, and the changes seen at these particular crucial stages of even normal development are significantly marked. However, it is clear from the remarkable recovery often seen in adult stroke patients that even though land-grabs in the brain may be less striking later in life, they do not cease with age. Even in adults, the various sensory systems can cross the official boundaries between one and another, as when the visual cortex of blind people is activated during the reading of Braille. By the same token, the neuroscientist Helen Neville has also demonstrated how auditory impairment induces specific compensation in enhancing vision, while conversely the blind process fast auditory stimulation better.[10]

The same fundamental brain mechanisms driving plasticity during learning in the intact immature brain are also pressed into service during relearning in the damaged or diseased brain. Recovery of function after brain damage falls into three stages: (1) *restoration*: restoring function to the residual brain area; (2) *recruitment*: recruiting new brain areas to aid in the performance of the original function; (3) *retraining*: training new brain areas to perform efficiently in the new function.[11] With language, the right hemisphere, which is not normally dominant for speech, can take over from the traditional left when it is damaged.[12] Meanwhile, in the case of a non-functioning hand in monkeys, just one hour per day of training will keep its neuronal representation in the brain from shrivelling to uselessness. This effect has also been demonstrated in humans. Many brain-damaged patients with a consequently malfunctioning hand will prefer to use the healthy counterpart, but such a strategy impairs recovery of function. So, a sleeve is often placed over the good hand, attaching it to the body to encourage disproportionate use of the impaired hand, and thereby making it as operational as possible.[13]

The brain does not tolerate vacant space, namely a situation where neurons would not be put to work. The over-quoted old idea that we only use 10 per cent of our brains is a complete myth, and easy to refute. Firstly, there is no area of the brain that can be damaged without loss of ability of some sort, but if the 10 per cent myth held true, we could afford for 90 per cent of our brains to be damaged. Secondly, the brain is the greediest organ of our bodies at rest, guzzling up 20 per cent of our energy supplies even though it constitutes only 2 per cent of body weight. Why would we use so many resources to maintain 90 per cent of neurons to do nothing? Thirdly, brain-imaging techniques reveal that, with the exception of cases of severe damage such as persistent vegetative state, no brain areas show up in scans as completely inactive and silent. Fourthly, all brain areas appear to contribute to functions: there is no structure in the brain that doesn't have a job, even though we may not understand exactly how the contributions from different brain areas all fit together to give rise to an ultimate net behaviour. Finally, as we've just seen, the brain operates an unambiguous 'use it or lose it' principle when it comes to neuronal survival and connectivity. Were 90 per cent of the brain to remain unused, autopsies would reveal large-scale degeneration of up to 90 per cent, but they don't.[14]

The harder specific neurons work away at a particular activity, the more brain territory they will take up. In one experiment, Michael Merzenich showed that owl monkeys trained to rotate a disk with two digits only had an enlarged area of the touch (somatosensory) cortex relating to those two digits.[15] This finding has a fascinating counterpart in humans: musicians who play string instruments exercise their left hands more than their right and, in string players, the section of cortex related to touch is accordingly larger for the left hand than the right.[16] Many other examples of plasticity in the sensory system of adults abound, and the impact of repeated experiences on brain functioning are the bedrock of Mind Change, so it's worth getting an idea of just how sweeping and dramatic plasticity can be.

First there are snapshot studies, rather like the one with the taxi drivers, where the brains of a group of people who do something unusual or excessive on a daily basis show differences compared to the rest of us. Quite generally, for example, brain structures differ between musicians and non-musicians. Anatomical scans of professional musicians (keyboard players), amateur musicians and non-musicians showed size differences in a range of structures: motor, auditory and visuospatial brain regions.[17] It's worth noting that there are strong relationships between musician status and practice intensity, suggesting the anatomical differences are linked to learning and not to a predisposition to music. Meanwhile substantial time spent at maths induces increased grey matter density in specific (parietal) areas of the cortex known to be involved in either arithmetic processing or visuospatial imagery/mental creation/ manipulation of 3-D objects.[18]

Then there's sport. Experience-dependent plasticity is detectable in the brains of basketball players:[19] when players were compared to healthy controls, there was an enlargement in the brain's 'autoplilot', the cerebellum. Comparable changes can also be seen in the skilled golfer's brain, albeit in a different cerebral structure, in contrast to those who were less proficient.[20] However, since there was also no linear relationship between a golfer's handicap level and the anatomical changes, it is impossible to say whether the skilled golfers were already predisposed to this particular talent. This chicken and egg conundrum is one of the big disadvantages, more generally, of snapshot studies of one-off scans of different groups of people.

An alternative type of experiment which can this time differentiate cause and effect, is to observe changes in the brain over time as normal human subjects with no particular skill or talent are trained from scratch in some standardised experimental task.[21] In one case, it was juggling. Subjects underwent daily training for three months to learn a three-ball juggling task, where perception and anticipation were key to determining upcoming movements accurately. Scans were performed before, after three months and after six months, with no juggling between three and six months, by which time performance had deteriorated back to baseline: use it or you will lose it. Meanwhile the brain scans over this time showed that structural changes occurred within seven days of beginning training and were most rapid during the early stages, when performance level was low. This result suggests that it is the *learning* of a new task that is pivotal in changing the structure of the brain rather than ongoing rehearsal of something already learned.

Most comforting of all is that such training can still induce brain structure changes in the elderly. In a juggling task like the one just discussed, the performance of the elderly wasn't quite as good as that of a younger population, but grey matter changes *did* occur in identical brain regions.[22] More generally, memory training can induce growth in the cortex in the elderly. When an intensive eight-week training program is deployed, memory performance improves and cortical thickness increases in the experimental group undergoing the memory training.[23] And if older people show brain changes as a result of increased mental activity, it should come as no surprise that younger people do too.

Preparation for the German 'Physikum' basic medical exam can have a demonstrable effect on the brain.[24] This exam 'includes both oral and written tests in biology, chemistry, biochemistry, physics, social sciences, psychology, human anatomy and physiology demanding a high level of encoding, retrieval and content recall'.[25] Structural changes related to learning occurred in a variety of brain regions related to memory: hippocampus, parahippocampal grey matter and posterior parietal cortex. But it's not just the acute and stressful experience of exam preparation that's key. Learning a second language increases the density of grey matter, the changes observed being correlated with skill level.[26] Five months of second-language learning, in this case with native English-speaking exchange students learning German in Switzerland, resulted in structural changes that matched up with the increase in second-language proficiency. Once again, the individual amount of learning achieved was reflected in brain structure changes.

The exciting and scary fact of life is that you don't have to actively engage in a specific training task to change your brain: it will happen in any case as a result of the experiences you have and of the environment you are in. In her revealing and fascinating book *The Plastic Mind*, Sharon Begley writes about how 'new synapses, connections between one neuron and another, are the physical manifestation of memories. In this sense, the brain undergoes continuous physical change . . . The brain remakes itself throughout life, in response to outside stimuli to its environment and to experience.'[27]

The earliest demonstration of the impact of the outside world was with what was eventually to be called an 'enriched' environment and dates back to the 1940s, when the visionary psychologist Donald Hebb did what would be impossible nowadays: he took some of his lab rats home.[28] The actual reason for this bizarre game plan is lost in the mists of time. However, astonishingly, after some weeks in the house, these 'free range' rats turned out to have superior problem-solving abilities, such as maze running, compared to the less fortunate creatures that had remained in standard lab cages.

Since then, more formal studies have shown just how powerful a factor the environment can be, especially when it is stimulating and novel and invites exploration. The very first mention of the term 'environmental enrichment' in a scientific article was by Mark Rosenzweig and his team at the University of California in 1964, when they demonstrated for the first time physical changes in neural circuits through experience. The scientists had actually set out to identify the neural mechanisms underlying individual differences in behaviour and problem-solving in different strains of rats, but quickly realised the enormous influence that experience had on the behavioural performance relative to their standard caged counterparts.[29]

Over the ensuing decades, neuroscientists have learned that an enriched environment leads to a whole host of physical changes in the brain, all of them for the good: increased cell body size of neurons, increased overall brain weight and increased thickness of cortex; a greater number of protuberances on branches of cells which increases surface area (dendritic spines); increase in the size of synaptic junctions and hence of connections; an increased number of glial cells (the housekeeping cells of the brain that ensure a benign micro-environment for neurons). These effects are more pronounced in younger animals but can still be observed in adult or old rats. There is also increased production of new brain cells in parts of the brain associated with memory and learning (hippocampus, dentate gyrus and cerebellar Purkinje cells), as well as a greater blood supply and an increase in the amount of growth factors and protein synthesis.

This type of stimulating environment, where there is no fixed task to perform but which nonetheless generates different types of experience, can have a surprising impact even when destiny seems otherwise to be determined strongly by genes. In an experiment done fifteen years ago which has now become a much cited classic, mice were deliberately genetically engineered to develop Huntington's disease, a neurological disorder which manifests in wild, involuntary movements known as chorea (after the Greek for 'dance').[30] The mice left in typical lab cages lived out their genetic fate as they aged, and scored worse and worse each day on a variety of movement tests, while a genetically identical group were exposed to an enriched environment: a world consisting of greater space to explore and more objects (wheels, ladders and so on) with which to interact. The study conclusively demonstrated that mice living in such a stimulating environment developed movement problems much later, and with a far more modest degree of impairment. Even here, with a single gene disorder and in the less complex brains of mice, nature and nurture interact.

Research since the early 1990s on 'enriched' animals have revealed a wide range of physical changes in the brain at the level of individual neuronal networks, as well as demonstrating that the *duration* of the enrichment experience is a significant factor. For example, in one study a single week of environmental enrichment had no effect, but four weeks of enrichment had behavioural effects that lasted two months, while eight weeks of enrichment led to behavioural effects lasting six months.[31]

Given all these physical changes in the structure and chemistry of the brain, it comes as no surprise that 'enriched' animals are superior in tests of spatial memory and show general increases in cognitive functioning such as learning ability, spatial and problem-solving skills, and processing speed. They also have reduced levels of anxiety. In addition, enrichment attenuates the enduring or persistent effects engendered by past negative experiences such as prenatal stress or neonatal maternal separation: the protective effects of enrichment are particularly apparent in animals that are highly anxious or when the task is extremely challenging for the subject.

Enriched environments can also be beneficial in animal models of recovery from brain injury. For instance, transfer to an enriched environment improves the outcome after an experimentally induced stroke, as well as significantly improving motor performance in spontaneously hypertensive rats previously housed in standard laboratory cages, compared with controls remaining in the less stimulating environment.[32] Moreover, an enriched environment will reduce spontaneous cell suicide (apoptotic cell death) in the rat hippocampus by 45 per cent. And if that were not enough, these environmental conditions can also protect against experimentally induced seizures.[33]

The beneficial and widespread effects of environmental enrichment also persist in aged rats and across a diverse range of species, namely mice, gerbils, squirrels, cats, monkeys and even birds, fish, fruit flies and spiders – every animal 'from flies to philosophers'.[34] There is still some controversy as to whether enrichment actually represents a super-special experience or is only a relative improvement over standard laboratory animal housing. However, the main point is the impact that a more stimulating and interactive environment can have, rather than which type of environment would be normal. That is, it is the differential between the two types of experience that counts.

But how can an external experience literally leave its mark on the internal brain? Just as muscle grows with exercise, so too do neurons respond to physical changes, by growing more branches. When it has more branches, a brain cell will have an increased surface area which makes it an easier target and leads to the possibility of more connectivity with other brain cells. Back in 1949 Donald Hebb came up with the startling suggestion that somehow stimulating the same chain of neurons so that they are active at the same time, or 'fire' together, as the result of an experience, will make them stronger, more effective: 'cells that fire together wire together'.[35] But how exactly? Spool on another few decades to when sophisticated techniques were available to monitor the activity of single brain cells by inserting microelectrodes inside them and recording the voltage, the 'activity' they generated. Using this technology, Swedish physiologist Terje Lomo and British neuroscientist Tim Bliss gained their place in the history of brain research for their breakthrough description of the actual step-by-step process of Hebb's idea.[36] Neuroscientists can now describe the specific physico-chemical steps by which signalling between two brain cells will become more effective as a result of repetition, that is experience.[37]

While it would be hard to impose a standardised enriched environment on humans, and even harder to justify an experimental 'control' group of people deprived of stimulation, the effect of different types of environment has been examined in older healthy adults by investigating the relationship between lifestyle and 'cognitive reserve',[38] namely 'the degree to which the brain can create and use networks or cognitive paradigms that are more efficient or flexible, and thus less susceptible to disruption'.[39] The findings, perhaps not surprisingly, indicate that a greater involvement in intellectual and social activities is linked with less cognitive decline. It seems that a mentally active lifestyle may defend against cognitive deterioration by increasing the density of synapses (thereby improving the efficacy of communication within intact neurons) and the efficiency of normal and alternative brain networks.[40] Then again, unless enrichment/stimulation is maintained, just as in animals, performance may decline after previously successful rehabilitation, leading to negative changes. This could be as a result of withdrawal from social situations or reduced levels of activity and/or communication.[41] Even when IQ, age and general health are all taken into account, older individuals living in community accommodation perform better in cognitive tests than those who are institutionalised.[42]

Most fascinating of all is that even brisk walking may stimulate the production of new neurons (neurogenesis). First, exercise increases the blood supply to the brain, and along with it the all-important oxygen it carries. Increased oxygen then enables stem cells (the universal progenitor cells from which different cells derive) to convert to neurons at maximum capacity, as well as stimulating the release of chemicals that help cells grow. But that's not all. While physical activity increases the manufacture of neural stem cells, additional stimulation from an enriched environment increases the connectivity and the stability of those connections.[43] Although it has only now proved possible to study cell production in the human brain,[44] changes in its processes and composition as a result of enriching social, mental and physical activities are now thought to help stave off cognitive decline as we age,[45] and in turn prevent the underlying loss of cells that characterises the remorseless cycle of death in Alzheimer's disease.[46]

If the environment can change thinking, in both the normal and the healthy brain, then could the reverse occur and might the mental process of thinking actually change the physical brain itself? Bizarre though this might sound, it *is* possible. One of the most cited examples of how a thought can drive a physical brain change was conducted by Pascual-Leone and his research group back in 1995 with three groups of adult human volunteers, none of whom could play the piano.[47] Over a five-day period, the control group were exposed to the experimental environment but not to the all-important factor of learning the exercises; a second group learned five-finger piano exercises, and over just five days showed an astonishing change in their brain scans. But a third group were more remarkable still. The subjects in this group were required merely to imagine that they were playing the piano: their brain scans showed almost identical changes to those undergoing physical practice!

Amazingly, the mere mental act of thinking somehow has a tangible impact on the physical brain. Many more examples have followed. Fred 'Rusty' Gage, professor at the Laboratory of Genetics at the Salk Institute has demonstrated that, in order for exercise to generate the appearance of new brain cells, that exercise has to be voluntary: the animal must *decide* to enter the exercise wheel and run in it.[48] Similarly, in humans, it appears that plasticity occurs only when movements are volitional and/or the subject is paying conscious attention. But if paying attention at the critical moment is essential for adaptive changes in the brain, then of still more importance is the individual's state of mind. Perhaps the most familiar but still seemingly improbable example would be the placebo effect whereby the simple belief that an inert substance has therapeutic properties is sufficient in itself to cure an illness.

We know that this effect somehow works through the naturally occurring morphine-like chemical system in the brain, the enkephalins; after all, a blocker of enkephalin, the drug naloxone, will correspondingly block the placebo effect. And it also turns out that the effects are not merely due to the presence of the enkephalin molecule itself just happening to be available; rather, it is necessary to have the actual belief about the action of the placebo drug.[49] Again, a conscious thought is all-important, not just the appropriate bottom-up landscape of brain cells and chemicals.

A further illustration of the key role played by conscious thought can be seen in clinical depression. It turns out that there's a big difference for depressed patients between bottom-up intervention of their condition with antidepressants such as Prozac, and the manipulation of their beliefs, their way of seeing the world, by various talking techniques such as cognitive behavioural therapy. Psychotherapy differs from antidepressant medication in that it encourages the patient to see the world in a new, more positive, way, as guided by the therapist. The cause of the depression, say the loss of a loved one, is not diminished but rather placed in a context that enables the patient to have a more positive outlook. Thus cognitive behavioural therapy for depression works in a similar way to inert placebo compounds. In both cases, the brain is operating from top-down, starting with a belief system on a macro scale of neuronal networking which will then trigger chemical changes in the brain – although understanding precisely how this happens is still a great puzzle in neuroscience.

Meanwhile, medication with drugs works differently, by directly modifying from bottom-up the availability of the chemicals, bypassing any personalised neuronal circuitry. And that personalised circuitry, what we can equate with the personal mind, could be all-important. A big difference between cognitive behavioural therapy and direct drug intervention is that the probability of relapse in depression is greater with drugs. Presumably the plasticity changes in personalised neuronal networking shaped by routine cognitive behavioural therapy are more enduring and powerful than a general but essentially transient change in the chemical brain landscape, where drugs are directly manipulating simply the individual's feelings and conscious state over a much shorter time window.

Interestingly enough, the mind-set of the clinic depressive can have a negative effect on neurogenesis: the brain region from where new neurons are created from stem cells (the dentate gyrus) shrinks in depression.[50] If these new cells would normally have made it easier to form new connections, then Sharon Begley has suggested that this physical change in the brain might account for why depressed patients are not so receptive to new things, why they persist in seeing the world in an unchanging, unexciting monochrome way.[51]

In summary, the brains of a whole range of animals are astonishingly plastic, and the human brain superlatively so. It is constantly adapting physically to repeated types of behaviours on a 'use it or lose it' basis. Such endless neuronal updating is particularly marked in critical time-frames during development, but continues throughout life into older age. Yet plasticity doesn't stop at the rehearsal of certain skills. The mere experience of living and interacting in a certain environment leaves its mark on the brain which in turn leads to a unique, changed, personalised brain circuitry (a 'state of mind') that can ultimately lead to further physical changes in the brain and body. But that leaves us with some exasperating riddles. How *can* an insubstantial thought modify a physical state? And, conversely, how can a drug that affects chemicals that modify physical states modify insubstantial thoughts? In short, what is the neuroscientist's story about the possible physical basis of the mind and consciousness?

HOW THE BRAIN BECOMES A MIND

7

When she had asked me 'how the brain worked', the little girl in the audience had posed one of the most difficult questions of all: it is so difficult because, even before we start to make sense of what all the powerful new neuroscience techniques are actually showing us, we immediately run into a problem with the question itself. After all, what does the phrase 'how the brain works' actually mean? The central nervous system achieves so many different functions, and on so many different levels of operations, that all this neuronal chicanery cannot really be subsumed under such a catch-all single word as 'works'. For example, on one level, everyone knows how Prozac 'works': a key action of the drug is to enhance the availability of a chemical messenger, the transmitter serotonin. But how an increased availability of serotonin 'works' in turn to alleviate the subjective misery of depression, remains a complete riddle.

Serotonin is, after all, just a molecule; it doesn't have happiness trapped inside it. Instead, the all-important issue is the context, the brain cell circuitry within which it is a bit player, a powerful one indeed, but only when it is operating in the right scenario. Like an actor reciting disconnected lines on their own in an empty dressing room, transmitters and other bioactive 'signalling molecules' need the other actors, the surrounding scenery, and a clear sequence of events for their lines to have any effect or relevance. In the case of serotonin and depression, we know that the crucial sequence of events involves at least some ten days, a 'therapeutic time lag' that is needed for Prozac to work. If cheerfulness were simply contained and released from inside a molecule of serotonin, then surely you'd experience an effect immediately. Having to wait means that the alleviation of depression is not just down to the transmitter itself, its immediate spatial surroundings, or even its direct action on the adjacent cells. Instead, something still more complex is going on within the wider neuronal network, and over a longer time-frame.

We've seen that the interlocking of a transmitter with its target molecule is a little like a handshake. Now imagine that handshake persisting, that someone keeps squeezing your hand. Eventually that hand becomes numb, less sensitive, and more pressure will be needed to achieve the same effect. And so it is with the molecular targets, the receptors that are now going to be bombarded by the unusually excessive amounts of serotonin released remorselessly day after day by Prozac. Slowly the receptors will become less sensitive - the technical term is actually 'desensitised', which suggests that desensitisation is a factor in alleviating depression. But how this, or any other physico-chemical brain mechanism, actually translates into a subjective sensation of either happiness or sadness is one of the biggest mysteries, if not *the* biggest mystery, of science.

Take another example. Henry Marsh is a distinguished neurosurgeon in London. Many of his operations are conducted while the patient is awake, so that he can see the precise functional effects of stimulating the brain in different cerebral locations before any surgical intervention. Gory though this might sound, there are no pain sensors in the brain, so it has been quite a routine procedure since the middle of the twentieth century to operate on brains that are fully conscious.[1] However, Henry now has closed circuit TV in theatre, and offers the patient the opportunity of watching the whole procedure. Think about it: the brain watching itself. What on earth can be going on?

What is going on, both in Henry's operating theatre and in anyone taking Prozac, is an enactment of the 'hard problem'. This is a phrase made famous by the Australian philosopher David Chalmers for referring to our current bafflement as to how the water of brain functioning is converted into the wine of subjective experience.[2] Yet in order to understand how the brain generates consciousness, we need at least some idea, however hypothetical, of what *kind* of answer would work as a satisfactory explanation: would it be a mathematical formula, a brain image or something more in the realms of science fiction? None of these possibilities seems anywhere near adequate or appropriate. Yet until we know what *kind* of answer we need to solve the hard problem, surely there can be little likelihood of our doing so.

Still, undeterred, some have looked to artificial, silicon-based systems for an answer. With the ever growing power of computational processing, the issue here is not so much the 'I' in artificial intelligence (AI), but the 'A': how would an artificial computer measure up compared with the real biological brain? Many still profess that the brain works 'like a computer'. This starting premise can then be developed in two possible directions: either we go from biological to artificial systems, or the reverse. If we start with a biological phenomenon, be it learning, memory or even consciousness itself, the usual idea is that we should be able to model it in a silicon-based device. But there's a problem immediately, since the idea of a model requires that you focus on the all-important salient features and jettison the extraneous features. A model for flight, as exemplified by a plane, would be the defying of gravity but without the requisite of feathers and a beak. So, in order to model consciousness, we would already have to know what the salient physical brain/body processes are, and what bits are extraneous and can therefore be ignored. And yet, if we knew that, we would have solved the problem already; there would be no need to bother with the model.

Travelling in the reverse direction and starting with an artificial system to elucidate the biology of cognitive processes, such as learning, memory or consciousness, can also be treacherous. A distinguished and diverse line-up of scientists such as Ray Kurzweil, Guilio Tononi and Christof Koch place a premium on the all-important issue being 'complexity',[3] that in the end it is sheer size that counts whether in neuronal networks or, as the philosopher John Searle once quipped, in old beer cans. In any case, the idea is that, by building machines of ever greater complexity, consciousness will emerge as a spontaneous and inevitable result, and that most overused of sci-fi characters, the conscious robot, will become a reality.

But this way of thinking overlooks the power of the underlying neuroscience that is normally at work: the trafficking of the huge variety of capricious and subtle compounds in the nervous system that work in different combinations, in different places, over different windows of time, with highly context-dependent and variable effects. The diverse neurochemistry of the central nervous system shows that quality cannot be reduced to quantity, that the complex dynamism of modulating chemicals and our brains is so much more than mere computation.

As we've just seen, neurons are highly dynamic entities capable of extraordinary plasticity, not a fixed component that can plug in and play with persistent and dogged regularity, independent of the surrounding micro-, meso- and eventual macro-scale environment in which it is located. The intense, ever changing dynamic interaction between coalitions of neurons is nothing like the rigid circuitry of computational devices.

No simple systematic building up of one silicon component after another could ever have the same effect, unless that unit were an exact simulacrum of the neuron, replete with all the chemicals and biochemical dynamics that make its characteristic restless plasticity and sensitivity possible.[4] Moreover, there's a whole body out there, beyond the brain, which receives and sends incessant feedback. Some time ago now, the neurologist Antonio Damasio pointed out the importance of these chemical signals that fed back and forth between the brain and the rest of the body, chemicals he referred to as 'somatic markers'.[5] The interplay between the three great control systems of the body, the immune, endocrine and nervous systems, should not be ignored. After all, if they were not interactive we would have biological anarchy; and, even if we didn't, it would be hard to account for the placebo effect where, as we saw, a thought (namely, some kind of neuronal event in the brain) can impact on health, an event in the immune system.

But just imagine that one day there *is* an artificial device, built in whatever material, 'complex' enough to be a strong candidate for having consciousness. Let's even imagine it has passed the Turing Test, the hypothetical test devised by Alan Turing, arguably the father of information technology.[6] In this test an impartial observer would not be able to distinguish between the responses of a human and those of the machine. I would still struggle to see how such an artificial system, feat of engineering though it might be, would help solve the hard problem. How might this ingenious conscious computer help us understand how the subjective 'feel' of consciousness is actually generated in an objective, physical system? Our inability to tell whether it is a computer or a human answering our questions tells us nothing about the elusive inner state of consciousness: what it is and how it comes about. In any case, it's all hypothetical: the Turing Test has still not been passed, although, apparently, there is a human being somewhere who failed it. Whatever their reasons for adopting this approach, perhaps for those fixated on building a conscious machine of some sort, the most exciting goal would be to strive to satisfy the late Stuart Sutherland's criterion: he would accept that a computer was conscious when it ran off with his wife.

Nonetheless, the conceptual impasse of the water-to-wine riddle hasn't stopped neuroscientists, myself included, from trying to make some sort of headway. A zig-zag way of progressing is to put the hard problem on hold and to ask a simpler question: can we lower our sights and just match up, 'correlate', certain subjective feelings with certain physical events in the brain, say the correspondence of Prozac-induced increases in serotonin and feelings of well-being, in a way that gives us a kind of consistent relationship between objective events and subjective experiences.

This game plan is the search for what has become known as 'neural correlates of consciousness'.[7] It's important to note here that no attempt is being made at establishing a causal link as to how the physical event could give rise to the mental, or vice versa. A mere correlation, just a humble matching up, is more feasible because it sidesteps the conceptual conundrum of the water-into-wine hard problem. But in order to come up with a convincing 'correlate of consciousness', we still need a way of describing subjective experience that serves as a kind of shopping list for what we're going to be asking the physical brain to deliver. Yet here's the snag: neuroscience, like all science, is ruthlessly objective, and everything we do, all experiments, are painstakingly impartial in their procedures and, most importantly, they are quantitative, all about measurement.

The catch is that conscious states are quintessentially subjective, qualitative and therefore anathema to conventional scientists, trained as we are to be impartially objective. So in order to come up with a consistent and persuasive correlate of consciousness, we need a way of describing subjective states that would be amenable to drawing direct parallels with brain processes. My own suggestion has been to argue that consciousness is not all-or-none but that it is indeed quantitative. Rather than the light being on during the day and off at night, I've proposed that consciousness is more like a dimmer switch, that it will grow as brains grow, both in evolutionary terms across the animal kingdom, and in individual development from a foetus onwards. Then, as an adult, this variability continues such that there are times when you are more aware than at others. In everyday jargon we talk about 'raising' our consciousness, or 'deepening' it; in my view, the actual direction doesn't really matter, but we should rather be talking about degrees of consciousness. And once we can do that, we can look in the brain for a physical something, a real process that also varies in degree from one moment to the next.[8]

As I see it, the most likely neurobiological candidates for consciousness are *neuronal assemblies*, large-scale coalitions of tens of millions of brain cells that can work in synchrony, and disband in less than a second. We also know that these highly transient, macro-scale phenomena can be dramatically reduced by consciousness-robbing drugs such as anaesthetics. The theory therefore runs that the more extensive the assembly profile at any one moment, the 'deeper' your consciousness. In turn, the extent of the assembly at any one time will be dependent on a variety of factors that determine how easily the transient coalition of brain cells can be recruited. One factor would be the sheer intensity of incoming stimulation, which is why an alarm clock will pull you out of unconsciousness into the harsh light of wakefulness.

But then what about when the alarm doesn't ring and you can carry on dreaming? Here's a situation where there's a weird consciousness of a sort, and yet you remain impervious to the external sensory outside world around you. I suggest the assemblies are very fragile and not very extensive, since they are driven by the happenstance of internal neuronal activity independent of the strong input of the senses and the external world. And if the assembly in dreams is small, so the corresponding consciousness will not be very deep, hence the lack of cause-effect logic and the disjointed, improbable narrative that constitutes and characterises the dreaming state.

If consciousness grows as brains grow, so we would also expect this small assembly mode to characterise the mind-set of those with still developing brains, young children whose behaviour is driven by the fleeting moment and instant emotions rather than by step-by-step consequences and planning. Yet there are further ways even the adult human brain could revert to this more basic small assembly mode, despite being fully awake. Many factors in the brain could contribute to the net result that ensues from a small assembly, not just lack of external stimulus (dreaming) or having insufficient brain connections in place (infants). What if there were an excess of a brain chemical that constrained the full spread of an assembly, or what if there were so many sensory inputs bombarding the brain that none had time to trigger an assembly to full potential before it was outcompeted by the next?

I've suggested that these two scenarios could occur in schizophrenia and fast-paced sports respectively, and that in many respects the resultant 'small' assembly, which occurs as a consequence of different factors, could nonetheless have a common net state characterised, as with dreaming and children, by high emotional content and a momentary consciousness unrelated to a past or a future.[9] If so, and if the human brain is indeed capable of different modes characterised by different brain states that match up, correlate with different types of consciousness, there will be important implications for the kind of consciousness that might result from continued cyber experiences. So what we need to do now is explore what normally happens in the human brain as infancy turns into childhood and matures into a full, unprecedented life story with a past and a future.

As the great psychologist William James described so beautifully around the turn of the twentieth century, you are born as a baby into a 'booming, buzzing confusion'.[10] You will evaluate the world around you in purely sensory terms, because all you have are your senses bombarding your brain: how sweet, how cold, how bright, how loud. The wonderful thing about being born a human as opposed to, say, a goldfish, is that although we are born with pretty much a full complement of neurons, it is the growth and connections between the brain cells that account for the astonishing growth of the brain in infancy and early childhood. We've just seen how the generic human brain is capable of very sensitive plasticity that will personalise it into a unique entity, and how a brain cell stimulated by the environment grows more branches, which in turn increase its surface area and thus make it easier to form connections. So we shouldn't be too surprised now that all these available connections can provide us with an adaptability that has important implications for each individual. If you have individual experiences, then you're going to become unique as your particular experiences start to rearrange and reorganise your synapses.

In humans, from about the age of 6 years, the supernumerary connections start to get selectively pruned back. This is not an impairment, but rather the development of particular patterns of responses and skills that enable you to navigate and thrive in your particular environment. Where you previously stood at a crossroads, with all possibilities open and unrealised, you now have to make choices, to take a clear direction: you are now becoming ever more different from everyone else as your brain still continues to adapt to each new experience. As the weeks turn to months and to years, connections between your brain cells will slowly grow to accommodate persistent patterns of, say, an abstract visual image of colours and blobs, perhaps accompanied by a consistent voice, texture and smell. And, as these connections form, you will gradually make the transition from an entirely sensory take on the world to a more cognitive one. Erstwhile abstract visual patterns and sounds will now be transformed into your mother. And if Mum features again and again in your life, then, as with the examples of plasticity we looked at earlier, so will your brain adapt with a unique configuration of brain cell connections and Mum will come to mean something to you that she means to no one else. Slowly your brain's relation to the outside world will progress from a one-way street to a two-way dialogue. Instead of your being constantly in a booming, buzzing confusion, incoming stimuli (a person, an object or an event) will carry a meaning wholly specific to you. You will evaluate these stimuli in terms of the existing neuronal connectivity, while at the same time the very experience of doing so will further update the status of those neuronal connections.

Take the example of a wedding ring. It may perhaps first be of interest to a small baby simply because of its conspicuous sensory properties: the gold gleam, the central hole, the smooth round surface that rolls. But as connections associated with the ring become established, the object will slowly gain a meaning as a particular type of object which you put on a finger, eventually further defined as something you put only on one particular finger and only under particular circumstances, then further refined still, as the neuronal connections proliferate, into a broad multifaceted meaning relating to love, weddings, commitment and so on that other merely generic rings do not possess. Eventually, if you acquire a wedding ring of your own, that specific object will have a specific meaning, a relevance that all otherwise very similar looking rings do not possess. The extensive, highly personalised experiences and hence unique neuronal connections of your brain will have given that object a deep, special significance, 'sentimental value', even though in purely sensory terms it is unexceptional. The difference between a generic wedding ring and what might be the most important object in your life is entirely in your head. In this way, the erstwhile one-way street now has traffic going in both directions. Everything you are currently experiencing from one moment to the next is read against the pre-existing associations, but at the same time that current ongoing experience will be updating the connectivity to change it forever. As you grow, the development of your mind will be characterised by this increasingly vigorous two-way dialogue between your brain and the outside world.[11]

So as you mature, the raw sensation of the outside world gives way to a cognitive take where objects, people and events have a personalised meaning for you. But that's not all. Being able to see beyond, literally, face value will enable you to evaluate and assess more accurately whatever is happening to you. Take the simple case of someone coming into a room on Halloween dressed up as a ghost. While an adult would be able to interpret the situation as benign, on the basis of prior experience and knowledge, a small child could well be very frightened. Younger children lack the checks and balances of a robust conceptual framework, based on prior experience that would enable them to interpret the new event appropriately. Without any frame of reference, however, this strange apparition could be life-threatening.

The more we can relate a phenomenon, action or fact, to other phenomena, facts or actions, the deeper, I'm suggesting, is the *understanding*. Here is an example. When my bother Graham was only 3 years old, and I was 16, I thought it great fun to give him a hard time, as is the way of adolescent elder sisters. One way was to get him to learn by heart great chunks of Shakespeare, and in particular the famous Macbeth soliloquy, 'Tomorrow, and tomorrow, and tomorrow. . .'. Graham obligingly learned it like a little parrot and was soon quickly reciting the famous lines on demand, much to the amusement of my giggling school friends. Had I asked him what the line 'Out, out, brief candle! Life's but a walking shadow' actually meant, the best he could have replied would have been something about blowing out the candles on his birthday cake. What he could never have grasped at that age, with his relatively paltry neuronal connectivity, was that the extinction of the candle was really about something else altogether. He could not place the phrase in a wider context and realise that the line was not so much about the extinction of a flame as the extinction of life, that it was a metaphor for death. He couldn't fully understand what Shakespeare had written, because he couldn't make the connection.

Understanding, then, is basically seeing one thing in terms of another, and surely this is what *intelligence* is really all about, going back to its literal Latin provenance of 'understanding'. It is a very different type of ability from the fast processing demanded of IQ tests towards a specified end, and which are far more appropriate for silicon systems.[12] The mathematician Roger Penrose pointed out long ago that it would be impossible to devise an algorithm for those key human abilities of intuition or common sense. Even further back in time the great physicist

Niels Bohr admonished a colleague with the withering put-down, 'You're not thinking, you're just being logical.'[13]

This distinction of the efficient processing of an input to come up with the right output (rote learning of Macbeth, say) in contrast to real understanding, fits well with a distinction that has been acknowledged for quite a while, of 'fluid' versus 'crystallised' intelligence. Psychologist Raymond Cattell first thought up these two distinct concepts back in 1963. Cattell defined fluid intelligence as 'the ability to perceive relationships independent of previous specific practice or instruction concerning those relationships'.[14] This skill is considered independent of learning, experience and education. Meanwhile *crystallised intelligence* involves knowledge that comes from prior learning and past experiences. Fluid intelligence peaks in our teenage years and then declines but, as we age and accumulate new knowledge and understanding, crystallised intelligence becomes stronger.

This well-established distinction in psychology could correspond directly to whether or not an extensive neuronal connectivity is being used. With fluid processing, the efficient input-output processing is free of context, as it was for my brother; there is no need for personalised neuronal connectivity to give a frame of reference. But the crystallised process that is dependent on prior information is an excellent metaphor for extensive neuronal networking. We could even think of the neuronal network structure more literally as a little like a crystalline structure, of intense interconnectivity. So a neuroscientific definition of the mind would be the personalisation of the human brain through its dynamic neuronal connectivity, driven in turn by an individual's unique experiences.

Now let's go one step further. I've often wondered how the one-off subjective state of you being *you* manifests in the physical brain.[15] How might an awareness of this unique you-ness be generated at the level of the physical brain? Through the lens of neuroscience, *identity* is best seen as an activity rather than a state: it's not a solid object or property locked away in your head, but a certain type of subjective brain state, a feeling that can change from one moment to the next. In order to understand how social networking sites, for example, might be changing our identities, we need to establish the basic criteria that the physical brain must deliver, in order for someone to 'feel' that they are a unique entity. As I see it, there are five basic requirements.

First you need to be fully conscious, that is, not asleep or anaesthetised. The actual subjectivity of the first-hand experience of the world that is unique to each of us currently defies an objective neuroscientific account. As we've seen just, the deal-breaker is that we still have no idea as to what kind of answer we would expect to answer the question satisfactorily. Nonetheless, this conceptual gridlock shouldn't prevent us moving on to work out further requisites. A rat can be conscious but not have a self-conscious sense of identity. So more is still needed.

Secondly, your mind has to be fully operational. In the default mode of the normal adult human brain, we've now seen that the mind will enable the individual to react in a certain way to objects, people and events in accordance with the checks and balances of previous beliefs and experiences. This unique mind, reflected in your unique neuronal connectivity, will enable you not just to make sense of what is happening around you at any given moment, but to make possible the third item on the shopping list.

The third criterion is that you will now react in a particular way that is determined not just by your past experiences and how they shape your current response to the context prevailing at any particular time, but also by how those earlier experiences have subsequently shaped your wider beliefs. The key distinction between memories and beliefs is that the former can be evoked independently. A memory is a memory and gains access into your consciousness without further justification, while beliefs can be appreciated only according to potential validation or resistance to validation. I have previously suggested that beliefs could be described along a spectrum, ranging from rational to irrational, in respective relation to this eventual independent validation, or resistance to evidence to the contrary.[16]

An *irrational* belief (say, all men are superior to women) through to a more *rational* belief (the sun will rise tomorrow) could be so defined in accordance with where they would sit along a crucial single scale of how much they resisted and/or depended on, additional evidence. In the brain this set-up could be realised in the extent of neuronal connections and, just as importantly, by their strength in persisting in the presence of contradictory inputs (say, the obvious prowess of women) that would, could or should either enforce them or cancel them out, as in the case of sexist beliefs. This potential validation, or refutation, could also be realised, in neuroscience terms, as associations or connectivity that have the potential to offset or cancel out the original association (the belief), but do not actually do so either because the original connection is too strong or the validation is still too weak. These real or hypothetical reactions, your beliefs, in turn will modify your memories and how you will respond differently next time around in whatever situations life flings at you.

But there is still more to identity than just having a mind, memories, and even a set of beliefs. Imagine being alone on a desert island. What happens to your identity? On a desert island, who would you actually *be*? I'm suggesting that the issue at stake here would be suddenly not having any context within which to express yourself. The difference between mind and identity is that mind is passive and does not depend on interacting with others, while identity is active, and depends on some kind of societal context. Mind is how you see the world, whereas identity is how the world sees you. And for this you need a world, a society, a context in which you do something in the eyes of others. The fourth requirement is therefore a context-dependent action–reaction.

Identity in the family, for example, would be inevitably based on strong associations from infancy initially with the colours, sounds, smells and visual pattern that gradually transform from a conglomeration of raw, abstract senses into say, the cognitive perception of your mother. Hence in these early years, identity will be strongly linked to momentary consciousness, and will not have much risk of being displaced by any competition, any alternative roles. But as we grow and other relationships and other contexts independent of your mother start to unfold, then identity within the family will recede to become one of many options and not, therefore, continuously present in your consciousness. However, when it is triggered in the context of, say, Christmas, weddings or funerals, it will come to the fore as the strongly dominant identity once again out of the background.

Identity in a team is, arguably, the opposite. The long-term associations are relatively weak, having been laid down over a much briefer period of time, much more intermittently and probably much later than infancy, well outside of the critical periods of development. But this time, unlike the family identity, the context of the moment will be the much more salient factor. The fast-paced thrill of a game, with heightened arousal, will emphasise the consciousness component of identity (item 1 on our list) relative to the mind component (item 2) which more strongly drives the sense of identity within a family.

Fifthly, this specific instance of action–reaction at any one time within a specific context replete with values and memories will now be incorporated into a still wider framework, a narrative of your cohesive past-present-future: you. It is this *subjective awareness* of your whole unique life story captured at any one particular moment but dependent on a hinterland of highly extensive and complex neuronal connectivity that could then constitute the moment-to-moment feel of your identity. The scenario of a lifetime of memories and beliefs being funnelled into a single moment of consciousness is reminiscent of William Blake's famous lines from the 'Auguries of Innocence':

> To see a World in a Grain of Sand
> And a Heaven in a Wild Flower,
> Hold Infinity in the palm of your hand
> And Eternity in an hour.[17]

Everything that happens has its own moment in time but can now be linked to all the other events as either preceding or anteceding them. Your identity is therefore a spatio-temporal phenomenon that combines the hard-wired neuronal network of the mind with momentary consciousness – the fleeting generation of macro-scale coalitions of neurons (assemblies) – in less than a second. The long-term generalised network of connectivity is your mind, which can now in turn play its part at any particular moment in time. If consciousness is indeed linked to the fleeting generation of macro-scale coalitions of neurons in less than a second, and if the enduring networks of neuronal connections (the mind) can drive a more extensive coalition (assembly), then the ensuing 'deeper' consciousness would be directly related to a deeper understanding of events, people and objects as you encountered them.

The crucial take-away from this neuroscientific attempt at a deconstruction of identity lies in the vital role of *the context in which the mind is operating* from one conscious moment to the next. So what happens in situations where this mind is 'blown' or 'lost'?

8 OUT OF YOUR MIND

Imagine a mature, carefully crafted, individual brain with connections that are responding to, activated by, strengthened and shaped by sequences of specific experiences that no one else has ever had, nor ever will have again: this is the physical basis of an individual's mind. But now imagine those highly individualised connections being slowly dismantled as the branches of the brain cells shrivel back. The person would return to a more childlike state since they would no longer have the requisite framework of the adult mind against which to evaluate ongoing experiences. People and objects would no longer have the highly personalised significance so carefully accumulated over a lifetime. We would see the sad and tragic symptoms of Alzheimer's disease, where the patient is indeed 'losing their mind', literally *dementia*. Yet we can also 'lose' our minds on a more frequent, temporary and positive basis, in situations where the lure of here-and-now sensation turns us into passive recipients rather than proactive thinkers. In this case we have, after all, 'let ourselves go'.

But, first, a word of caution. We need to be careful, when we talk about 'blowing' or 'losing' the mind, not to confuse it with what has been called 'mindless' crowd behaviour, such as was seen in the Nazis' Nuremberg rallies,[1] where a collective mob identity derived from political and racial ideologies of the twentieth century, just as a collective identity derives from a religious fundamentalism in the twenty-first.[2] In all cases, the overheated and often violent mob are not just blindly emotional, as in road rage, or the French *crime passionnel* (where you 'see red' and are not accountable for your actions/crimes). Far from being 'out of their minds', the mob will have a very specific narrative, albeit an utterly repugnant one: they know whom they are targeting in order to enact their revered story-line. They are not mindless at all.

If the mind is the personalisation of the brain through its individual neuronal connectivity, driven by personal experience, then truly losing your mind would occur when those carefully personalised connections are not fully accessible. For example, drugs and alcohol will impair the chemical communication between neuronal connections, while recreational environments filled with rave music or the rapid-volley stimuli of fast-paced sports do not require a complex cognitive infrastructure, as they are primarily 'sensational'. Often, the more the raw senses dominate, the greater the magnitude of pleasure, it seems. The very word 'ecstasy' in Greek means 'to stand outside' of oneself. It has often intrigued me that it is this emotional, unreflective state that we seek out through diverse pursuits that have one thing in common: an absence of self-consciousness, an abnegation of a sense of self in favour of becoming the passive recipient of the incoming senses, indeed of being 'abandoned'. So you can lose, or be out of, your mind while still being conscious, hence the importance of distinguishing the two terms 'mind' and 'consciousness'.

What could be going on in the brain when someone remains conscious yet 'blows' their mind? The most obvious tool at the brain's disposal here are the chemical messengers, the transmitters and other modulating chemicals released when neurons are active. One naturally occurring substance in particular is a likely candidate for helping to mediate a 'sensational' experience: the transmitter dopamine. Dopamine is the final common conduit for all psychoactive drugs of addiction, regardless of their primary site and mode of action; the dopamine system has also been linked to processes in the brain relating to feelings of pleasure. For over half a century now, brain scientists have been fascinated by the phenomenon of 'self-stimulation'. Classic experiments by the psychologist James Olds revealed that if electrodes were implanted in certain parts of the brain but not others, rats would work at pressing a bar to stimulate these key brain areas to the exclusion of all else, even feeding.[3] The brain areas that, when stimulated, presumably caused the rats to feel good were those releasing dopamine. In a short-hand but rather inaccurate way therefore, dopamine has sometimes been simplistically referred to in the popular press as the 'molecule of pleasure'.

When you are highly excited, aroused or feel rewarded, or indeed if you are taking drugs, this same single transmitter will somehow play a key part in delivering these different subjective experiences. In all these cases, dopamine plays a pivotal role by being released like a fountain from the primitive region at the top of the spine (brainstem) outwards and upwards throughout the brain, where it then changes the responsiveness of neurons in many different areas. But there is one area in particular that is crucial to human cognition that is targeted by dopamine: the prefrontal cortex.

The *prefrontal cortex*, as its name suggests, sits at the front of the brain behind the forehead. While no one exclusive brain area makes us human, the prefrontal cortex is the key brain region that shows a huge quantitative difference between our species and the rest of the animal kingdom, comprising 33 per cent of the adult human brain but only 17 per cent in chimps, our nearest relatives. The prefrontal cortex has more inputs to all the other cortical areas than any other part of the cortex and therefore plays a key role in operational brain cohesion. So, if this key area is damaged or underactive, there could be a profound effect on holistic brain operation, as indeed there was, famously, some 150 years ago.

The classic example of this is the case of one Phineas Gage who, in the mid-nineteenth century, was working as a foreman on a railway gang in Vermont.[4] His job was to clear any obstacles in the way of the railway track that was being laid across America at the time. One day, as he was pressing down explosive with a large rod, a 'tamping iron', an alarming accident occurred that earned Gage his place in medical history. The explosive went off prematurely and drove the formidable rod through his brain, more specifically through his prefrontal cortex.

After this terrible event and the reason why the story is now so famous there were, amazingly, no obvious or immediate signs of problems with either Phineas's senses or his movement. Only as the weeks turned to months did it emerge that he had more subtle cognitive problems, such as excessively reckless behaviour – not a good trait in someone working with explosives. Surprising though it now seems, Phineas seemed sufficiently unimpaired to return to work, but he had become unbearable as a team player. He was proving to be not only reckless but also, in the words of his physician, Dr Harlow, 'exceedingly capricious and childish . . . particularly obstinate; he will not yield to restraint when it conflicts with his desires'.[5] Gage was a living example of the parallel between an underactive prefrontal cortex and childhood. In biology a well-known mantra is that 'ontogeny' reflects 'phylogeny' – individual brain development reflects evolution – so the human prefrontal cortex becomes fully matured and functional only in the late teenage years and early twenties.[6]

Adolescence is exemplified by intense social behaviour, novelty and attention seeking, as well as tendencies towards risk-taking, emotional instability and impulsivity; relationships take on a greater significance and seeking out fun and exciting experiences are a high priority. There is also the likelihood of pervasive negative moods, of complaints and boredom, which may also drive the teenager to search for stimuli offering more thrills. Research shows that adolescents apply greater reward value and show greater sensitivity to the reinforcing properties of pleasurable stimuli, where, in particular, the enhanced release of dopamine displays a lifetime peak.[7] In addition, imaging studies of the adolescent brain commonly reveal widespread activity unrelated to any specific task.[8] Such generalised activity decreases as adulthood is reached, suggesting a more organised collection of networks resulting in more efficient processing. As the adolescent brain matures into that of the adult, there is a shift into a more integrated network activity pattern, connecting more distant brain areas; the result is long-range synchronous activity across the brain, enabling improved communication between all the different regions, as the prefrontal cortex is fully operative and thus able to coordinate activity in diverse brain regions.

The subsequent onset of more restrained, inhibitory adult behaviour could be due to the fact that more evolutionary primitive brain regions (in particular the ventral striatum, which releases dopamine) are fully operational much earlier than the evolutionarily newer ones, in particular the sophisticated prefrontal cortex. So teenagers will be more inclined towards risk and reward as a result of an inability of their cortex to inhibit the primitive areas.[9] Meanwhile, in addition to this delayed shift in power balance between older and newer brain areas, there are changes in the levels of various chemicals: shifts will be occurring in the 'significance' of reward as a result of altered connectivity in systems using the now familiar dopamine, as well as oxytocin, a powerful hormone which enhances feelings of well-being; this in turn leads to increased sensation seeking and risk-taking in adolescence.[10]

There are other, very different, groups of people that fit this living-for-the-moment profile who are characterised by an underactive prefrontal cortex. In schizophrenia, for example, there is a chemical imbalance, in particular a functionally disproportionate level of dopamine:[11] the world shifts from the cognitive towards raw sensations driven from the outside. Like children, those suffering from schizophrenia are easily distracted or baffled by proverbs such as 'People who live in glass houses shouldn't throw stones.' A typical attempt at explanation might be: 'If you live in a glass house, and someone throws a stone at it, your house will break.' The child and the schizophrenic both take the world literally. To them, it is a vibrant world that can implode on and crush the fragile firewall of the vulnerable inner world.

Yet another – completely different – group of those with an unusually underactive prefrontal cortex are those with a high body mass index (BMI),[12] who are heavy relative to their height. Interestingly enough, we now know from a recent study using a gambling task that obese people take more risks.[13] What could possibly be the common factor between these very different outward states of gambling, eating, schizophrenia and indeed childhood that have in common an under-functioning prefrontal cortex?

Anyone who eats knows the consequences of eating too much, and anyone who gambles is always aware of the possible outcome. But the thrill of the moment, be it the sensation of the taste of the food or the excitement of the roll of the dice, trumps the consequences. The press of the senses, the here-and-now environment, is unusually paramount, as it is for the schizophrenic and for the child. So here are three very different states or activities – overeating, gambling and schizophrenia – all characterised by an emphasis on external stimulation and an underactive prefrontal cortex: the small assembly mode of consciousness, which we saw just now, could be described as a here-and-now state driven by sensation and, among other things, high levels of dopamine.

If so, then another example of this brain state could also include dreaming, already flagged as an example of a shallow, childlike consciousness of the small assembly mode. In fact, a review of imaging studies by Thien Thanh Dang-Vu and colleagues in Liège, Belgium, highlights how dreaming leads to inactivation of the prefrontal cortex.[14] When this key area is under-performing, there is a corresponding drop in holistic coordinated brain operations. Nothing 'means' anything, it just is what it is: the small assembly mode of consciousness where what you see is what you get, and you get it immediately.

Normally, when you are fully awake and accessing your personalised neuronal connections, and therefore using your mind, you are able to understand the world in your own special way. For example, the banner of stars and stripes may have a profound meaning for a US Army veteran, but be merely a piece of coloured cloth with a strange pattern to a young child raised in Papua New Guinea. For the veteran there would be a myriad of different events and experiences all covertly contributing to a highly personalised and extensive network of association, as well as symbolising certain abstract values. Your neuronal connectivity, therefore, gives you the ability to appreciate symbolism, to see one thing as standing for something else, which could never be guessed from the sensory features of the object alone.

Sometimes we make inappropriate or excessive associations that over-interpret an experience or object, discerning a hidden meaning that to most others would seem neither realistic nor accurate, or even a little crazy. Seeing faces in cloud formations, or attributing luck to an object may be everyday examples of such idiosyncratic associations. Similarly, the pairing of two otherwise unrelated events may seem to some to be a silly superstition, but to others it may be a deeply significant sign or portent. Not only do your neuronal connections allow you to imbue objects, events, people and their actions with your own personalised 'meaning', but they also enable you to understand the world as you live in it. The very act itself of making these associations, of being aware of a meaning beyond face value, can be regarded as *understanding*. In all cases the person, object or event would be read off against the checks and balances of your particular neuronal network associations, a conceptual framework that is constantly evolving and expanding as you develop. The more extensive the associations, the greater the conceptual framework in which you could embed the new arrival of the moment and the more deeply you can be said to understand it.

This mind can be distinguished from consciousness, as any dementia patient stands testament. Moreover, the various diverse states where you can, tellingly, 'let yourself go' can give clues as to what might be happening in the brain when the mind is not fully operational but you are simply the passive recipient of the senses. We've seen that various extreme states of overeating, gambling and schizophrenia place an emphasis on stimulation comparable to childhood, and that where the prefrontal cortex under-functions most recreational pursuits are also associated with the transmitter dopamine mediating feelings of pleasure. These literally sensational experiences might be characterised by the small assembly correlate of consciousness, a correlate that characterises non-human animals and the dreaming adult brain, where thought plays less of a role. But how does a thought differ from a raw feeling?

Remember from earlier the comment that 'Thinking is movement confined to the brain'? We saw that any thought, be it a hope, a memory, a logical argument, a business plan or a grievance, all share a fixed sequence of cause and effect: a beginning, a middle and an end. You end up in a different place to where you started. So in physical brain terms perhaps the bases of thoughts are connections between relevant neurons or neuronal groups. Thinking, that superlative talent of the adult human brain, requires enough neuronal circuitry to take a series of steps, to make connections, and a correspondingly longer time-frame. Meanwhile emotions can be characterised by their focus on feeling something right now and only now. Conscious thought extends beyond the immediacy of the moment and is not readily trumped by any new here-and-now stimulation.

While information processing is just that, the appropriate response to an incoming stimulus, *understanding*, in contrast, requires that the stimulus be embedded in a conceptual framework. We've seen that a conceptual framework of the type required for understanding can be interpreted, in brain terms, as the growth of the connections between brain cells that are formed postnatally and are subsequently driven, shaped and strengthened by individual experience. Hence every individual human will have a uniquely personalised brain, as well as a mind that is constantly evaluating the current world in terms of existing associations while simultaneously being updated by it.[15] 'Knowledge' would be the embedding of a fact or action within a conceptual framework so that it makes sense, that is, can be understood. Meanwhile 'wisdom' requires still further and widespread connectivity whereby the associations made are drawn from an ever wider range of experience and/or individual memories that enable the assignment of more generalised values.

As we survey the impact of twenty-first-century technologies as the drivers of Mind Change, constantly recurring themes will

Table 8.1 Two basic modes for the human brain?

Mindless	**Mindful**
Sensation	Cognition
Strong feelings dominate	Thinking dominates
Here and now	Past–present–future
Driven by external environment	Driven by internal perceptions
Little meaning	Personalised meaning
Not self-conscious	Robust sense of self
No time or space frame of reference	Clear episodes that are sequentially linked
Children, schizophrenics, gamblers, drug takers; those with high BMI; those engaging in recreational pursuits, e.g., fast-paced sports, sex, dancing, dreaming (driven by chance neuronal activity)	Normal adult life
High dopamine	Less dopamine
Prefrontal under-function	Normal prefrontal activity
World meaningless	World meaningful
Small assembly correlate of consciousness	Larger assembly correlate of consciousness

be that of 'narrative', one personal life story, and of 'mind' as a real physical entity, namely the unique configuration of neuronal connections in each individual brain. Table 8.1 summarises, in an extremely simplified way, how we could think of this mind in relation to the subjective conscious state, as well as various features in the physical brain, which we can use as a guiding frame of reference when we come to consider how the digital technologies could be impacting not just the generic brain, but the individual mind, beliefs and states of consciousness. We have come a long way from the pink plastic model but the journey is really only now just beginning.

9 THE *SOMETHING* ABOUT SOCIAL NETWORKING

> People forgetting about my existence is what really gets to me. If I went to a party or on a vacation and didn't document it on my Facebook, did it really happen? Does it just chip away at my presence as a human being and force me to wear an invisibility cloak? . . . I have almost 800 friends on Facebook, but only hang out with a handful of people in real life. Isn't that bizarre? Who are these 790 friends of mine? When's the last time we actually hung out? Do I even know them? If I don't, why would I want them to know me? All of this rhetoric is making me want to simultaneously delete my Facebook and check to see if I have any new messages. Regardless of my decision, I think we can all agree that Facebook has messed with my generation's lives in a very real way. It has dictated our day to day lives by creating new social rules and etiquette we must abide by. It's basically turned us into paranoid neurotic messes who are afraid of a real human connection. Mark, why do you have such contempt for us?[1]

This is from Ryan O'Connell, writing in *Thought Catalog* back in May 2011. Although his words are spoken tongue in cheek, this mind-set might be vividly reflecting the colossal impact of social networking sites on our current way of life. If so, is it a sinister sign of a dysfunctional society to come, or does socialising online merely provide a more frequent and accessible version of what we have all always done? Either way, there will be important implications for our lives and culture in the future. Never before have so many had the opportunity to share freely music, photos, videos and opinions as they blog away with ease, and often with almost instant feedback.

While social networks have existed as far back as 1997, sites such as Myspace, Bebo, Instagram, Tumblr, Facebook, Twitter and LinkedIn remain the most used worldwide, with Facebook dominating the Western social networking market. Compared with other social networks, Facebook users are the most engaged: 52 per cent visit Facebook daily, with other popular sites such as Twitter (33%), Myspace (7%) and LinkedIn (6%) trailing behind.[2] The average smartphone Facebook user checks their profiles fourteen times a day.[3] Thus, while there are numerous social networking sites, given the popularity of Facebook worldwide and the subsequent amount of research into Facebook use, much of the discussion here will focus specifically on Facebook. The 'Mark' rhetorically challenged by Ryan is, of course, Mark Zuckerberg, founder of Facebook and *Time*'s Person of the Year 2010. It's hardly surprising that the horizons, as far as he's concerned, are unequivocally clear and bright:

> There is a huge need and a huge opportunity to get everyone in the world connected, to give everyone a voice and to help transform society for the future. People sharing more even if just with their close friends or families creates a more open culture and leads to a better understanding of the lives and perspectives of others. As people share more, they have access to more opinions from the people they trust about the products and services they use. This makes it easier to discover the best products and improve the quality and efficiency of their lives.[4]

I doubt if the primary reason for someone going on Facebook, especially a teenager, will be, as Zuckerberg suggests, the earnest goal of improving the efficiency of their existence. Over 1 billion people in the world are signed up, and of these just over half are visiting the site daily.[5] For social networking to be as popular as it is with individuals from such a vast range of cultures and backgrounds, it must be meeting a very basic human need and doing it really well.

The most common reason put forward to explain the immense popularity of sites like Facebook is that they help us connect online with our offline (real-world) friends and make it easier to maintain long-distance friendships.[6] However, alternative and still popular forms of computer-mediated communication, such as emails or Skype, are effective and easy for communication over long distances. So connecting with friends cannot, on its own, account for the appeal of cyber socialising. Additionally, recent research has found that those who use Facebook to collect a large network of virtual friends report *more* life satisfaction, compared to those who use it to maintain close and enduring real friendships.[7] Alarmingly, this study found that Facebook users are more satisfied with their life when their Facebook friends are regarded as their own personal audience to whom they transmit unilaterally, rather than when they have mutually reciprocal exchanges or more offline relationships within their online networks.

Perhaps it all boils down to that most simple driver of all: the desire to feel good. In one survey, results suggested that the opportunity to develop and maintain social connectedness in the online environment is linked with less depression and anxiety as well as with a greater satisfaction with life.[8] Zuckerberg would presumably agree:

> Personal relationships are the fundamental unit of our society. Relationships are how we discover new ideas, understand our world and ultimately derive long-term happiness . . . We have already helped more than 800 million people map out more than 100 billion connections so far, and our goal is to help this rewiring accelerate.[9]

Already, Zuckerberg is gesturing here at a new type of existence, one that is now more joined up, where your identity is no longer so much internalised as constructed in close conjunction with others. His use of the word 'rewiring' implies that we're functioning together as nodes in some complex machine, that we were already all previously connected ('wired' in a different way) and that this new rewiring is superior. None of these three assumptions are valid. Firstly, although the concept of a global network of thought (the noosphere) was developed, as we saw earlier, by a Jesuit monk named Pierre Teilhard de Chardin almost a century ago,[10] it has never been regarded by anyone else as the potential apotheosis of humanity. Secondly, we have never actually been constantly 'wired' together, hence the popularity of this novel condition of connectedness. And, thirdly, why should we automatically assume that whatever Facebook offers is superior to all previous forms of communication? We need to look at what's going on a bit more closely.

The opposite state of being in some way connected to someone else is not to be connected at all, to be alone. In evolutionary terms, there would be a survival value and hence a basic subjective 'pleasure' in any behaviour that combated solitude. And it turns out that loneliness is really bad for your health. For example, women with fewer social relationships have experienced strokes at twice the rate of those with more, after adjusting for all other possible factors.[11] Moreover, DNA analysis has identified 209 genes relating to immune system function for combating response to illness, which are differentially expressed in subjects reporting high levels of social isolation.[12] Evolutionarily ancient immune system defence cells appear to have evolved a sensitivity to socio-environmental conditions that may allow them to shift basal gene expression profiles, to counter the changing threats of infection associated with hostile social conditions. Moreover, changes in the expression of inducible genes relate more strongly to the *subjective* experience of loneliness than to objective social network size. And if that weren't enough, loneliness can increase the incidence of cardiovascular disease through reduced levels of oxytocin, the naturally occurring hormone we met earlier, which normally reduces and stabilises heart rate.[13] Because oxytocin surges during close physical contact and is associated with well-being, clearly isolation will inactivate this natural defence mechanism.

The number of people living alone has doubled over the last twenty years, such that in the United Kingdom an unprecedented one-third of all adults are single-member households.[14] This trend is particularly pronounced in the age group 25–44 years of age. More people living alone equates with a greater potential for loneliness, so the subsequent arrival of social networking sites will have met a clear demand among a growing group of immediately receptive customers. The subsequent shift in how adults socialise has fundamentally transformed social interaction in two decades. In 1987, according to one estimate, we spent on average six hours per day in face-to-face social interaction, and four via electronic media.[15] In 2007 the proportion had reversed, with almost eight hours a day spent socialising via a screen, and only two and a half hours in face-to-face social interaction. The advent of social media not only met an existing need but did so even more effectively than normal interpersonal communication.

The neuroeconomist Paul Zak has suggested that social networking itself will increase levels of oxytocin.[16] Perhaps the cyber simulation of being close is the same as the real thing, as far as the body is concerned. But this special experience of sharing involves a trade-off of sharing information about yourself and your feelings to an unprecedented degree. So what's wrong with that? Surely, if we are boosting our oxytocin levels, feeling close to others and fending off the health-threatening effects of loneliness, what's not to like?

The data on the relationship between feeling lonely and social networking is surprisingly complex.[17] Research shows that all those who are actively engaging in Facebook via messaging friends and posting on friends' walls report lower levels of loneliness, while those who primarily engage in passive observation of friends' profiles report higher levels.[18] Loneliness also apparently predicts emotional attachment to Facebook,[19] indicating that only the most solitary use the site to compensate for their lack of offline relationships, whereas those with healthy, already established real-life networks simply turn to Facebook as an additional nice-to-have. Interestingly, students with higher levels of loneliness also report having more Facebook friends than those who are in reality more sociable.[20] Thus, while social network use might be used to deal with feelings of loneliness, it may not have the desired effect after all. For example, the futurologist Richard Watson has serious reservations:

> I believe that one of the main reasons that Facebook and Twitter are so successful is that we are lonely . . . Universal connectivity means that we tend to be alone even when we are together. You can see this when couples go out to dinner and spend most of their time texting or when kids get together for play-dates and end up sitting next to each other on separate gaming consoles for hours on end.[21]

Some researchers suggest that escaping online to avoid real-world problems may actually exacerbate them.[22] One study examined Facebook use from the perspective of adult attachment theory, which emphasises the role of the primary caregiver during infancy.[23] Attachment theory was developed by psychiatrist John Bowlby in the mid-twentieth century, when he was treating emotionally disturbed children. Bowlby proposed that attachment was 'lasting psychological connectedness between human beings' and showed that babies were either 'secure', 'anxious' or 'avoidant' in their attachment styles.[24] The secure baby might cry when the mother left the room but, as soon as she returned, would start to play again. In the case of anxious babies, however, when the mother came back, they would push her away and burst into tears. In contrast, the avoidant baby would act as if nothing had happened, despite a rise in heart rate and levels of the stress hormone cortisol.

Adults behave like babies too. While secure people feel comfortable with intimacy, avoidant individuals struggle to establish emotional connections. They are more likely to be socially isolated and to attempt to shut down their emotional needs in relation to others. In contrast, anxious attachment individuals are anxious about being alone; they fear rejection and will engage in behaviours to strengthen their relationships. The researchers found that individuals with high levels of anxious attachment used Facebook more frequently, were more likely to use it when feeling negative and were more concerned about how others perceived them on Facebook.[25] So it would seem that Facebook fills a need for those with maladaptive early experiences. However, it's still unclear whether Facebook use could help those with high levels of anxious attachment by combating feelings of loneliness and reinforcing their relationships.

But it's not just the lonely and the anxious who are drawn to social networking. Research has also shown that individuals with higher levels of openness spend more time on Facebook and have more friends there.[26] Openness signifies an active imagination, a willingness to try new experiences, an attentiveness to inner feelings, a preference for variety and having a curious mind.

Thus, having a large number of Facebook friends, paradoxically, is associated both with higher openness levels and also with being more lonely. Although it might seem counter-intuitive, openness and loneliness are not incompatible: openness is a personality trait, whereas loneliness is a state. A combination of the 'pull' of wanting to be open and the 'push' of loneliness is a potent factor in determining just how much you give away about yourself. It is this self-disclosure that is crucial to understanding the real appeal of social networking sites.

As a species, we seem to have such a craving for self-disclosure that we could see it as a very basic part of the human psyche. Harvard scientists have actually demonstrated that sharing personal information about oneself, as promoted on social networking sites, activates the reward systems in the brain the same way as food and sex do.[27] Astonishingly, the participants in this particular experiment were even willing to give up monetary rewards for the opportunity to talk about themselves. The results also suggested that the existence of a cyclical feedback for self-disclosure rewards and perpetuates the sharing of personal information on a basic biochemical level. Consequently, the appeal of social networking is rooted in a biological drive of which we are unaware and which we find difficult to control voluntarily.

The conscious need for personal expression and self-disclosure could be the crucial key to what so many find compelling about Facebook and other types of cyber socialising. Although social networking sites will, of course, make such communication easier, the socialising itself may not be the key issue. Instead, the *real* hook may be the experience itself of transmitting personal information on an unprecedented scale, because Facebook and other comparable sites encourage you to divulge information about yourself to others in a way you may never have done before. When someone updates their status with something personal, they share it with their hundreds of Facebook friends. Just think about it. Of course we have shared personal information with each other since the dawn of time, but now we do it with 262 people (the average number of Facebook friends across all ages and demographics) instead of just our close friends.[28] The point is that, when you share personal information on Facebook, whether through your profile or as a status, you share it with an immediate audience that is the largest ever in human history.

If so, then the next question is why are we willing to give away so much personal information on such an unprecedented scale? Perhaps social networking sites and the psychological disposition for self-disclosure can interact reciprocally and reinforce each other. One of the most consistent outcomes of computer-related research shows that the lack of face-to-face communication leads to a corresponding rise in self-disclosure, because we don't have visual cues or access to the appropriate body language to discourage us or to make us second-guess what we might disclose.[29] When we meet people in the flesh, shake their hand, look them in the eye and pick up on cues through body language, we gradually build trust and rapport and gradually feel that we know that other person before we let our guard down. Until then the defensive body language, the averted eyes, the physical distance, even the interruptions and voice tone as we speak, may all act as warnings not to give too much away too soon. Body language is an ancient evolutionary mechanism for not letting our defences down prematurely. If there are no such cautionary signs, nothing to prevent us talking or writing on and on and on, then disclosure is far easier. People who want to disclose more will use social networking sites more, which only encourages them to disclose even more.

For example, 488 users of social networking sites were surveyed in Germany twice within a six-month period.[30] Individuals with a stronger disposition to self-disclose showed a higher tendency to network socially. At the same time, frequent social networking use increased the wish to self-disclose online, because self-disclosing behaviours are reinforced through accumulating social capital within Facebook and similar environments. The $64,000 question then is: why? If loneliness is the main driver of social networking use, there are far more effective, reciprocal and personal ways to communicate with individuals than the ubiquitous status update online. Yet the lonely are the most attracted to the screen. Just why is it so pleasurable, as the Harvard study[31] clearly demonstrated, to divulge all your feelings and thoughts not to a single confidant occasionally, but to an audience of hundreds or thousands, on such a grand scale and on, say, an hourly basis?

Arguably, with time and distance to hide behind, you can portray yourself as someone completely different and more interesting. The opportunity to avoid the awkwardness of hesitating and stumbling over your words seems wonderful, especially as you won't have a chance to say anything you don't mean or might regret. You are secure and inviolate as you derive tactile pleasure from tapping the keys, and see the writing on the screen dance to your precise command and control. Another part of the excitement of being online comes from being constantly connected. Someone somewhere is always available to interact with you right now; after all, you are globally wired. But, at the same time, you can say anything you like without the embarrassment or discomfort of a face-to-face interaction. No wonder such an experience makes you feel good.

In 2011 a joint Italian and American investigation aimed to dissect the type of experience people have while using Facebook.[32] Is it primarily a relaxing or a stressful experience? Thirty students aged 19–25 took part in short exercises where they first looked at panoramic landscapes (the relaxing experience), then spent three minutes navigating their own Facebook account and finally spent four minutes completing a stressful task, such as solving a mathematical problem. During these tests, their physiological stress levels were recorded to measure how stressful or relaxing the participants found each trial. During the stressful experience, activation of the fight-or-flight system was triggered, namely increased respiration, sweat and pupil dilation, whereas the relaxing experience led to activation of the parasympathetic nervous system, which resulted in an opposite scenario. What was most interesting was that the results showed that navigating your Facebook page offers an experience that is neither relaxing nor stressful, but a more active positive state. Participants showed a mixture of physiological responses that were found in both the relaxing and the stressful conditions. The researchers concluded that the success of social networking sites 'might be associated with a specific positive affective state experience by users'. *In short, going on Facebook is physically and/or physiologically exciting*. But what biological process actually triggers this experience of feeling good, of enjoying Facebook more than you would, say, looking at a painting or going for a walk?

We saw previously how brain scientists have long been fascinated by the phenomenon of 'self-stimulation', where rats will work at pressing a bar to stimulate key brain regions, to the exclusion of all else including feeding. The areas that, when stimulated, presumably caused the rats to 'feel good' were those releasing the transmitter dopamine. As well as contributing to feelings of pleasure, dopamine plays another role in the diurnal rhythms of sleep-wakefulness, where it is linked to heightened alertness. Just think of the hyperactivity caused by 'speed' (amphetamine) which releases abnormally high levels of dopamine in the brain. It's not difficult to see an overlap between feeling excited and feeling happy. Many activities in life that are arousing, such as fast-paced sports, are also rewarding. Suffice it to say that if various brain states relating to arousal and reward are consistently linked to raised levels of dopamine, and if social networking sites are rewarding and exciting, it is very likely that social networking might serve as another trigger for the release of dopamine in the brain.

Dr Susan Weinschenk is a behavioural psychologist who has published five books on user experience in computer systems and lists the specific features of Facebook and other social networking sites that might make them particularly appropriate triggers for dopamine release.[33] First, *a need for instant gratification*: you can now connect to someone immediately and probably get a response in a few seconds. Second, *anticipation*: neuroimaging studies show higher stimulation and activity when people anticipate a reward than when they actually get one.[34] Similarly, the anticipation of whatever new tweets, updates or comments on your profile you might find drives the fascination of many social networking sites more than the actual information you receive. Third, *small pieces of information*: the dopamine system is most powerfully stimulated when the information coming in is modest enough not to satisfy entirely. The limited capacity of a tweet or a 'like' is therefore ideal to activate the dopamine system. Finally, there's *unpredictability*: this is the long and much studied reward/punishment mechanism involved in intermittent or variable schedules of reinforcement. When you check your email or text, or use Twitter or Facebook, you don't know exactly who is contacting you or what you'll receive. This feedback mechanism is largely unpredictable and exactly what stimulates release of dopamine in your brain. The posting and receiving of entries on Facebook or Twitter could trigger the release of small blips of dopamine, possibly encouraging such activity to become not only rewarding but also compulsive.[35]

This almost instant feedback from others, which is unlike any real-world interactions, is much more prevalent when there are so many more people out there in cyberspace who can oblige. The sight of a name flashing up presents a little burst of excitement, a little blip of dopamine that will ensure anticipation for the next fix: you can never actually be satiated. But then why should the mere sight of a response on your particular site, irrespective of what it actually says, trigger that blip of dopamine in the first place?

Attention and approval from adults are among the strongest rewards we experience as we are growing up. Infants need a meaningful relationship with a caring and involved adult in order to survive, grow and thrive. Astonishingly, the human growth hormone is thought to be released in proportion to the amount of caring attention a child receives.[36] When babies cry to announce their hunger or other discomforts, they rely on the world, particularly adults nearby, to correct the problem. These demands are necessary for survival, and when they are met the existence of the child is acknowledged. A hungry baby that yells until someone comes with the right source of nourishment *knows* that they have an effect on the world. The world acknowledges that they exist. This tiny human already has significance. A baby whose needs are ignored eventually gives up and 'ceases to exist'. In extreme and, fortunately, very rare cases of neglect, such infants stop crying when they are hungry and literally starve to death. A child's emotional well-being begins with attention paid to their basic physical needs. Yet the need goes further: the caregiver has to approve and to show approval. Once the physical needs are met, this drive for further validation is one of the strongest motivating forces in our nature. When we aren't met with positive feedback, we no longer feel safe and protected. And over time we become conditioned to crave approval not just from our parents, but from others as well.

The importance of such recognition does not diminish with age. Unlike the real world, Twitter and Facebook can always be relied on to provide an almost instant response to even your adult demands for attention. Facebook may readily be filling a gap that friends and family do not fill so comprehensively.[37] This in turn may explain why the obsessive social networker relies on the illusion of cyber intimacy, despite the inevitable price of a loss of privacy. Many of us take privacy for granted until we feel it is being invaded, whether by an intrusive personal question or the extreme scenario of a helicopter from Google Maps hovering outside the bedroom window. As film star George Clooney quipped: 'I don't like to share my personal life . . . it wouldn't be personal if I shared it.'[38] Until now, most of us most of the time have felt in control of our private lives, of how much we confide, to whom and when. But now such assumptions no longer hold.

It is impossible to give an operational definition of privacy, but most of us, until now, have had a strong instinctive sense of it. In his first non-fiction book, *The Blind Giant*, novelist Nick Harkaway weighs up the balance between the blessings and the threats of the Internet:

> Privacy is a protection from the unreasonable use of state and corporate power. But that is, in a sense, a secondary thing. In the first instance, privacy is the statement in words of a simple understanding, which belongs to the instinctive world rather than the formal one, that some things are the province of those who experience them and not naturally open to the scrutiny of others: courtship and love, with their emotional nakedness; the simple moments of family life; the appalling rawness of grief.[39]

In contrast, at a technology conference in 2010, Mark Zuckerberg defended his controversial decision of the previous year to change privacy settings that pushed users to reveal more personal information, saying, 'We decided that these would be the social norms now and we just went for it.' Zuckerberg told his audience that Internet users don't care as much about privacy anymore: 'People have really gotten comfortable not only sharing more information and different kinds, but more openly and with more people and that social norm is just something that has evolved over time.'[40]

Already privacy appears to be a less prized commodity among the younger generation of Digital Natives: nearly half of teenagers have given out personal information to someone they don't know, including photos and physical descriptions.[41] Meanwhile over half of young people send out group messages to typically over 510 'friends' at a time (the number of Facebook friends an average youth has),[42] fully aware that each of these contacts could then pass on that information to *their* network of further hundreds. The trade-off for more attention and the possibility of fame is, and always has been, loss of privacy and it was always a tough call on how to achieve the appropriate balance. So how is it that we previously treasured privacy so much, yet now hold it in increasing disregard? Until now, privacy was inextricably linked to an internally generated sense of identity; the one always entailed the other. But if identity is now constructed externally and is a far more fragile product of the continuous interaction with 'friends', it has been uncoupled from the traditional notion of, and need for, privacy.

Of course, for many, social networking is a fun adjunct to a normal life that enhances the communication between existing friends made in the real world. Yet there is more to the popularity of these sites than their trendiness and ability to make life easier would suggest. Social networking sites could be viewed as a kind of junk food for the brain: harmless enough in moderation, but deleterious when over-indulged. It seems that the *something* about social networking harnesses and promotes a potentially vicious biochemical cycle, whereby evolutionary biological forces ensure that humans feel good when they are combating loneliness by sharing personal information with others, mediated by the release of dopamine in the brain. As a result, self-disclosure creates a hit of pure pleasure as direct as that derived from food, sex, dancing or sport. And, until now, this natural urge to let it all hang out has been counterbalanced by the rigours and constraints of body language in face-to-face communication, which makes you all too aware of your private self. This awareness of being a private individual can serve the very valuable role of ensuring that we are not manipulated or taken over from the outside. So, by constraining the natural urge to disclose information about ourselves to everyone and anyone, the opposing desire for privacy will ensure that only trusted individuals access the 'real', vulnerable, you.

However, social networking removes these constraints, allowing individuals to disclose more through this medium than ever before. The consequent trading in of the age-old birthright of privacy may mean that others will think less of the 'real' you that is now revealed. But imagine if this mode of constant self-disclosure and feedback were to become the norm. It may become increasingly difficult to protect the 'true self', with all of its weaknesses and failures, from being reshaped and supplanted by an exaggerated, ideal self that is presented to an audience of hundreds of 'friends' and 'followers'. So what would happen if such a cyber-airbrushed persona started to elbow out the real you?

10 SOCIAL NETWORKING AND IDENTITY

'Over the next 10 years, people's identities are likely to be significantly affected by several important drivers of change, in particular the rapid pace of developments in technology.'[1] So reads the opening salvo of *Future Identities*, a report commissioned by Sir John Beddington, Chief Scientific Adviser to the British government. His starting point at the time was that 'The emergence of hyper-connectivity (where people can now be constantly connected online), the spread of social media, and the increase in online personal information, are key factors which will interact to influence identities.' Is this all just scaremongering by a high-profile establishment figure or is it a serious and urgent wake-up call?

Social networking sites evolved from the 1990s version of the Internet, which was already providing many new ways to communicate and socialise. Computer-mediated communication back then was dominated by forums, early online games, chat rooms, bulletin boards and so on, all of which had a default setting of anonymity; it was up to the user to make it personal.[2] Individuals logged on and could select any name they wanted to use as an alias, for example, John_Smith9000. Those who've researched this earlier style of computer-mediated socialising have suggested that it was this potential for anonymity that was all-important: it allowed individuals to discover their repressed identities and learn more about themselves, presumably in a fairly safe way.[3]

Thus, initial investigations into online self-presentation mostly focused not so much on identity, but rather on its absence in anonymous or pseudonymous online environments. These investigations found that individuals tended to engage in role-play games and unusual behaviours in an environment that was arguably healthier than that of the real world.[4] In contrast, nowadays, anonymity is no longer an inherent part of socialising online. The interesting question then is what happens when you are 'nonymous' (i.e., not anonymous) in an online environment:[5] the identities that result are very different.

Technology researchers Nicole Ellison and danah boyd (who prefers her name in lower case), have defined present-day social networking sites as sites that enable a user to (1) 'construct a public or semi-public profile within a bounded system'; (2) 'articulate a list of other users with whom they share a connection'; and (3) 'view and traverse their list of connections and those made by others within the system'.[6] Revealing personal information is now part of setting up a social networking profile: Facebook requires a user's real name.[7] While there are always ways around this, the point is that social networking sites have transformed computer-mediated communication by tethering it to your real-world identity. Additionally, a significant proportion of a user's 'friends' are people that they know or have met in real life. That's a massive and important shift: socialising on the Internet has become fiercely personal. Identity, and any shifting notions of identity in relation to social networking sites, is therefore a central issue.

But how *you* see yourself need not be shared with everyone else: your online self and your 'true self' are not necessarily the same. This notion of a 'true self' was first introduced as long ago as 1951 by the influential American psychologist, the late Carl Rogers, widely considered to be one of the founding fathers of psychotherapy.[8] His theory was that the true self is based on existing characteristics which need not necessarily be fully expressed in normal social life, perhaps because there are not necessarily occasions when they'll be manifest, but rather imagined as particular reactions in hypothetical situations. Fifty years later, the digital age saw John Bargh and his team developing the concept of the 'true self on the Internet' to refer to an individual's tendency to express the 'real' aspects of the self through anonymous Internet communication rather than face-to-face communication.[9] The claim is that the Internet provides individuals with a unique opportunity for self-expression that encourages people to reveal their true self, including the aspects which are not comfortably expressed face-to-face. Because of this effect, cyber communication could be regarded as more intimate and personal then face-to-face communication. Those forming friendships in this way through social networking sites are more likely to put a premium on self-disclosure, in the hopes of expressing their true self.

According to Katelyn McKenna at New York University, people who believe that they are better able to express their true self on the Internet are more likely to form close relationships in cyber space.[10] Moreover, people with a higher tendency to express their true self in this way in the cyber world are more likely than others to use the Internet as a social substitute.[11] Using the Internet as a social substitute involves establishing new relationships with strangers and having Internet-only friends. Such people are more likely to develop a compulsive passion for their Internet activities.

In a survey of university students exploring their motives for Facebook use,[12] a particularly interesting result was that individuals with a high tendency to reveal their true self on the Internet reported using Facebook for establishing new friendships and for initiating or terminating romantic relationships more frequently than individuals who were less concerned about expressing their identity. So it would seem that, for some though not all, the use of Facebook as a vehicle for self-expression goes hand in hand with it being the main conduit of friendship. Wanting to express one's true self through Facebook is also linked with obsessive Facebook use.[13] Once again there is a paradox: those who most keenly desire to express their 'true' identity are precisely those who rely most heavily on relationships in cyberspace. So it's not so much that Facebook is inherently good or bad, but rather how it is used, and the role and importance it plays in one's life.

Unlike in the real world, a Facebook identity is implicit rather than explicit: users show rather than tell by stressing their likes and dislikes instead of elaborating on their life narrative, their strategies and attitudes for coping with problems and disappointments, and all the other baggage of a normal life.[14] If someone posts a picture of a chocolate cake without any meaningful accompanying explanation, they leave it up to their audience of 'friends' to infer what they will. In a real-life relationship, the cake might be a physical tie-in to a much deeper and personal story: it could bring back fond memories of a shared excursion or the sense of triumph that comes with mastering a new recipe. But without special shared experiences or interests, namely shared associations, the cake will 'mean' nothing. And the same could apply to people. As one Facebook user, a female student I spoke to, described it:

> When you get to know people on Facebook, whom you've hardly met, you may think at first that you know them; but it turns out that you only really know the artificial things, bands and movies they like – you'll not know how they react to situations and crises in a way that reveals their 'real' identity to others and, even to themselves.

The most interesting question, however, is this: might this new and different way of expressing yourself actually mean that you see yourself differently?

Whether or not a social networking profile expresses a distorted 'true' self, or displays something more comparable to the real self, there is no doubt that, whatever identity a person is most comfortable promoting, it is likely to be the best possible version. Untagging unflattering photos, or deleting regrettable posts are just two examples of micro-managing the types of information to be seen by colleagues, family and friends. Unsurprisingly, looking good in a photo is the most important factor reported by teenagers when considering which profile picture to select on a social networking site.[15] Canadian sociologist Erving Goffman described how in general we human beings are always on the alert to how others react to us, continuously adapting our outward demeanour to ensure the best possible image.[16] Goffmann died in 1982 and therefore never lived to see the advent of Facebook and Twitter. Yet he understood how we long to promote our 'front stage' self, while the real 'backstage' self pedals away furiously to ensure the most impressive performance. These are desires which sites like Facebook and Twitter now cater for superbly by providing the widest audience ever.

Adapting this dichotomy of front stage versus backstage to the Facebook culture, we can think of a 'networked identity', a term first coined by danah m. boyd, who described it as follows:

> On MySpace for example, you have to write yourself into being: in other words, you have to craft an impression of yourself that stands on its own. Is it the end-all and be-all in developing your sense of self? Of course not. But online expressions are a meaningful byproduct of identity formation.[17]

Research is showing that the identity portrayed on Facebook is neither the uninhibited real self, previously displayed in anonymous computer-mediated environments, nor is it the self that is presented in three-dimensional, face-to-face interactions.[18] Rather, it is a deliberately constructed, socially desirable self to which individuals aspire but have not yet been able to achieve.[19] Astonishingly, social networking has now resulted in three possible selves: the *true self*, expressed in anonymous environments without the constraints of social pressures; the *real self*, the conformed individual who is restricted by social norms in face-to-face interactions; and, for the first time, the *hoped-for, possible self* displayed on social networking sites.[20]

But perhaps this is splitting hairs. It turns out that there is little difference between a displayed Facebook page personality as rated by an observer and the Facebook page owner's actual traits.[21] Nonetheless, although the observed personality profile may be recognisable as the same individual, the possibility of online identity management allows for distortion. Researchers agree that, like a funhouse mirror, the online self is likely to be an exaggerated version of the real self. And this exaggeration could get out of hand. It's not that social networking sites have provided the first ever opportunity for us to distort our identity and hence relationships, but they are now providing an unprecedented opportunity to do so. Creating, managing and interacting through an online profile is a chance to advertise yourself unchallenged by the constraints of reality, to be an idealised, edited version of the 'real' you. Although this online self is 'an invention that, for most people, is a continual approximation of presenting our sense of self to the world',[22] the clinical psychologist Larry Rosen fears that a dangerous gap could grow between this idealised front stage you and the real backstage you, and lead to a feeling of disconnection and isolation.

One direct outcome could be an exaggerated obsession with the self, since many researchers have commented on how social networking sites provide the ideal platform for narcissists.[23] Given the extent of control one has over one's online presentation and the scope of audience that can be reached, a bi-directional relationship might come as no surprise. Social networking can demonstrably increase narcissism levels. In the meta-analysis mentioned earlier, Jean Twenge and her colleagues investigated over 14,000 college students[24] and found that twenty-first-century students scored substantially higher on questionnaires for narcissism, compared to those from 20 years previously. However, Facebook use did not become widespread until after 2006, which means that in this study any screen-based effects on indulging the ego would have to be attributed to earlier forms of social networking sites. True, but Facebook could now be tapping into this existing predisposition which is another reason for its popularity, thereby feeding the trend for self-obsession in a self-perpetuating cycle.[25]

This relationship between heightened narcissism and social networking, though well documented,[26] appears to be confounded by a number of different factors, such as the number of friends, status updates and photos, and the types of interactions with other users. The link needs to be unpacked further as narcissism itself can be unpacked. Narcissism is a complex phenomenon that can be broken down into a range of characteristics: exhibitionism (showing off), entitlement (believing that one deserves the best), exploitativeness (taking advantage of others), superiority (feeling that one is better than others), authority (feeling like a leader), self-sufficiency (valuing independence), and vanity (focusing on one's appearance).[27]

Research shows that adults high in superiority have a preference for posting on Facebook. For the younger generation of students, it is posting on Twitter that is associated with superiority, with Facebook activity linked to exhibitionism.[28] In contrast, for adults, Facebook and Twitter are both used more by those focused on their own appearance but not as a means of showing off, as is the case with college students. These findings are important as they reveal just how many factors are involved, on the one hand, in different types of social networking and, on the other, in the very different groups of people who are all users. Most interesting of all for Mind Change is the generational difference between students and adults, which suggests that a lifetime of early exposure to the influences of Facebook and Twitter are developing a cultural mind-set that is different from previous generations.

But the basic fact remains across different age groups and irrespective of the particular characteristics that predominate: enthusiastic use of social networking sites is linked strongly to narcissism. Of course, human beings have always been vain, self-centred and prone to bragging, but now social networking provides the opportunity to indulge in this behaviour unabated, around the clock. Interestingly enough, such behaviour may also be linked to low self-esteem.[29]

For those of any age with an existing network of friendships built up in the three-dimensional world, social networking sites can be a happy extension of communication, along with email, Skype, or phone calls, when face-to-face time together just isn't feasible. The danger comes when a fake identity is both tempting and possible through relationships that are *not* based on real, three-dimensional interaction, and/or when the most important thing in your life is the second-hand lives of others rather than personal experiences. Living in the context of the screen might suggest false norms of superlative lifestyles awash with friends and parties. Inevitably, as the ordinary human being follows the activities of these golden individuals, so self-esteem will plummet: yet the constant narcissistic obsession with the self and its inadequacies will dominate. We can imagine a vicious circle where the more your identity is compromised as a result of social networking, and the more inadequate you feel, the greater the appeal of a medium where you don't need to communicate with people face-to-face.

Individuals with low self-esteem perceive Facebook as a safe, appealing place for self-disclosure and they spend as much, or more, time using Facebook than people with high self-esteem.[30] A world of airbrushed online portraits may appear to be a low-risk environment ideal for enriching relationships by sharing things which they might otherwise be too inhibited to share. However, people with low self-esteem tend to make updates that emphasise their negative features at the expense of the positive, compared to those with high self-esteem. Sadly, as a result, they are 'liked' less than people who have a higher opinion of themselves.[31] When asked the reasons why people unfriended others on Facebook, 41 per cent nominated their annoying status updates as reasons.[32] Ironically, the conviction that it is safe enough to disclose their feelings on Facebook may encourage people with low self-esteem to reveal things that then lead to the very rejection they fear.

Moreover, given that the majority of a Facebook user's 'friends' do not spend time in face-to-face interactions, the impression many Facebook user 'friends' have of someone with low self-esteem is likely to be negative, and this leads to further rejection.[33] In contrast, expressing negativity in face-to-face interactions typically takes place in a trusting and intimate fashion, when a close friend can be trusted to be honest and you can feel flattered that they would confide their insecurities to you. In contrast, the unique platform of social networking sites can lead other users to perceive as distasteful the negativity of an effective stranger with low self-esteem. This creates a situation where Facebook contact may be the only way that many 'friends' communicate, yet people with low self-esteem who 'over-share' on Facebook will, ironically, deter others from becoming close to them.

While many see Facebook as a harmless tool to maintain existing friendships, a recent study found that avid users attach too much significance to the type and amount of attention they receive on their Facebook page, and hence are disappointed.[34] The conclusion is depressing: 'Facebook appears to be a tool for transforming both close connections and unknown others into audiences for individualistic self-displays . . . public self-displays on social network sites may be one way young people today enact increasing values for fame and attention . . . new communication technologies augment an individualistic focus on the self.'[35]

Data from both self-report and observer rating show that individuals are more likely to express more positive emotions and present better emotional well-being on Facebook than in real life.[36] Moreover, Facebook can open up an alternative world in which people can escape from reality and be the person they would like to be. We are also being exposed to 'perfect' lives as we read about people who seem to have it all and are always smiling. These apparently wonderful lives increase the pressure on us to be perfect, admired and fulfilled: a goal that is inevitably doomed to failure. Perhaps it's more than a curious coincidence that, over the last twenty years, the number of people saying there is no one with whom they can discuss important matters, has nearly tripled.[37] In summary, the culture of social networking may predispose users to a narcissistic mind-set that in turn enforces low self-esteem. By relying on Facebook to satisfy this need for approval, users not only think less and less of themselves but also long desperately for others to notice and to interact with them. This in turn encourages the development of an exaggerated or completely different identity: the hoped-for, possible self.

Although this scenario may seem far-fetched, it is precisely what might now be happening. Kidscape, a British charity that helps prevent bullying and protects children, conducted a survey in which they assessed young people's cyber lives through an online questionnaire.[38] Of the 2,300 or so respondents aged 11–18 taking part from England, Scotland and Wales, one in two say they lie about their personal details on the Internet. Of those, the one in eight young people who speak to strangers online are the most likely not to tell the truth, with 60 per cent lying about their age and 40 per cent about their personal relationships. This suggests that many young people adopt a different identity online. Although this particular survey was specifically concerned with children's safety online, it also highlighted the fact that children often create a different persona when they interact with others, especially strangers, in a way that they wouldn't or couldn't in the real world. The survey found that young people start to change their identities and to act differently online at just 11 years of age, and to create identities which allow them to be more rude, more sexy, more adventurous, and which generally indulge in inappropriate behaviour. However, knowing that people may be viewing your input and judging you accordingly could encourage young people to edit their material and be overly self-conscious. This new trend might well be just harmless fun, but then again it also might herald a society where relationships are based on ephemeral connections between imaginary identities.

Social networking sites seem to be enabling, for the first time, some kind of unreal, idealised self in the words of one 21-year-old girl, that of an 'alter ego'. People sometimes actually talk of a split personality, an online self as opposed to an offline self, like a Dr Jekyll morphing from time to time into a cyber Mr Hyde. For Mr Hyde there are no constraints on behaviour and new possibilities are therefore opened up beyond the mere 'fun' Dr Jeykll could ever have just being himself.

As far as the brain is concerned, as we've seen, it is impossible to disentangle identity from environment and context: so it is inevitable that the identity of the next generation will be formed in the context of a pervasive, ever changing cyberculture. The very structure of our lives means that friendships in the real world face competition from those we develop using constantly present and convenient social media. For those who do not have persistent and stable relationships, obsessive indulgence in cyber friendships might have a negative effect on identity. Most worrying would be the dominance of the front-stage mentality of living primarily to gain approval and recognition in the eyes of others, where whatever you might be doing is assessed as to whether or not it's Facebook-worthy. There is the risk that those with impressionable minds and relatively little experience of the real world may become overly concerned with their social lives and define success or achievement in terms of how many friends they have on Facebook or followers on Twitter.

There is even the suggestion that social networking maps directly onto the physical brain: Professor Ryota Kanai of University College London has claimed that the size of an individual's online social network is closely linked to physical brain structures implicated in social cognition.[39] By identifying brain regions associated with an individual's online social network size, Kanai and his colleagues found that the number of social contacts publicly declared on a major web-based social networking site was strongly associated with the structure of focal regions of the human brain. Specifically, they found that variation in the number of friends on Facebook strongly and significantly predicted the size of certain brain structures. The team also found that the grey matter density of one particular brain region, the amygdala, was linked to social network size in the real world, and also correlated with a subject's online social network size.

But what does this scientific-sounding result actually tell us? Could it really be the case that using social networking sites can change brain structure, or that those who already have a certain brain structure will have a larger online social network? The difficulty lies not so much in what the scans themselves show but in the danger of over-interpretation. However fascinating this study may be, a simple brain scan does not tell us whether an activated area is an effect, a side effect or even a cause of the behaviour being observed. The imaging of different brain areas is excellent for revealing a match-up, a correlation between brain and behaviour, but it does not mean that that area is the centre *for* that behaviour. The light on your iron does not mean that it's the centre for the function of the iron: it is just a corollary, a side effect of the iron working.

Remember that brain regions don't have single jobs that map one-to-one onto behaviour in the outside world. Apart from the most primitive brain regions, such as the specialised cells controlling respiration, most areas of the brain participate in many different functions. There is no big boss or hierarchy of command. So what does it actually mean when a particular brain area is comparably larger or denser in a scan? Interpretation, and the validity of that interpretation, will depend very much on just how precise the activity is that is being matched up to the scan.

Think back to the London taxi drivers exercising their working memory of the streets of London and exhibiting changes in size of different brain areas in scans. The skills involved in knowing the best routes for navigating the metropolis are far more specific and definable, and less vague, than those in forming friendships. And again, the rookie pianists who imagined playing the piano were nonetheless still performing in their mind the preludes to a specific set of movements, whether or not the actual contraction of muscles then actually ensued. A network of friendship is a far more abstracted concept and thus harder to define operationally.

Still, we shouldn't throw the neuroscience baby out with the bathwater of simplistic interpretations. Instead, let's think about the complex ways in which the delicate, malleable brain responds to social networking, from the instant a pulse of dopamine is triggered by a response to the latest tweet, through to the long-term shaping of brain cell connectivity, which will ultimately result in a lifelong rearranging of synapses in the brains of those who might eventually be regarded as narcissistic or low in self-esteem.

Sherry Turkle has laid out a convincing case in her book *Alone Together* for the argument that the more connected you are, paradoxically, the more isolated you feel.[40] If you are constantly connected, you are a kind of commodity that can be compared to others and found wanting. This scenario was described in Oliver James's *Affluenza* in relation to material goods and a dysfunctional lifestyle in a capitalist society: if you believe that you need to be more beautiful and richer than the next person in order to have significance, and if you see other people also as commodities for enhancing your perceived significance still further, you will be incapable of having the kind of human relationship essential for well-being.[41] Each person is reduced to a series of ticks in boxes, with no independent worth despite being in a constant state of comparison. It is precisely these qualities of connectivity and comparison that have come to define the quintessence of social networking.

Social networking sites provide an unprecedented platform for social comparison and envy.[42] One 2013 study investigated the relationship between envy, life satisfaction and Facebook use, and found that Facebook had triggered over 20 per cent of all reported incidences of envy or jealousy. This envy was primarily caused by self-comparison with the social lives or holidays of others, which subsequently decreased life satisfaction. However, since previous research indicates that most individuals portray an exaggerated or falsified state of contentment, a vicious cycle may result of portraying exaggerated happiness, feeling envious of others' happiness and experiencing a subsequent stronger need to increase the portrayed levels of one's own well-being.

This cyclical arms race driven by the basic brain mechanisms of addiction and reward would be a far cry from the identity and narrative of a life story that has until now given us our purpose, and mandates an elaborate cognitive context developed throughout life. That is not to say that envy and unhappiness, part of our *cognitive* make-up, don't interact with the *biological* hook of the dopamine cycle. They have to. And if so, paradox though it might seem, are we becoming weirdly addicted to constant comparison with others, even if it ultimately makes us unhappy? Perhaps the unhappiness, that flat, let-down feeling of disappointment, is simply because you didn't win this time around, so try again: spin the wheel or roll the dice again and next time you may just be lucky and impress everyone else. And if you could do that, it would mean you were 'cool'.

So what defines 'cool' on social networking sites? In the past, status was proclaimed by your watch, your car, your achievements. Now status for the Digital Native is measured not by possessions or a prestigious job, but by how 'cool' you are, with 'cool' being informally and loosely defined as how 'famous' you can be. Interestingly enough 'coolness' has now been democratised. Wealth, gender and age are no longer relevant. Achievements are no longer required. It's the simple networking that counts. Those who do decide to keep only close friends on their Facebook profile may lose out in another way, since the number of friends is seen as related to physical and social attractiveness. The number of friends on Facebook is proportionate to how socially attractive you are judged by others and your subsequent social status,[43] and just in case you need reassuring the optimum number of friends in relation to social attractiveness has been found to be 302.[44]

For those seeking a quick and painless way of combating low self-esteem and promoting the self, a San Francisco-based company named Klout could be the answer. It provides social media analytics to measure a user's influence across their social network. The analysis takes data derived from sites such as Twitter and Facebook and measures the size of a person's network, the content created and how other people interact with that content. This information is blended with data from a number of other social networks, such as comment, likes and the number of friends in your network, to come up with a Klout score that reflects your online influence.[45]

And just in case you're thinking that a Klout score would be an irrelevance when it comes to the mainstream real world, ponder the following disturbing comment from a recent article: 'Just as a SAT score is used to judge students and a credit score is used to judge financial standing, Fernandez (The Klout creator) hopes that the Klout score will become an "ingredient" in job interviews.'[46] Since he's the founder, perhaps Fernandez's predictions are a little biased and overly enthusiastic. Still, Klout makes me feel unconditionally queasy. Firstly, impact according to Klout is based entirely on the cyber lifestyle activities of social networking sites; secondly, it is the quantity rather than the quality of your messages that is evaluated; thirdly, the response you generate provides an opportunity for you to use your 'influence' to draw attention to different brands. Although Klout claims, 'You have no obligation to talk about the product. You're welcome to tell the world you love it, you dislike it, or say nothing at all', the possibility of perks such as free laptops and airline tickets even if you don't have a high Klout score means that your friendships have become advertising space. And the fact that importance is measured through social networking, that it depends on how much attention you attract and that this attention can be rewarded, is unlikely to bring out the best in anyone. What kind of lesson are you learning about relationships, and indeed how you see yourself?

For some with a robust background of experience of real-life relationships, spending time updating social networking sites and communicating with friends may improve well-being, just as a good gossip on the phone might, but there is the danger that 'well-being' could now be achieved simply by being 'popular' or approved by other Facebook users or having a high Klout score. While in the short term well-being is obviously a good thing, in the longer term you may question such a superficial reason for feeling happy as a high Klout score: so you begin to feel that something is still missing from your life, such as the sense of fulfilment typically gained from hard work, a real life challenge, sporting achievement or other creative skills. In any event, taking things to the extreme, consider the question: how would any of us feel living in a future society where the end point for achieving a feeling of contentment was simply the sheer number of people noticing you in cyberspace?

'I deleted Facebook,' a friend (from the real world) confided, 'because it was just like high school all over again, where every girl is more popular and beautiful than you are.' While some individuals may be ready to break this false happiness cycle all together, they remain in the vast minority. In 2011, 100,000 UK Facebook users deleted their profiles.[47] In a study of Facebook quitters, the main reason cited was privacy concerns. Individuals with higher excessive Internet use were more likely to quit Facebook, indicating that they had been concerned about their obsessive social networking use.[48] The very fact that quitting has been termed 'virtual identity suicide' by social networking researchers indicates the importance some place on their Facebook profile.

When we were looking at the neuroscience of identity, I suggested that it entails the carefully constructed and unique mind interacting with a large number of momentary external contexts over time. Those contexts and that interaction will be hugely significant in determining who you are and how you see yourself. Until now, the adult mind was the product of a dialogue between environment and self, and this dialogue allowed for pauses, self-reflection and the slow but sure development of a robust internal narrative. In contrast, an unremitting environment lived out on social networking sites will present the polar opposite: a scenario that displaces a robust inner sense of identity in favour of one that is externally constructed and driven. And because identity would in this case be so strongly dependent on the responses of others, it would be recapitulating the insecurity and fragility of a child's lopsided, still nascent sense of self.

Until now, the continuing dialogue between the individual and the environment has been weighted in favour of an internalised, personalised life story and inner commentary which, I've suggested, amounts to what we call identity. As we've just seen, the very basic drive to try to share this narrative with anyone and everyone has traditionally been offset by the biologically based constraints of face-to-face interaction, where friendships are consequently formed gradually and highly selectively. However, social media removes these evolutionary precautions, and presses the accelerator on unfettered self-disclosure in a context where the usual brakes applied by normal interpersonal feedback are absent. So instead of a small circle of friends, the self is now publicised to an audience of hundreds and, like all public performances, it is held up to endless scrutiny and comment. How will this overly self-centred yet fragile identity fare in interpersonal communication and relationships?

SOCIAL NETWORKING AND RELATIONSHIPS 11

Even in ancient Greece, the importance of face-to-face interaction over mere words on a page was recognised. Socrates warned: 'Every word, when once it is written, is bandied about, alike among those who understand and those who have no interest in it.'[1] Nowadays, the screen provides the opportunity for abandoning interpersonal interaction on an unprecedented scale, and with it a wholesale reduction in the risk of social interaction and hence embarrassment. No one can see you blush, hear your voice go squeaky, feel your damp palms, nor can you pick up on these all-important cues for working out how the other person might be reacting.

In 2012, the British communications watchdog, Ofcom, produced their ninth annual Communications Market report. The director of research for Ofcom, James Thickett, was acutely aware of the significance of the decline that they found at the time in the number of mobile calls by 1 per cent and of landline calls by 10 per cent. He concluded:

> In just a few short years, new technology has fundamentally changed the way that we communicate. Talking face-to-face or on the phone are no longer the most common ways for us to interact with each other. In their place, newer forms of communications are emerging which don't require us to talk to each other, especially among younger age groups. This trend is set to continue as technology advances and we move further into the digital age.[2]

Ofcom reported that the average person was now sending 50 texts a week.[3] A staggering 96 per cent of young people aged 16 to 24 were using instant message (non-oral) communication, be it email, text message or a social network, every day to contact friends and family. Meanwhile, verbal communication over the phone or in person has become correspondingly less popular, with only 63 per cent talking face-to-face with friends or family daily.[4]

Although Digital Natives may prefer non-oral communication, through text messaging or the Internet, the type of emotional support that can be provided by these forms of communication turns out to be very inferior. Researchers at the University of Wisconsin–Madison asked the following question: could the content alone of an emotionally supportive conversation between a parent and a teenager convey reassurance, or would the tone of voice and/or physical presence of the parent also play a role?[5] In the experiment, teenagers performed a stressful task, and were then comforted by their parents over the phone, in person or through instant messaging, or had no parental contact whatsoever. Salivary levels of cortisol (a marker of stress) and oxytocin (an indication of bonding and well-being) were measured after the comforting conversation. Teenagers who spoke with their parents over the phone or in person released similar levels of oxytocin, and showed similar levels of low cortisol, indicative of a reduction in stress levels. In comparison, those who instant-messaged their parents released no oxytocin and had salivary cortisol levels as high as those who did not interact with their parents at all. Thus, while the younger generation may favour non-oral modes of communication, in regard to providing emotional support, messaging appears comparable to not speaking with anyone at all.

The extent to which this increase in communication online is not just a symptom but a cause affecting young people's ability to socialise and empathise in face-to-face conversations has not yet been empirically established. Such reluctance to make human contact with someone, especially a stranger, may be through a fear of, or simply a lack of practice in, this most basic of human talents. However, neither alternative bodes well for society. Imagine that you've never had much practice at face-to-face communication because, from an early age, you've interacted with others mostly through a screen. Instead of body language, tone of voice and physical contact, the dominant vehicle for expression is words. It's hardly surprising that many people complain that they've been misinterpreted when chatting through social media. However much you may discuss your emotions, the statements just cannot live up to true facial expressions.

And scarier still is the idea that real, non-verbal communication might be subverted by a parallel cyber universe in which the skills of interpersonal interaction are not sufficiently rehearsed; and if they are not rehearsed it is unlikely that you will be any good at them. So perhaps many younger people, brought up with the safer option of communicating offline, prefer not to risk looking someone in the eye, giving them a hug or taking a chance that their voice may rise up an octave. In turn, this might mean that cyber relationships are indeed very different from real ones. Professional matchmaker Alison Green has found she faces unique problems when dealing with Digital Natives: they appear to struggle to communicate face-to-face, and have shifted the development of romantic relationships online, with couples preferring to get to know each other first through the distance and safety of their smartphones.[6]

The big question is whether such a trend is to be welcomed or not. Sherry Turkle has suggested that Facebook gives 'the illusion of companionship without the demands of friendship'.[7] But in a relatively recent review, Paul Howard-Jones concludes that, all in all, the Internet 'can benefit self-esteem and social connectedness'.[8] Reaching a similar conclusion, Moira Burke from Carnegie Mellon University surveyed over 1,000 English-speaking adult Facebook users for two months around the world, recruited through an ad.[9] The results showed that Facebook increased bonding and decreased loneliness with direct communication. But, tellingly, as users passively consumed news they felt they had less access to new ideas being generated by others. Most important of all, loneliness was experienced in proportion to the amount of content that they consumed. These findings highlight a possible crucial difference between actively supporting existing friendships and the passive consumption of other people's social news. Favourable outcomes from relationships on social networking sites *appear only to apply to those communicating with existing friends*. It turns out that using the Internet to make new friends actually has a very different result. A long-term study of the relation between adolescent boys' and girls' computer use and their friends and quality of friendship reveals that using the Internet to make new friends is now linked to lower levels of well-being.[10]

Along similar lines, drawing from a sample of pre-adolescents and adolescents, researchers found that online communication was positively related to the closeness of friendships.[11] No surprises there. However, this effect held only for respondents who communicated online primarily with already existing friends and not for those who communicated mainly with strangers. It was the socially anxious respondents who perceived the Internet as more valuable for intimate self-disclosure, and this perception in turn led to yet more online communication. So it seems that real-world social intimacy and Facebook intimacy are far from being the same thing: a distinction borne out by a recent survey.[12]

This crucial dissociation between number of cyber friends and real-life emotional ones also applies to older generations. This time a study examined the relationships between use of social media (instant messaging and social network sites), network size and emotional closeness in individuals ranging in age from 18 to 63 years.[13] Perhaps not surprisingly, time spent using social media was associated with a larger number of online social network 'friends', but it was *not* linked to larger offline networks or with feeling emotionally closer to offline network members. So, in general, how might online socialising differ fundamentally from that in the real world? One difference might be in the development of interpersonal communication skills, and consequently in empathy.

The human ability to care about and share other people's emotional experiences is something that clearly differentiates us from most of the rest of the animal kingdom. However, chimpanzees famously have 'mirror neurons' at work in their brains, cells such as the ones related to eating which can be nonetheless activated by simply observing another chimp eating.[14] It seems that the observer chimp has 'empathised' with the luckier counterpart actually enjoying a real grape. So the ability to empathise is quite a basic component of the tool-kit of the primate brain. Studies have found that babies and toddlers also show empathetic behaviour. One investigation with 34-hour-old infants showed that even very young babies cry to the sound of another newborn's cry, and that the cry is a response to the vocal properties of the other's cry.[15] The babies exposed to the crying of another newborn cried significantly more often than those exposed to silence or those exposed to a synthetic newborn cry of the same intensity.

However, full-flowering empathy is not necessarily guaranteed as part of our birthright. It would be hard to imagine a complex trait like empathy being encoded completely and independently in strands of DNA, not least because it is such a culturally dependent phenomenon. For example, although work by Ariel Knafo and his team at the Hebrew University some five years ago indicated a significant genetic contribution, the actual ability to empathise with others keeps maturing well into our twenties.[16] While an array of genes will inevitably be necessary for the realisation of the diverse cognitive traits of the healthy human brain, that contribution will be very indirect and far from sufficient: nature and nurture are inextricably linked. So there is ample time for the environment and the experience of relationships to play a significant part in determining our ability to empathise, especially when the environment is the all-pervasive one of social networking.

The term 'emotional intelligence' has increasingly crept into everyday language to define the 'the ability, capacity, skill or a self-perceived ability, to identify, assess, and manage the emotions of one's self, of others, and of groups'.[17] Whether or not emotional intelligence is part of, or different from, more general intelligence is an interesting question – but not our immediate priority here. Suffice it to say that if it's something that, like intelligence itself, varies from person to person, then emotional intelligence cannot be a feature that is determined and guaranteed from birth. As we saw earlier in the survey of 14,000 Michigan college students, levels of empathy may be declining.[18] While this survey, like all surveys, cannot provide a causal link, the somewhat eerie correlation between the soaring popularity of social networking sites and the decline in empathy is undoubtedly worth considering.

A particularly interesting approach by Miller McPherson was to compare ideas of friendship in 1985 with those in 2004.

McPherson's team discovered that the 2004 subjects had fewer people they could really talk to, with the number of available confidants down by about a third. Even more alarming, the proportion of those actually having no one at all with whom they could discuss important matters had nearly tripled.[19] While there were losses from both within the family and in friend groups, the largest deficits in confidants occurred in the community and neighbourhood. McPherson and his colleagues raised the possibility that respondents might have interpreted the question as pertaining to strictly face-to-face discussion, and if so the shift from oral to online communication may account for the apparent decline.

It is easy to see how these two trends, a decrease in empathy and an increase in online relationships, could actually be linked. As the psychologist Larry Rosen has pointed out, if you hurt someone's feelings but cannot see their reaction, you'll lack sufficient cues to understand, apologise or take otherwise compensatory action.[20] The increase in feelings of isolation may be the result of an increase in opportunity, thanks to the ease and speed with which personal information can be posted, which may encourage thoughtless and possibly damaging information to go out to the world with insufficient forethought. If empathy arises from experience of interpersonal face-to-face communication, and we are good only at what we rehearse, then empathetic connecting in the real world could be a good analogy for the networking between individual neurons which, when they 'fire together' – in Hebb's famous words – 'wire together'. However, if you have no one whom you feel cares about you, you might be all the more tempted to be uncaring to others or just care less about being so. And what effect might this indifference have on our own view of what is important and appropriate to share?

Beyond empathy, excessive Internet use could lead more generally to a reduced ability to communicate effectively, as it has been associated with a lack of emotional intelligence, including poor performance on interpreting facial expressions.[21] Perhaps it is unsurprising that excessive Internet users have deficits in face processing. One particular study used a visual detection system to compare the early stages of the processing of face-related information in young excessive Internet users by analysing their EEG.[22] By presenting subjects with images of faces and objects, researchers had discovered that the brain waves elicited by the viewing of faces were generally larger and peaked sooner than the same responses elicited by objects. This meant that the faces had more significance for the average observer than the objects. However, excessive Internet users generally had a smaller brain wave response than normal subjects, whether they were looking at faces or at tables. This result suggests that for heavy Internet users faces were of no more importance than everyday inanimate objects. Although it's still unknown whether these impairments would extend to deeper processes of face perception, such as face memory and face identification, these observations indicate that excessive Internet users have deficits in the early stage of face-perception processing, an impairment which is in turn associated with a range of disorders including psychopathy and autism.

In the United Kingdom alone, over half a million people, around 1 per cent of the population, have a form of autism. Autistic spectrum disorder is characterised by a 'triad of impairments': (1) difficulty with social communication, both verbal and non-verbal, so that patients often find it hard to 'read' other people; (2) difficulty recognising or understanding other people's emotions and feelings, as well as expressing their own; (3) difficulty with social imagination, namely understanding and predicting other people's behaviour, making sense of abstract ideas and imagining situations outside their immediate daily routine. Nonetheless, the terminology surrounding autism continues to be a problem. In clinical practice and almost always in general discussion, 'autism', 'autism spectrum disorders' and the very clumsy catch-all 'pervasive developmental disorder, not otherwise specified' are terms often used interchangeably.

Traditionally, autistic spectrum disorder is diagnosed within the first two years of life, and hence has been dismissed by some specialists as impossible to link to social networking since very young children won't be accessing the sites. Yet, while an individual obsessively using social networking may well not have a formal diagnosis of autism spectrum disorder, Dr Maxson McDowell, a psychoanalyst, has pointed out that they could still develop autistic-*like* traits, such as avoiding eye contact. Infants who cannot track their mother's face often become autistic, and early eye contact initiates the ability to connect with others' subjective experiences, so essential for social communication and interaction, which is impaired in autism.[23]

Meanwhile, three academics at Cornell University, Michael Waldman, Sean Nicholson and Nodir Adilov, have explored possible associations between technology use and the later development of autism. They considered a variety of screen activities including watching television, watching videos and DVDs, watching films in a cinema and using a computer. A link emerged between early TV watching and autism. If TV can be a factor, it would hardly be surprising if the screen world of the Internet didn't turn out to have an impact as well.[24]

So if we accept the broadening of the term 'autistic-like trait', the Cornell findings might suggest that we shouldn't, after all, exclude environmental factors in some cases. Rates of autism diagnosis have been increasing rapidly in the past two decades.

This increase cannot be attributed solely to genetic causes, yet may well be explained by a more astute diagnosis. However, the possibility that triggers in the environment, such as prolonged and early exposure to a world of the screen where no one looks you in the eye, cannot be dismissed out of hand. One study by Irva Hertz-Picciotto and Lora Delwiche at the University of California showed that, even after taking into account changes to diagnostic criteria and the broadening of the spectrum, a significant proportion of the rise in autism cases was still unexplained.[25] Even if you are never formally diagnosed, your evolutionary mandate to adapt to an environment that does not rehearse the interpersonal skill essential for empathy might result in the development of autistic-like difficulties with empathy.

Interestingly, David Amodio at New York University and Chris Frith at University College London have shown that one of the symptoms of autism is an underactive 'prefrontal cortex'.[26] Remember how the prefrontal cortex sits behind the forehead and comprises 33 per cent of the adult human brain but only 17 per cent of that chimps, our nearest relatives? We saw that this newest evolutionary area has more inputs to all other cortical areas than any other region of the cortex, and therefore plays a key role in ensuring that the brain functions cohesively. So, if this key area is underactive, there could be a profound effect on holistic brain operations, creating the mind-set suggested earlier where the sensory trumps the cognitive, where nothing 'means' anything: it just is what it is. A laugh, a frown, a blush, a smile, anything might 'mean' a lot less: what you see is what you get simply at (almost literally) face value.

Whether or not screen technologies could ever increase the possibility of autistic-like behaviours, it is well accepted that the reverse holds true, and autistic people are most comfortable in cyberspace. Catrin Finkenauer and her team at the University of Amsterdam investigated the link between autistic traits and Internet use in a longitudinal study and showed that people with a tendency towards autistic traits, especially women, were more prone to compulsive Internet use.[27] This evidence suggests some kind of link between an attraction to the Internet and impairments in empathy, as revealed by the lack of distinction between faces and tables or a diagnosis within the spectrum of autistic disorders.

This affinity for the screen has been already exploited for therapy, one notable example being the UK-based ECHOES Project which helps schoolchildren with autism experiment with difficult social scenarios. ECHOES is 'a technology-enhanced learning environment where 5-to-7-year-old children on the Autism Spectrum and their typically developing peers can explore and improve social and communicative skills through interacting and collaborating with virtual characters (agents) and digital objects. ECHOES provides developmentally appropriate goals and methods of intervention that are meaningful to the individual child, and prioritises communicative skills such as joint attention.'[28]

But why should the screen hold such appeal for someone who has problems with empathy? The most obvious answer is that, in such a world, there is no need to understand what might be going on inside the minds of others. What you see is what you get, and actions can speak louder than words. Perhaps when anyone goes online, given the absence of all the valuable non-verbal cues, we are all autistic-like.

To sum up: there is a link between atypical brain wave responses in problematic face recognition, characteristic of autism, and also of heavy Internet users; a link between autistic spectrum disorders and an under-functioning prefrontal cortex, indicative of a more literal take on the world; a link between early screen experiences and later development of autistic spectrum disorders; and a link between autistic conditions and the appeal of screen technologies. While it is impossible to establish cause and effect between these various links, and indeed impossible to draw any firm conclusions, there appear to be some parallels between heavy Internet use and autistic-like behaviours that deserve further exploration.

This line of thinking inevitably brings us to question what we mean in any case when we talk of a relationship. Surely, to be a true friend, you need a real understanding of a person, of how they will react in a host of different contexts. The big difference between online and offline relationships is that in the former you only show what you want, often just cataloguing what you like and dislike. No one sees how you really deal with problems or suffer in stressful situations that have real and permanent consequences, which therefore have a real and long-lasting significance. By contrast, you cannot so successfully hide from a real friend in a face-to-face situation what you may be truly feeling, especially if they are adept at using all the three-dimensional and the five sensory clues needed for real empathy. The lack of rehearsal of social skills might well foretell a decline in deep and meaningful relationships. An important consideration is that a preference for online rather than face-to-face communication could result in greater distrust of people. After all, trust grows from empathy, which in turn is best established through face-to-face communication and body language.

Surely it is when time spent on cyber relationships reduces or replaces time spent on real human interaction that the potential to miss out on deeper intimacy with others is more likely. So we need to think about the impact of Facebook relationships on lifestyle in general. Too much social networking can cross the line into interpersonal dysfunction and damage, even demolishing careers and marriages. It can displace time spent on relationship maintenance, and lead to an increased opportunity to communicate with ex-partners or potential future partners, either of which leads to temptation or to jealousy in current relationships. A 2013 study found that high levels of Facebook use were associated with negative relationship outcomes, leading to more cheating, break-ups and divorces, and this effect was influenced by how much conflict the couple experienced in relation to Facebook.[29]

Social networking sites now expose users to information to which they wouldn't otherwise have access, such as photos of new boyfriends with ex-girlfriends or of ex-boyfriends with new girlfriends, suggesting that Facebook can feed the insecure and jealous side of human nature.[30] One friend told me that she left Facebook because it started making her feel paranoid, even though she wasn't an inherently jealous type: 'But suddenly there was this information that I could know about my partner, that I didn't want to know, but I couldn't help myself looking for.'

And there are more formal studies evaluating and recognising just this reaction. One investigation was based on an earlier finding that continuing offline contact with an ex-romantic partner may disrupt emotional recovery.[31] Results from 464 participants revealed that those who remained Facebook friends with their ex-partner, compared to those who did not, reported sexual desire and longing for the former partner, combined in a toxic mix with lower personal growth. The researchers concluded that, 'Overall, these findings suggest that exposure to an ex-partner through Facebook may obstruct the process of healing and moving on from a past relationship.'[32]

Of course this is true in real life as well. It's hard to get over people whom you continue to see routinely. But Facebook makes this unhealthy perseveration so much more accessible and more difficult to resist. Historically, our relationships would be periodically pruned, through the demise of an intimate relationship, a fall-out with a friend, a change in jobs, schools or residence, or simply losing contact with someone. Now, thanks to Facebook, we can so much more readily cart around all that emotional baggage from the past into our present.

Moreover, greater access to others' personal information has led to a culture where snooping on individuals is not only allowed but expected. The Facebook vernacular is 'stalking', but social networking site researchers have softened the term to 'social surveillance'. Regardless of the semantics, the ability to pry freely and anonymously into the lives of others is a serious issue. You only have to look at the popularity of the gossip celebrity magazines to realise that humans are inherently nosey; but this tendency can now be amplified through using social networking, where interpersonal surveillance is a fairly common practice: 70 per cent of college students reported using Facebook to check up on their romantic partner, with 14 per cent reporting doing it at least twice a day,[33] and the behaviour occurs irrespective of gender.[34] Indeed, an increased level of Facebook use predicts jealousy linked to the social networking site. Investigators argue that this effect may be the result of a feedback loop: Facebook use can expose people to ambiguous information about their partner that they may not otherwise have access to, and this information incites jealousy and further Facebook use.[35]

One law firm which specialises in divorce claimed that almost one in five petitions they processed cited Facebook.[36] Flirty emails and messages found on Facebook pages are increasingly being used as evidence of unreasonable behaviour. According to law firm Divorce-Online, Facebook was implicated in 33 per cent of marriage break-ups in 2011, up from 13 per cent in 2009. Mark Keenan, managing director of Divorce-Online, commented:

> I had heard from my staff that there were a lot of people saying they had found out things about their partners on Facebook and I decided to see how prevalent it was. I was really surprised to see 20 percent of all the petitions containing references to Facebook. The most common reason seemed to be people having inappropriate sexual chats with people they were not supposed to.[37]

Time spent using technology is time spent away from the real world and real people. It is through seeing others, or hearing their voice, that we can try to understand how they feel. Too much time focused on the two-dimensional world of social networks may, as we saw earlier, be affecting young people's ability to empathise with others, form meaningful bonds and ultimately get the best out of their relationships.

In a debate in London in February 2012, I locked horns with Ben Hammersley, the editor of the magazine *Wired*. The motion was 'Facebook is not your friend'. It would be unfair to Ben, who has no voice in these pages, to try and summarise the entire interchange of views. However, the reason I raise the occasion here is that, in our summing up, Ben conceded that Facebook was indeed your friend because it was 'just fun', and obviously it was no substitute for real friendships. Inevitably I launched into a heated riposte but, in retrospect, wish that I had simply acknowledged that Ben had just proved my point. Social networking sites could be as much fun, as insubstantial and as potentially compulsive as junk food. What seems irrefutable, however, is that such sites are having a significant impact on interpersonal communication and hence relationships. And if that is so, then, as with junk food, there will inevitably be still wider repercussions for society as a whole.

12 SOCIAL NETWORKING AND SOCIETY

The whole point of the term 'Mind Change' as opposed to, say, the sci-fi sounding 'brain change' is that it explores many more aspects of how we as individuals think and feel and interact with each other the longer we live in this unprecedented digital environment. In order to gain the bigger picture, it's important to think not just about the neuroscience underpinning these transformations, but also about the psychology, social science and even philosophy. From the seventeenth century onwards, great thinkers such as Thomas Hobbes, John Locke and Jean-Jacques Rousseau promoted the idea of the *social contract* which explains how individuals have consented, either explicitly or tacitly, to surrender some of their individual freedoms, or *rights*, for their own ultimate protection and well-being. So how will social networking sites impact on the accepted moral values of a society?

Megan Meier was a 13-year-old living in Missouri when, in 2006, she started communicating with someone she thought was a boy named Josh Evans.[1] 'Josh' at first seemed caring but then became increasingly critical and insulting: he told Megan that she was such a bad person she should kill herself. In fact 'Josh' was the mother of an ex-friend of Megan's. This story not only demonstrates how easy it is to adopt a completely different persona but, much more significantly, also illustrates the effects that such bullying can have. Megan did as she was told and hanged herself. Alarmingly, this type of tragic story is becoming increasingly common.

The vulnerability of teenagers to sanitised yet minimised communication, their age-related propensity to take risks, the twenty-four-hour availability of social networking, plus an unedited and unrealistic snapshot of what everyone else is up to, are all factors that might prove to be a heady cocktail for some individuals, who could then behave in a dysfunctional way with eventual implications for society as a whole. In 2012 a survey in the United States, Canada, the United Kingdom and Australia showed a stark increase in the number of suicides resulting from cyber bullying, with 56 per cent of cases occurring over seven years and 44 per cent of cases in the most recent fifteen months of the study.[2]

Cyber bullying is when someone uses the Internet, mobile phone or other electronic device to threaten, tease or embarrass another person. Various studies report that 20–40 per cent of young people have been victims.[3] In a survey of US teenagers in 2011, 33 per cent of girls aged 12 and 13 who use social networking sites said that peers' interactions on social networking sites are 'mostly unkind', and 20 per cent of girls aged 14–17 reported the same thing.[4] Often these bullies will set up a website or form a group on Facebook and get others to join in and make comments about another person. But it isn't fair to blame the Internet for this. Bullying has long cast its dark shadow over the playground and workplace, and seems deeply engrained in our psyche.

'Perhaps it is only human nature to inflict suffering on anything that will endure suffering, whether by reason of its genuine humility, or indifference, or sheer helplessness.' This suggestion came from Honoré de Balzac in his 1835 novel *Le Père Goriot*.[5] It's even been hazarded that bullying has evolutionary value as a stabilising factor in the shifting struggles for hierarchical status in primate colonies.[6] But, while bullies have blatantly been a blemish on society ever since Flashman, for example, strutted his stuff in *Tom Brown's Schooldays*, the vehicle for them to express their nasty predispositions so effectively and easily, has not. Now that the Internet and social networking have removed most constraints on accountability, it is possible that this technology could cause behaviours in people and in situations which wouldn't previously have been possible.

Some will argue that the effects of the digital culture on cyber bullying is a non-issue, because the medium is irrelevant. For example, Dan Olweus, who runs a bullying prevention programme at Clemson University, found in a large sample of younger teens that there was a high degree of overlap between those who traditionally bully and those who cyber bully. However, 12 per cent of new victims or bullies in the US sample were cyber bullying only, and had not been victims or bullies in the traditional way. Olweus argues this is a 'very small percentage' and goes on to say, 'These results suggest that the new electronic media have actually created few "new" victims and bullies. To be cyberbullied or to cyberbully other students seems to a large extent to be part of a general pattern of bullying, where use of the electronic media is only one possible form and, in addition, a form with a quite low prevalence.'[7]

However, the 12 per cent of young teenagers who participate in bullying or are victims of it is hardly a 'very small percentage'! Moreover, we need to ask not only whether the Internet encourages this behaviour but also, more importantly, whether cyber bullying can affect a victim more seriously than traditional bullying. After all, the scale of the audience that can witness the bullying, and the permanency of it on the Internet, are far greater than would have been the case with traditional bullying. A recent study found that both cyber bullies and their victims experienced significantly greater levels of internalising problems, such as depressive symptoms and suicidal behaviour, compared to traditional bullying. So the medium can affect the bully *and* the victim much more seriously.[8]

Experts have argued that the Internet creates a unique world which adds extra 'disengagement' from immoral actions.[9] The process of moral disengagement describes how an individual is able to deactivate internal moral controls that otherwise inhibit their behaviour,[10] and this disengagement may be needed to cyber bully: visual cues such as the victim's distress are absent, while the distance created by a screen suppresses any feelings of guilt and shame. Furthermore, because young people associate the use of technology with online games, chatting with friends and exchanging photos, cyber bullying is often closely connected with other means of entertainment.[11] This finding is in line with research showing that cyber bullies have less remorse, which may be due in part to the lack of direct contact between the bully and the victim. However, two investigators, Sonja Perren and Eveline Gutzwiller-Helfenfinger at the University of Zürich, found no relationship between moral disengagement and cyber bullying.[12] Their finding suggests that the screen may dehumanise victims to such an extent that bullies do not even need to suppress any moral values to harm others online; such values are absent in the first place.

Diffusion and dilution of responsibility are other drivers.[13] Although cyber bullying does not mandate the physical presence of a gang within which the responsibility will be diluted, bullying within the virtual crowd occurs more often than traditional real-world bullying. The Internet offers mob anonymity and thus the opportunity to behave in a more shameful way than one would in person. Dr Graham Barnfield, a media researcher and lecturer at the University of East London, told the British TV programme *Tonight with Trevor McDonald* that 'happy slapping' when bullies film and upload bullying onto their phones can be seen by the 'slappers' as a short cut to 'fame and notoriety'. This is an example of a completely new kind of mentality made possible only by the Internet.

There's also another phenomenon which, like bullying, seems also to bring out the worst in human nature and, like happy slapping, could only really happen on the Internet. 'Trolling' is prevalent in chat rooms, Twitter streams and blogs. The concept of 'trolling' generally describes someone who adopts an offensive or controversial stance in order to annoy others or to provoke an emotional response.[14] Mature and seasoned Internet users may take trolls' comments, especially if they are more witty than spiteful, with the appropriate pinch of salt, but more sensitive users or impressionable younger victims may take offence or have their self-esteem and confidence demolished.

It could, of course, be that a certain unpleasant type of person naturally enjoys causing offence no matter what and, if so, they might have found another outlet. But then it is hard to imagine how a troll might truly express themselves face-to-face with their victim in the real world. For example, in one terrible case Internet trolls contacted a bereaved mother pretending to be her dead young daughter getting in touch from hell.[15] Extreme though this example may be, it illustrates how an environment of widespread global access, diminished responsibility and anonymity, combined with a lack of experience of interpersonal relationships, have pushed trolling to new heights, or more accurately lows.

John Newton, head of a school in Somerset, wrote of his concerns in a national British newspaper, the *Daily Telegraph*, suggesting that social networking websites pose a serious threat as they blur the lines between gossip and fact before schoolchildren learn to appreciate the difference.[16] Dr Newton has warned that social networking sites are 'a far more powerful weapon in the hands of our children than we appreciate'. Of Facebook in particular he asks:

> Is it a meaningful social hive generating goodwill and reuniting old friends, or is it a gossips' paradise infesting the world with innuendo, half truth and insult?

If they flippantly post comments on-line, young people especially may not realise the irreversible consequences to someone's reputation

> . . . They have not necessarily understood what constitutes gossip, nor appreciate the exocet quality of a hurtful word; half-formed opinion is all that counts.

This picture of a more malicious and less moral society driven by social networking sites varies in different societies. One investigation compared social networking site use in a collectivistic culture, China, and in an individualistic one, the United States.[17] Over 400 college student participants were recruited from a southwestern university in China, and a comparable number from a midwestern university in the United States. The participants completed a survey about their use of social networking, namely time spent on it, its importance to them and their motives for use. There were clear cultural differences. US users spent more time on social networking sites, considered them to be more important and had more virtual friends than their Chinese counterparts. These findings suggest that in collectivistic cultures the importance of the family and of friends may be partly responsible for Chinese users' weaker ties to social networking. In contrast, individualistic cultures may support less close and enduring friendships, resulting in US users' greater use of Facebook and the like. Given the evidence so far that social networking promotes an individualistic focus, it's surely unsurprising that the Western world seems to use social networking in ways not paralleled in Eastern cultures. However, a further important factor is that the Internet is very heavily censored in China with the government not only blocking website content, but closely monitoring individuals' online activity.

Despite accumulating evidence of the dark side of social networking, with cyber bullying,[18] the potential to spread information at breakneck speed in countries where information may be repressed or controlled is a vital tool. Facebook and Twitter use among activists played a key role in the Arab Spring uprisings in 2011.[19] Moreover, social networking may be an effective means of raising global consciousness among users, for example, to engage young people in the United States to vote and to impart awareness of humanitarian plights. In turn, large sums of money can and have been raised by crowd funding, the collective effort of individuals who network and pool their money via the Internet to promote efforts initiated by others in support of a wide variety of activities, from disaster relief to start-up companies; recently termed 'clicktivism'.

What effect is this clicktivism having? For example, did liking or sharing the *Kony 2012* video to stop war criminal Joseph Kony change a user for the better? The rate at which individuals participated in the Cover the Night activism proposed by *Kony 2012* was significantly lower than would have been predicted, based on the immense popularity of the video. An outstanding issue in clicktivism is how to translate the download on the screen into real-world actions.[20] Social networking sites can provide us with all this information about world issues, and clicktivism requires next to nil effort while making users feel good. Others have termed this kind of passive, easy concern 'slacktivism'.

Indeed, given the research we've discussed showing that the screen can sanitise issues and dehumanise individuals, viewing humanitarian crises through a social networking site may have less impact than if a user were exposed to the situation offline. Clicktivism could well reduce the incentive to make a credible impact on humanitarian issues, because a user feels that liking and sharing a cause has been enough.

Drawing on interviews with teens and young adults, one study explored the extent to which young people's approach to online life included moral or ethical considerations.[21] The data revealed that individualistic thinking was the primary focus when making decisions online; community-focused thinking was least prevalent. Moreover, nearly all individuals in the study had at least one instance where they had trivialised the moral elements of online activities, indicating that individuals have a 'greater tolerance for unethical conduct online'. Perhaps we are indeed in danger of forgetting Donne's famous lines:

> Any man's death diminishes me,
> Because I am involved in mankind,
> And therefore never send to know for whom the bell tolls;
> It tolls for thee.[22]

Facebook, Twitter and similar sites deliver the promise of being constantly connected, wanted, admired, even loved. They have brought into our society interpretations of identity and relationships that challenge current values and morality, in a way that would have been inconceivable even just a decade ago.

13 THE *SOMETHING* ABOUT VIDEO GAMES

There's no point in having fun. But surely that *is* the point: to focus entirely on an activity in the here-and-now present, an end in and of itself. Yet there may be more to it than that. Since the dawn of time human societies have appreciated the importance of fun, in culturally institutionalised events like parties and feasts. Wine, women and song, and their more modern reincarnations, sex, drugs and rock and roll, free us up to live for the moment, to have our raw senses directly stimulated, with no time for abstract thoughts and self-conscious introspection. And all this fun could actually have evolutionary value. Immersion in a sensory-soaked present would favour participating in the material, immediate joys of reproduction and nutrition that are essential to survival.

And it needn't stop there. Talents rehearsed across the card table or playing charades in a rainy winter drawing room translate directly to becoming proficient in the interpretation of body language, in how to employ eye contact, in learning to empathise generally with thought processes and emotions, as well as in developing important cognitive skills such as reasoning and memory. Playing with dolls anticipates caring for babies, while all types of sports develop the team-work, physical health and competitive skills that in the primeval savannah would have ensured the continuation of the fittest. Yet video games could, for the first time, be dissociating fun from any of the survival-value requisites that traditional games have met. Rather than serving as a twenty-first-century answer to age-old needs, the video-gaming experience could be an end in itself rather than a means for thriving in the real world.

The advent of the smartphone has further transformed the experience: 36 per cent of American gamers access games on their smartphones,[1] and it seems that this trend will grow in the future as phones become increasingly personalised to your own thinking and your tastes. These vast technological advances make video games richer and more diverse experiences, and have all contributed to their soaring popularity. Interestingly enough, and contrary to earlier trends, games are rapidly becoming popular with the older generations. The average age of a gamer is now estimated at around 30 years old, with 45 per cent of gamers being women.[2] Nonetheless, video games readily offer something that appeals to all ages, backgrounds and cultures, which the real world and traditional games only rarely do.

Nicole Lazzaro is the founder and president of XEODesign, 'the world's first player experience design consulting company' and a leading researcher 'on emotion and the fun of games'. As an authority on emotions and video games, Lazzaro identified four different types of fun, with the best-selling video games offering at least three out of four on the list. *Hard fun* gives you challenge combined with the promise of eventual mastery; *easy fun* provides the sheer joy of the gaming experience itself; *serious fun* enlivens your otherwise dull tasks; while *people fun* is the inevitable result of hanging out with your friends.[3] Real life rarely provides more than one or two of these opportunities at the same time and certainly not on tap, whereas video games are meticulously designed to do just that.

However, not all games are created equal. They can vary not only in their platform (e.g., PC, gaming console, mobile phone) but, most significantly, in their mode (e.g., single player, multiplayer, offline, online). First-person shooter games remain popular in both online and offline modes where one of the most sought-after titles, the latest version of the *Call of Duty* series, sold over 27 million units within the first six months of release.[4] While incentives to play differ according to gender, age, personality attributes and mood of the gamer, a few common elements in the appeal of video games rank consistently high as factors. Players most frequently cite the opportunity 'to achieve' and 'to escape', as well as 'to socialise', as reasons for entering these unreal worlds.[5]

Video games have existed for over half a century, but only in the past two decades have they become endless collaborative online experiences, often with thousands of other human players interacting simultaneously. These 'massively multiplayer online role-playing games' focus on the progression of the gamer-controlled character, an avatar, in a fantasy world. Unlike typical first-person shooter games, massively multiplayer online role-playing gamers have entire control over the physical features, development and attributes of their avatar. Avatar progression is realised through combat, exploration, item acquisition, skill development, socialisation and narrative. The massively multiplayer online role-playing world in which this action unfolds is much larger in scope than first-person shooter games, with ever more thousands of human players able to interact in the same virtual world simultaneously. Furthermore, this global game is persistent, in that, regardless of whether or not a gamer is logged in, the world continues to turn in the cyber sphere, updating and evolving. In contrast, first-person shooter games are typically made up of purely 'instance' scenarios, in which the plot only exists for the duration of the game and can be restarted at the original point an infinite number of times.

This distinction is important. In a review of the current findings on video gaming, authors Daria Kuss and Mark Griffiths conclude that, given the endless possibilities of the new worlds of massively multiplayer online role-playing games, their social nature and the possibility for the gamer to develop an attachment to their avatar, they are the most addictive type of video game.[6] A friend whose son had become hooked on video games to the exclusion of much else and who can himself see the appeal of, and vulnerability to, gaming tried to explain: 'The games are designed to pull the player in, to ensure that each level is rewarded by the next level, that play never naturally stops and that if you take a break you either suffer in the game play or you feel desolate as a result of the lack of exciting and rewarding game play.'

This personal attachment to, and emotional investment in, an alternative gaming self adds to the lure. Experiences are designed to provide excitement and meaning so that behaviour can then be manipulated. As the designer of Gamasutra, a website founded in 1997 that focuses on all aspects of video game development, John Hopson has been able to analyse the attraction in terms of established 'behavioural theory', where conditioning is used to learn new information and behaviours in both humans and animals. For example, rats can be controlled by being rewarded with food pellets or punished with shocks in accordance with a simple behaviour such as pressing a bar. Hopson has described how, like a rat, a gamer too can be manipulated into continuing to play when reward is given only under specific circumstances. In certain schedules, not only are the rats avoiding the unpleasant, but they are also hooked by the uncertainty of not knowing when a reward will appear; they just know that one will eventually come along.[7] For human gamers, there may be a reward after a number of actions have been completed (*fixed ratio schedule*) or, alternatively, a specific number of actions required, with the number changing every time (*variable ratio schedule*). Then there are *chain schedules*, multiple stages to the goal, where the player needs to respond quickly. Hopson has also analysed how to make players play 'hard' with a variable ratio schedule where each response has the chance of producing a reward, or to play 'forever', where there is always a reason to play. Avoidance behaviour leads to something seemingly rewarding, simply by postponing something aversive. Games are thus excellent vehicles for manipulating brain processing at a very basic level.

Back in 2002, social scientist Nick Yee conducted seminal research on nearly 4,000 players to gain more insight into gaming behaviour.[8] He found that well over half of all the gamers confessed to playing massively multiplayer online role-playing games for ten hours continuously or more in a single sitting, and over 15 per cent reported feeling anxious, irritable or angry if they were unable to play. Nearly 30 per cent admitted they continued to play even when they became frustrated or upset or had stopped enjoying the game, while 18 per cent claimed that gaming had caused them academic, health, financial or relationship problems.

Many of us have our own stories to tell.

> Having had a son who lost a year of university through playing *World of Warcraft*, I nevertheless believe that the fact that he has moved on from that game and is now in a successful career (for the moment touch wood!) does not mean he is free of the gaming addiction. He is not, and I doubt if he ever will be.

This father was almost in tears the first time he told me of his son's plight, and for quite a few months it was the sole topic of conversation. The parents, my friends, felt guilty and out of their depth: when and how had this happened?

Although no substances are ingested, any behaviour might have addictive qualities that is characterised by a compulsion to engage over and over in an action until that action has a serious and persistent negative effect on an individual's physical, mental, social and/or financial well-being. 'Internet use disorder' has, as of May 2013, been included in the fifth edition of the *Diagnostic and Statistical Manual of Mental Disorders* (*DSM-5*) as a condition 'recommended for further study' within Section III, where uncertain illnesses are classified. This move effectively postpones full recognition and inclusion until uniform criteria needed for a robust psychiatric diagnosis can be agreed on.[9] For over a decade, numerous studies have produced evidence that excessive use of the Internet, and of related features such as gaming, may be considered a behavioural addiction comparable to pathological gambling.[10] But herein lies a snag: not all Internet activity involves gaming, and vice versa.[11]

Then again, when researchers study specific features of excessive Internet use, (online) video gaming is the most frequently explored. Despite the multiple ways we might conceptualise excessive gaming and measure the behaviour, two symptoms appear consistently: significant problems as a result of overuse of games, and an inability to control use. Some hallmarks of gaming addiction include lying about how much time is spent gaming; intense feelings of pleasure or guilt; spending more and more time gaming to get the same enjoyment; withdrawing from friends, family or spouse; experiencing feelings of anger, depression, moodiness, anxiety or restlessness when not gaming; spending significant sums of money on online services, computer upgrades or gaming systems; thinking obsessively about gaming even when doing other things.[12]

Some argue that these screen-based experiences are just a medium through which an addictive activity is accessed.[13] In other words, the gambler who drives every day to the casino isn't addicted to driving. They are addicted to gambling. Similarly, the person who uses the Internet to gamble isn't addicted to the Internet but to gambling. However, while online gambling has a real-world alternative option, video gaming, by definition, does not. Unlike gambling, it's a phenomenon specific to digital technology. Hence any abnormal behaviour associated with video games cannot be divorced from the medium of the screen and the unique experience it gives. So, while much Internet activity might encompass video gaming, we need to remember that an addiction to video gaming will be an addiction to video gaming, and not to anything else.

Statistics on Internet addiction vary widely across cultures and depend on the form of evaluation used:[14] however, the numbers for video-gaming addiction specifically seems to be much more consistent. Drawing on a US sample, Douglas Gentile found 8 per cent of video gamers aged 8–18 were classified as addicted,[15] while another recent review gives an estimate of 2–12 per cent.[16] Moreover, a ballpark figure of just under 10 per cent seems to be consistent across continents: in a two-year longitudinal study performed with a general elementary and secondary school population in Singapore, including some 3,000 children in grade 3, the prevalence of 'pathological gaming' was similar to that in other countries, 9 per cent.[17] But leaving aside questions of definition, conflation with other Internet activities, statistics and the additional appeal of online interaction, can we say with any certainty that gaming is addictive?

Aviv Weinstein at the Hadassah Medical Organization in Jerusalem believes that the craving for online gaming and the craving for substance dependence could well share the same neurobiological mechanism.[18] Weinstein argues that teenagers may play for longer, prioritise their time in thinking about games, game to escape emotional problems, have difficulties with academic work and socialising, and conceal gaming activities from their family. Individuals with this behavioural pattern who then experience intolerable irritability when they stop gaming are displaying the classic hallmarks of an obsessive, even an addictive, profile. But can these behavioural commonalities of traditional addiction, intense gaming hours spent, emotional attachment and inability to control usage, all be linked to the same single brain state?

In one particular brain-imaging study, healthy control subjects had a reduction in the molecular target (receptors) for the transmitter dopamine in a key brain region (the ventral striatum) after playing a motorbike riding computer game. In striking contrast, ex-chronic Ecstasy users showed no change in the status of their receptors after playing this game.[19] For the non-addicts experiencing the thrill of gaming, there was a surge in the release of dopamine which 'desensitised' its receptors (remember the handshake analogy and how a hand would become numb when pressed for too hard or too long). But the brains of the Ecstasy addicts told a different story. Here chronic use of the drug had accustomed the brain to vast amounts of dopamine. The video games added no excitement because they worked via the same common mechanism. *It seems that as far as the brain was concerned, taking Ecstasy and video gaming were comparable experiences*.

Another way of showing that gaming releases excessive levels of dopamine in the brain is through looking at changes in the actual size of brain structures. Remember how the hippocampus was bigger in London taxi drivers because they constantly relied on their working memory while driving? It seems the same principle might apply to video gamers and their dopamine systems. In young gamers, brain imaging shows an enlargement of the area of the brain (the ventral striatum[20]) where the transmitter dopamine is released.[21] Interestingly enough, a similar feature is also characteristic of the brains of pathological gamblers, another behavioural addiction.[22] So it seems that, whether we're talking about addiction to drugs, gambling or video games, all three conditions are linked to excessive dopamine release in the ventral striatum.

The next question is whether individuals with brains that happen to have an enlarged ventral striatum are predisposed to gaming, or whether excessive gaming has literally left its mark on the brain. This presents a tricky chicken-and-egg conundrum that in general bedevils brain research: does an unusual brain feature cause an unusual behaviour, or does an unusual behaviour change the brain, thanks to its plasticity?

Let's start with the chicken: that video gaming, as with all life experiences, leaves its mark on the impressionable, plastic brain. The work of Simone Kühn's team at Ghent University in Belgium would suggest that this is the case: they showed that video gaming could be linked to a higher volume of a key brain region (the striatum), thereby reflecting adaptive neural plasticity through the sustained release of dopamine.[23] In other words, the more time spent playing, the more pronounced the expansion of the striatum. This suggests the former caused the latter.

Then there's the egg: the idea that a pre-existing brain state might predispose individuals to compulsive video gaming. Kirk Erickson at the University of Illinois found a correlation between the volume of a key brain area, the dorsal striatum, and later training success in a video game.[24] Erickson has also described a link, again seen with imaging, between activation of the striatum before training, and subsequent later skill acquisition during video gaming. These findings highlight the importance of the striatum, a rich source of dopamine, and how this might be consistent with the idea that some brains are more susceptible to the lure of games. Individuals who happen to have a larger striatum might experience video gaming as more rewarding in the first place. This neurological set-up in turn could facilitate skill acquisition and lead to further reward resulting from playing.

So what came first, the chicken or the egg? Did a strong and sustained experience shape the brain, or was a special type of brain already predisposed to respond readily to that experience? An important clue to the right answer is the anatomical make-up of the striatum itself, in that it can be divided into two compartments, an upper (dorsal) and a lower (ventral). It turns out that the latter releases more dopamine than the former.[25] So it may not be surprising that the two regions are associated with different kinds of functions: the dorsal striatum coordinates sensorimotor functions for attaining a goal, while dopamine released from the ventral part enhances the impact of the actual reward that then ensues.[26] So one way of resolving the chicken-and-egg problem might be to say that a brain predisposed to effective sensorimotor coordination, an active upper (dorsal) striatum, will have a predisposition for gaming, while it is the games themselves that change the way the brain (the lower/ventral striatum) reacts to reward; yet neuroscience is rarely so simplistically cut and dried, and certainly research in this area is still in its infancy.

In any case, the chicken scenario, where obsessive gaming directly impacts brain states, does not necessarily rule out the egg scenario of a particularly predisposed type of brain. The most significant issue here is the contribution of dopamine. Neuroscientists at Hammersmith Hospital in London have shown that playing video games directly results in a release of this transmitter.[27] However, just as it is impossible to establish the causal link, say, between the known biochemical actions of

Prozac in enhancing serotonin availability and in alleviation of depression, so the translation of the objectively observed release of dopamine in the brain into the subjective effects of feeling wildly happy is very difficult to conceptualise.

There is nothing magical locked inside the dopamine molecule. Rather, it is the particular site in the brain, together with the environmental context in which it operates, that determines the final net effect. Suffice it to say that raised levels of dopamine are consistently linked to various brain states relating to arousal, reward and, indeed, addiction. Moreover, the idea that the chicken and egg are not mutually exclusive but may actually be reinforcing one another would be a great example of how the brain and the environment are in an intense and continuous two-way dialogue.

So why do some people and not others become addicted to video games? Perhaps an individual's capacity for excitement could be pivotal. Since dopamine is linked to high arousal, as can be seen with the drug amphetamine, this idea is quite logical. One investigation identified two types of gamers: the excessive first-person shooter video gamers had significantly higher levels of arousal during gaming, which dropped off immediately after gaming.[28] By contrast, non-excessive gamers stayed 'high' even after gaming had finished. Massively multiplayer online role-playing gamers who were excessive in their play displayed significant *decreases* in physiological arousal, which rose again immediately after gaming. Meanwhile, massively multiplayer online role-playing gamers who weren't excessive showed normal increases during gaming and then reached a plateau after their session.

These differences in arousal seeking for video gamers of different genres are comparable to those reported in the scientific literature on pathological gambling. First, there's the thrill-seeking, impulsive addict who takes stimulating substances or engages in high-risk behaviours; then, by contrast, there is the escapist, the often depressed addict who is not seeking high levels of arousal. So, even without a dopamine high, for the second type of player, who experiences low arousal, the time spent in massively multiplayer online role-playing games, and the meaningless nature of the activity, could have long-term implications for their mental state. Of course, once again the chicken-and-egg complication applies. These disturbances in arousal regulation could either be a cause of gaming addiction or a consequence of it. Nonetheless, the discovery that the activity physiologically affects excessive gamers differently from non-excessive gamers is an important consideration to bear in mind.

Yet, at the end of the day, what finally determines whether or not an individual has these different levels of arousal and, one way or another, becomes addicted to one or other type of video game? This is impossible to answer, as is the question why certain individuals and not others are predisposed to being kind or shy or funny. There may be some extremely indirect, genetically based predispositions. For example, a possible inherited vulnerability to video game addiction has been reported in studies on the genes encoding for a subtype of dopamine receptor.[29] This in turn might influence the effects of dopamine released in the brain, but even here the causal link is impossible to establish. Remember that it is very unlikely that there is just one single gene *for* any complex cognitive trait.

It is impossible to tease out a cause-and-effect sequence of events as the brain interacts with the environment, and therefore it is hard to predict with any accuracy whether someone will become addicted to video games. There are likely to be the cumulative effects of risk factors, such as low socio-economic status, parental depression, parental criminality, domestic violence and parental alcohol and substance abuse, offsetting protective factors. But, in the case of my middle-class friend and his expensively educated son, none of these factors applied.

A more plausible view would be that what goes on in the brains of those addicted to video games is not *qualitatively*, but rather *quantitatively*, different from the brains of those who are less obsessive. Why else would video games be rewarding, by definition, to every single person who plays them? It seems that video gaming can induce enough brain dopamine to keep the user feeling good, but not enough to desensitise the effect completely. However, the lure of gaming doesn't just operate at the mechanistic biochemical level of brain dopamine, but also at the more cognitive one of social relations too.

A compulsion for gaming must involve not just the internal machinations of the brain, *but the brain interacting in an ongoing two-way relationship with the screen*. The very nature of this screen environment is crucial in keeping the individual playing. Games are noisy and have visually rich scenes, just like an action film. In addition, they are immersive, offering not just strong sensory stimulation but 'flow', or the capacity for a gamer to lose themselves in the game world and become utterly involved.

'Playing *World of Warcraft* makes me feel god like . . . I have ultimate control and can do what I want with few real repercussions. The real world makes me feel impotent . . . a computer malfunction, a sobbing child, a suddenly dead cell phone battery, the littlest hitch in daily living feels profoundly disempowering.'[30] So claimed English professor Ryan Van Cleave, recalling a time when he was playing video games for some 60 hours a week. Note that Ryan never even mentions 'having fun' and that his mind-set is signifying something much more profound. *World of Warcraft* was, for him, a refuge from a real world where he felt inadequate.

Olivia Metcalf from the Australian National University, who has studied the psychology of excessive video gaming, makes the distinction that the appeal may not be a positive consequence of the video games themselves, but that they provide an escape from purposeless, directionless 'real life':

> Perhaps video games are more than just escapist fun; they give disillusioned youth the chance to fulfil those needs so intrinsic to being human: competency, purpose, success, achievement, and so on. Research indeed suggests that these are some of the motivations to play video games: the chance to be outstanding when in real life we are probably average. (Personal communication, March 8, 2013)

The 'human' challenge projected through cyberspace as you're simultaneously navigating the real world in three dimensions perhaps creates an even greater compulsion for many gamers. As such, online video games have a higher addictive potential than offline games. Specifically, massively multiplayer online role-playing games are thought to have a number of unique characteristics that give them higher addictive potential then other genres. Dr Daniel King, a senior research associate in the School of Psychology at the University of Adelaide, conducted an extensive review of worldwide research into 'pathological' or harmful video game playing behaviour and found that social interaction is important in the development of excessive gaming. Games with avatars that players can identify with are associated with higher addictive potential. These qualities account for why excessive gaming is most commonly seen in massively multiplayer online role-playing games. The subsequent rewards and social interaction are part of the game, with gamers controlling their avatars. King also found that excessive gamers value the achievements gained through video gaming:

he proposes that the reward structure built into the game influences the development of excessive gaming, while the once clear lines between genres of video games are becoming more blurred.[31]

Massively multiplayer online role-playing games are only accessible online, have intricate reward systems built into the games, with gamers constantly trying to reach the next level: but it is the social interaction that appears to be the real extra hook. Perhaps the appeal is that the player is now not just playing a game, but playing out an idealised life that is simultaneously exciting and safe, both physically and mentally. The real world is messy and ambiguous. Real people are never either wholly good or bad and devoid of any inner thoughts or secrets. Actions always have consequences, however indirect, with long-term repercussions that cannot be reversed. In the real world, feedback, especially positive feedback on your achievements, is all too hard to come by. And, as for life goals, they are for most of us far from clear and usually too complex and provisional to define categorically. According to Nicole Lazzaro (who clearly likes lists of four items), video games remove much of what is difficult and confusing about real life since they should (1) simplify the world; (2) suspend consequences; (3) amplify feedback; and (4) set clear goals.[32] This inventory may add up to the crucial *something* about video games that makes them such a compelling escape from the uncertainty and complexity of the real world.

More generally, sometimes the real world is not the best place to be. In some cases games can provide calming routines for people who are unable to cope with the frenetic uncertainty of the real world. Unlike traditional real-world games, video games offer a total escape from the dull, difficult world to one that is not just more exciting and sensational (i.e., appealing to the senses), but where there are reassuringly definite and predictable outcomes in which the player can participate as a better self. Research shows that, when people are unhappy or dissatisfied with their lives, they create avatars that are very different to themselves.[33] Happy people create avatars just like themselves. Game enjoyment is inversely related to the avatar-person similarity, that is, individuals who are unhappy and create an avatar very different from themselves end up enjoying the game world more. They are literally exploring a new identity for themselves in this game world that is better, faster, fitter, stronger, thinner, taller, prettier and smarter than they are or probably *can ever be.* Perhaps that's the crux of why video games may be so pernicious. For most people they remain a form of entertainment, but they open up an entire new world where everything is better than real life, including for the psychologically vulnerable themselves. And that could be pretty much all of us.

We saw earlier that identity is not just about having a fully fledged mind, which enables you to make sense of the world, but also involves a crucial next step: the reaction you would show, as a result of how you interact with the world, in a specific context at a specific time. Instead of *your* family, *your* football team, *your* choir or *your* colleagues, the all-important *momentary context* that is accumulated through the cause-effect chain of a unique life story will now be more standardised. Gamers become extremely emotionally dependent on their avatars. They are as attached to their avatars, their guild, their team as someone in the real world may be attached to their real-world relationships or objects. In these instances, the momentary context has shifted online into an artificial world. And what if so much of your life story isn't a story at all, not a sequence of events but, as is the case with first-person shooter games, an atomised, fragmented set of experiences that have no consequences in the real world?

In either case, you might start to feel uncertain about who you actually are.

This insecurity could be compounded by a sneaky feeling that what you are doing lacks any real significance or meaning. Meaning, as I've suggested already, can be interpreted through the prism of neuroscience as making connections, of seeing one thing in terms of another. And this can also apply to causal connections over time. This connectivity, as we've seen, has a corresponding parallel in the physical brain as neuronal connections are forged and strengthened through the remarkable plasticity of the human brain. So just as a wedding ring, a simple gold object, can acquire a complex meaning or significance by the associations that develop around it, so significance can be attached to a cause–effect linkage.

If you climb a tree and then fall out and break your leg, which in turn takes time to heal, the whole episode will be a meaningful one, not least because it is irreversible. Of course, your leg may well revert to its erstwhile healthy condition, but the event of the breaking itself cannot be airbrushed out. It has enduring consequences in changing forever, one way or another, your view of tree climbing. But if you drop a bit of paper on the floor and pick it up again immediately, perhaps that's the nearest you'll get to turning back the clock in the real world. It would also have been a pretty *meaning*less thing to do.

So if meaning can be directly related to consequences over time, but if video gaming has, by definition, and according to Lazzaro, no consequences, it could be regarded as a meaningless way of spending time. And if someone is going to spend all their spare time engaged in a meaningless activity, it may jeopardise in the long term any significance they eventually attach not just to that activity but, most importantly, to themselves. Yet, for the player untroubled by such possible long-term existential concerns, there is the opportunity to simplify and improve instantly on the immediate environment and how they feel within it. The *something* about video games is that they create a world where you feel good not only because you're having fun, but also because you're shutting out the kinds of experiences that would normally make you feel sad, anxious or worthless. You enter a world designed to cater to your psychological needs; therefore there will be a complex and wide range of effects on how you think and feel over the longer term. 'What we do know' concludes Daphne Bavelier, an expert in this field at the University of Rochester, 'is that, in technology, we have a set of tools that has the capability to drastically modify human behaviour', inevitably by modifying the brain.[34] What is needed, she feels, is a way to ensure that technology is specially designed in order to achieve desired outcomes. But this might be easier said than done.

We've seen here that video games can be affecting mental processes in a complex and diverse range of ways. There are a host of different questions that have to be unpacked separately. For example, if the gaming reward schedules are locked into a fast iteration of stimulus and response, then what effect might prolonged gaming have on attention? Moreover, given that violent games account for 50 per cent or more of all sales, will playing these games increase aggressive behaviour in the real world?[35] Finally, if, as we've seen, there is no permanent meaning in the escapist gaming world because actions don't have real consequences, will it result in people becoming more generally reckless in real life? Let's explore each of these issues in turn.

14 VIDEO GAMES AND ATTENTION

'The sounds of silence are a dim recollection now, like mystery, privacy and paying attention to one thing or one person at a time.'[1] *New York Times* columnist Maureen Dowd looks wistfully back to another era. Perhaps we shouldn't be too surprised that if nowadays we end up engaged for hours in activities bombarding us with fast-paced stimuli, then our exquisitely adaptable human brain will obligingly adapt to that environment, an environment that does not require sustained attention. And the more stimulation flooding in, the shorter the attention span that can be allocated to each input. So could video games, given their fast-paced and vivid content, be affecting attention in a way that is unprecedented and unique compared with all the usual, more muted distractions of real life?

Before we can even think about answering this question, we need to sort out the common and understandable complaint that the Internet in general, and video gaming in particular, is to blame for a range of problems that could be justifiably generalised to human nature, the modern world as a whole or at least any screen-based culture, such as the good old TV. Such critics have a fair point. For example, at the Seattle Children's Hospital, Dimitri Christakis examined over 1,000 children at 1 year of age and a similar number at age 3 years.[2] Surprisingly, 10 per cent of the children sampled had attentional problems at 7 years of age that were linked to hours of television that had been viewed per day between the ages of 1 and 3. So, while shortening the attention span is obviously not a good thing, video gaming can't have any *additional* impact compared to other, older screen-based experiences or can it?[3]

Edward Swing and his team at Iowa State University have conducted the first long-term study on the specific effects of video game use by elementary school children.[4] The project involved 1,323 6- to 12-year-olds who, together with their parents, recorded their television and video game exposure at four time points over a thirteen-month period. Teachers measured attention problems by reporting difficulties the participants had staying on task and paying attention, and whether a child often interrupted another child's work. It turned out that those who had more than two hours of 'screen time' (television and video games combined) per day were more likely to be above the norm in showing attention problems. However, the results also revealed that playing games was linked specifically to a greater risk of developing attentional problems, and that it was in fact a more robust predictor than television viewing. Even after allowing for the effect of TV exposure, as well as any earlier attention problems the child already had, *the amount of time spent playing video games by each child accurately predicted increases in problems with attention just over a year later.*[5] So video gaming would seem to have a specific detrimental effect.

Subsequent research has investigated in more detail the relationships between gaming and attentional problems and reached similar conclusions. At Iowa State University Douglas Gentile and his team followed up with a sample of over 3,000 children and adolescents measured over three years.[6] Children who spent more time video gaming had more attention problems, even when earlier attention problems, sex, age, race and socio-economic status were statistically controlled for. Interestingly enough, children who were more impulsive or had more attention problems subsequently spent more time playing video games, indicating a possible bi-directional effect of video gaming on attention problems: the one enhances the other, and vice versa.

These investigations provide the strongest evidence to date that the association between video game play and attention problems is not coincidental but causal. This possible inter-relationship has potentially interesting implications for Mind Change. It demonstrates clearly how the brain and the environment are in such constant dialogue with each other that it's often hard to tease out the chicken and the egg, as we've seen already. Someone who is impulsive and readily distracted might find in video games the perfect vehicle for their disposition, while, conversely, habitual time spent in a world mandating quick reactions and instant feedback will guarantee that the brain adapts to that fast-paced environment.

Modern video games, with their visually rich and fast-paced play, are likely to place significant visuospatial and cognitive demands on a gamer, and this will in turn leave its mark on the plasticity of their brain and hence on subsequent behaviour – but not necessarily with negative consequences. Research shows that young gamers make excellent drone pilots, and even outperform real pilots on certain tasks.[7] In the same spirit, scientists at the Duke School of Medicine have investigated just how effectively skilled video gamers can become highly proficient drone pilots, compared to their student colleagues who didn't play action games.[8] Greg Appelbaum, an assistant professor of psychiatry, set the subjects a visual memory task to see how efficiently they could recall information they had just seen for the first time. The experienced gamers beat their rookie counterparts, proving that they could respond to visual stimuli much more quickly, thanks to the skill, particularly in first-person shooters, where gamers need to decide what to 'blast' every second: 'Gamers see the world differently. They are able to extract more information from a visual scene.' Appelbaum concludes: 'They need less information to arrive at a probabilistic conclusion, and they do it faster.'[9]

Interestingly enough, some researchers have suggested that it is in fact the *motivations* of gamers that can create differences between gamers and non-gamers, rather than superior visuo-spatial skills.[10] Just think about it: gaming enthusiasts spend their free time using computers for the enjoyment and competition of game tasks, whereas non-gamers recruited into different studies obviously will not have a preference for such activities if other options are available. Thus perhaps it's simply that gamers have a certain mind-set to be more competitive, to enjoy computer tasks or to be more incentivised to do well in the scenarios that result in the visuospatial improvements.

A whole host of different processes and functions, such as vision and motor control, appear to be enhanced by regular video gaming.[11] Compared to non-players, seasoned action video gamers have demonstrably better hand–eye coordination and visuomotor skills, such as resistance to distraction, sensitivity to information in the peripheral vision and an ability to count briefly presented objects. With the development of the PlayStation Move, Kinect and Wii, video games can also lay persuasive claims to developing motor skills by encouraging full body movement.

One of the key studies showing the beneficial effects of gaming took place as long ago as 2003, when Shawn Green and Daphne Bavelier at the University of Rochester investigated the impact of action video game playing on vision. They were interested in seeing if learning could improve performance in different tasks other than those on which the training was focused.[12] Initial experiments indeed confirmed the expected improvements, that in different aspects of visual attention (the ability to focus on one part of the visual field) the habitual video game players outperformed the rookies: but, most significantly, in a final experiment the non-players who had been trained on an action video game showed a marked improvement that transferred to skills well beyond the training task. Bavelier and Green concluded, 'Therefore, although video game playing may seem to be rather mindless, it is capable of radically altering visual attentional processing.'

Subsequently multiple investigations have confirmed that playing certain video games confers on the gamer a wide range of diverse benefits, including enhancements in low-level vision, visual attention and high speed of processing, among others.[13] The fact that other properly controlled training studies have repeatedly demonstrated a causal link between video game playing and these subsequently enhanced abilities proves that the video games, and not any preternatural gifts of the players themselves, are causing this improvement. Nor does the video game experience just have to result in an immediate advantage in current tasks. Instead a real benefit of playing appears to be the even more impressive ability to improve on how gamers will learn completely new tasks. These newly found talents have subsequent real-world applications. They include, for example, a superior ability to see small details, faster processing of rapidly presented information, higher capacity in short-term memory, increased capacity to process multiple objects simultaneously and flexible switching between tasks - all useful skills in a variety of precision-demanding jobs. Laparoscopic surgeons who are habitual video gamers turn out to be 'better' surgeons than their non-gaming peers in terms of speed of execution and reliability.[14]

Time spent on video games is not a simple rehearsal of a specific skill but, remarkably, can be generalised to other situations and a wide range of unforeseen skills and behaviours. It is hardly surprising, therefore, that Nintendo advertises *Big Brain Academy* as a game that 'trains your brain with a course load of mind-bending activities across five categories: think, memorise, analyse, compute, and identify'.[15] Moreover, one of the promises is that, compared to traditional training methods, it can be engaging and entertaining.

And it is not just the normal, healthy Digital Native brain that appears to flourish. The evidence is convincing that games can have beneficial, remedial effects over a wide range of impairments, including a reversal of cognitive decline in the elderly. In one study, the researchers trained older adults in a video game for a total of 23.5 hours.[16] They assessed their subjects with a battery of cognitive tasks, including tests for executive control and visuospatial skills before, during and after video game training. The subjects improved significantly within the game but, most importantly, also showed clear improvement in 'executive control functions', such as task switching, working memory, short-term visual memory, and reasoning. Specifically, participants trained on the video game were able to switch between two tasks with less effort or cost to their attention than the control subjects, and showed short-term memory improvements for recall in the executive function tasks they were tested on before and after the training period.

When used to treat patients with a wide range of brain disorders, it seems video games can offer a truly beneficial and enjoyable experience. For example, they have been used effectively to reduce delusional symptoms in schizophrenic patients after just eight weeks.[17] Moreover, in a pilot study in adolescents with autistic spectrum disorders, there were visible changes in brain scans in response to emotional words and emotions during a six-week period of 'prosocial game playing'.[18] Meanwhile, in the rehabilitation of the victims of motor vehicle accidents with post-traumatic stress disorder, the virtual-reality experience of driving or riding in a car in a computer game improved symptoms and promoted recovery.[19] In addition, video games catering for specific psychological needs in certain disorders can offer effective complementary treatment options, such as those with impulse control problems.[20] Meanwhile, neuroscientists have been using popular iPhone games such as *Fruit Ninja* (where you simply slice fruit in half with your finger) to rehabilitate stroke victims.[21]

Playing video games could also have potential positive effects on more abstract aspects of brain function, such as social development and psychological well-being. For example, co-playing video games with parents has been linked with decreased levels of aggression and increased levels of prosocial behaviour, albeit only in girls.[22] However, the same research found that the length of time spent gaming, in general, was associated with increased aggression and lower prosocial behaviour. Therefore, the beneficial effect here could be due more to the joint activity with parents than to the actual action being played out on the screen. Even gender stereotyping might play a part. The authors speculate that, because boys play more video games than girls, the time the boys spent playing on their own may have diluted the beneficial effects of time spent co-playing. Additionally, they suggest that boys typically play more age-inappropriate video games than girls, and this may also offset the benefits of gaming with parents.

We've already seen, with social networking, that video game worlds may also be a realm where gamers can freely explore their identities.[23] Research also shows that tapping into leadership potential in massively multiplayer online role-playing games can spill over into workplace potential.[24] On the one hand, virtual games could help develop new organisational training techniques; but, then again, it could just be the case that a gamer who has the potential to be a leader in a video game ends up as a leader in the real world, while losers in the real world remain losers in a game. It's still debatable whether video games serve as a useful lesson for real life or as an escape from it. Games may indeed demonstrate to the gamer that choices are sometimes hard to make when they are trying to achieve a goal, as they weigh up their consequences and benefits, and decide whether to confront or to avoid a problem based on their individual skill set. Yet on the other hand, real-life experience in the real world will teach that anyway. After all, if there were no difference between real life and gaming, what would the point of the game in the first place? But, if there *is* a difference, would the game experience actually be that useful in terms of real-life applications?

Almost all other real-life tasks could be considered dull in comparison to well-designed, highly stimulating games and the consequences may be seriously negative. Kira Bailey and her research group at Iowa State University cautiously note that, while some video games may have positive educational and therapeutic effects, overall their data suggested 'that high levels of video game experience may be associated with a reduction in the efficiency processes supporting proactive cognitive control, that allow one to maintain goal-directed information processing in contexts that do not naturally hold one's attention'.[25] Or, to put it more simply, gaming could be bad for sustained attention.

While extensive research has shown how action video gaming can improve focusing on the screen, this gain may indeed come at a cost. Video games reward players for quickly modifying their behaviour when conflict is experienced, and this specific feature of action games may have differential effects on proactive and reactive control. Think of *reactive control* as the just-in-time type of response to a stimulus that is used only when needed, whereas *proactive control* would be deployed consistently and in anticipation of future stimuli, so that it indicates an individual's capacity to choose what they pay attention to and what they ignore.[26] While high-frequency gamers (playing more than 40 hours a week) are well rehearsed in responding instantaneously to suddenly presented stimuli (reactive control), their ability to maintain proactive attention over an entire task is less impressive. Video games may train an individual to respond rapidly to suddenly presented stimuli, but provide no advantage in being able to maintain focus over mundane tasks.[27]

In contrast, other recent work suggests that frequent video gamers may be more persistent than infrequent gamers in sticking at complex puzzles involving anagrams and riddles.[28] Frequent video game players spent longer times on unsolved problems relative to infrequent video game players. These results were taken as proving that video game use can lead to more perseverance across a variety of tasks: surely the attention span of gamers must have been beneficially protracted? Once again, it could be the case that different character traits are making the crucial difference. Gamers may be more competitive than non-gamers, and a laboratory assessment task measuring skill of any type will automatically motivate a frequent gamer to win. Moreover, the gamers in this study may have seen the puzzle as a game itself and not as a boring task. So the question is still open as to whether, irrespective of the task in hand, frequent video gamers will have the ability to pay more attention generally.

How can we square the circle to reconcile conflicting conclusions as to whether gaming improves or impairs attention? The answer may lie in the *type* of attention required to be successful at 'action' games. There are a number of taxonomies that attempt to describe the human attention system. *Selective or focused attention*, defined as the ability to focus on a specific set of stimuli, is a kind of attention that is typically driven by internal motivations. Then there is *sustained attention*, the ability to maintain vigilance over longer periods of time, often required during a tedious activity. While video games might rehearse and therefore be beneficial to the type of attention requiring the processing of *selective* stimuli, the *maintenance* of attention over long periods in the absence of fast-paced moment-to-moment stimulation could well be diminished. So, while video gamers excel at attending to a specific stimulus, their concentration suffers if that stimulus is competing with other distractions; nor are they able to pay attention for long periods of time. They have a problem not with selective attention – but rather with sustained attention.

One interesting question about these impairments in attention is their possible connection to the prevalence of attention deficit hyperactivity disorder (ADHD).[29] For some, the idea that attentional disorders could be linked to gaming is mere speculation. In the Nominet Trust review of *The Impact of Digital Technologies on Human Wellbeing*, Paul Howard-Jones concluded that 'We do not know [if] the use of digital technology by young children is a causal factor in developing ADHD.'[30]

Subsequently, Alison Parkes and her team at the University of Glasgow surveyed over 11,000 children and reported no effect of video games on their psychosocial development, including on attentional problems.[31] The size of the cohort studied here might seem impressive and hence the findings reassuringly conclusive. But there are some serious drawbacks. First, the study investigated 5–7-year-olds, while almost all the rest of the research literature focuses on older children who have greater opportunity for playing stimulating, violent or reckless action games not typically available to the very young. Secondly, the possible symptoms for ADHD were assessed solely by subjective report of the far from unbiased parents, hence the unusually large sample size; in contrast, other studies have used more comprehensive, time-consuming and objective assessment tools. Thirdly, the Glasgow project only measured weekday video game use, whereas there may be many more hours of video games played on the weekend, so the study does not provide a complete picture of the total gaming profile.

In any event, before we can be sure of a link between attentional problems and video gaming, various other issues need to be unpacked. A number of studies have investigated the relationship between excessive Internet use generally and ADHD symptoms.[32] A huge caveat, however, is that video gaming on the one hand and excessive Internet use on the other are two distinct activities: one might be related to ADHD, while the other might not. A further complicating factor is that, in ADHD, certain genres of games may have different effects. Massively multiplayer online role-playing games are actually associated with lower levels of impulsivity and ADHD symptoms, and in turn are linked to higher levels of anxiety and social withdrawal.[33] Moreover, the relationship between ADHD and video gaming might hinge on the actual frequency of playing, which will not necessarily have been taken into consideration. In addition, any relationship between excessive Internet use and ADHD may be attributable to an addictive state and not to the activity itself. That said, given that so many excessive Internet users are Internet video gamers, the relationship between excessive Internet use and ADHD needs to be explored.

Taking all the above considerations into account and bearing in mind that there is no single 'cause' of ADHD, there is still persuasive evidence that excessive amounts of video gaming can indeed be associated with these disorders. In 2006 Jee Hyun Ha and his colleagues investigated large numbers of children in Korea in two stages. The first consisted of screening all participants for Internet addiction disorder and then, from those who screened positive, randomly selecting a smaller group for a thorough psychiatric assessment.[34] Tellingly, the Internet-addicted children used the Internet primarily for Internet gaming. Over half of these youths aged 9–13 years, randomly selected from this group at the second stage, qualified for a diagnosis of ADHD. A year later a psychiatric comorbidity survey of over 2,000 Taiwanese high school students aged 15–23 years reported that 18 per cent of students were classified as Internet addicts and that Internet addiction was strongly associated with ADHD symptoms.[35]

As well as the finding that restriction of children's exposure to TV and video games reduces the likelihood of attention problems in class,[36] a study by Philip Chan and Terry Rabinowitz at Rhode Island Hospital found that, if teenagers played video games for more than one hour per day, they displayed more features of ADHD, including inattention. The most insightful conclusion from the authors highlighted the now familiar chicken-and-egg problem: 'It is unclear whether playing video games for more than one hour leads to an increase in ADHD symptoms, or whether adolescents with ADHD symptoms spend more time on video games.'[37]

While there is a significant association between the level of ADHD symptoms and the severity of Internet addiction in children, it also appears that the presence of ADHD in a child might predict the likelihood of developing gaming addiction. In a study of young people with and without ADHD, aged 6–16 years, there were no differences in the frequency or duration of video gaming between the two groups.[38] However, the ADHD group had significantly higher gaming addiction scores, indicating that ADHD children may experience such addiction with more intensity than non-ADHD children. It appears that children with ADHD may be particularly vulnerable to gaming addiction. So, if Internet use and/or obsessive gaming are influencing each other, it may not be that one is causing the other, but that both are symptomatic of the same single common brain state: two sides of the same mental coin. A clue as to what that brain state might be comes from looking a bit more closely at the current medication used to treat ADHD.

Methylphenidate, perhaps best known by one of its brand names, Ritalin, is a stimulant drug given widely to treat attentional disorders. In the United Kingdom, figures reveal the number of prescriptions of methylphenidate soared in England from 158,000 in 1999 to 661,463 in 2010.[39] In the United States, Benedetto Vitiello of the National Institute of Mental Health documented stimulant prescriptions between 1996 and 2008, and found that the number of prescriptions for children younger than 19 years increased significantly during that twelve-year period.[40] Those aged 6 to 12 had the most prescriptions, but teens aged 13 to 18 had the biggest *increase* in prescriptions. A similar trend was also found in Australia, where the use of stimulant drugs to treat ADHD in children has escalated dramatically, with prescriptions for Ritalin and its equivalents up 300 per cent between 2002 and 2009.[41]

Of course, it could be that these colossal increases in prescriptions across at least three different continents have nothing to do with an increase in ADHD itself, but owe more to a current clinical trend to medicalise a particular behaviour, and/or to prescribe the appropriate drug more readily.[42] Nonetheless, the current association between ADHD medication and abnormally short attention spans brings into play our old friend, the chemical messenger dopamine, which is released in the brain by methylphenidate/Ritalin. And yet it has proved a continuing riddle to neuroscientists why such a drug should be effective in treating someone with a short attention span.

When dopamine goes to work in the brain, you become more aroused, more excited, so drugs such as amphetamine are appropriately classified as stimulants. The apparent paradox of a stimulant drug effectively combating hyper-arousal can be explained by the ability of methylphenidate to desensitise dopamine's normal chemical targets. As we've discussed already, the interaction of these chemical targets (receptors) with their respective brain transmitter resembles a molecular handshake. But if the handshake is persistent and strong, then the hand (the receptor) will become numb, less sensitive (desensitised). The result will be that the dopamine now released in the brain will be less effective and you will be less hyperactive. So, in a healthy individual, attention spans can be prolonged and this could be viewed as desirable for thinking, more generally 'cognitive enhancement'.

Modafinil, a novel wakefulness-promoting agent, has a similar pharmacological profile to that of conventional stimulants such as methylphenidate. Psychologist Trevor Robbins and his team in Cambridge were interested in assessing whether Modafinil might offer similar potential as a cognitive enhancer in those who were perfectly normal.[43] Sixty healthy young adult male volunteers received a single oral dose of either a placebo (an inert substance that they thought could have beneficial effects) or of Modafinil prior to performing a variety of tasks designed to test memory and attention. Only Modafinil significantly enhanced performance on various cognitive tests including visual pattern recognition memory, spatial planning and reaction time. The subjects also said that they felt more alert, attentive and energetic on the drug and a further effect seemed to be to reduce impulsive responding. So might the excessive dopamine released by anti-ADHD drugs like Modafinil, and its beneficial effects on attention, give us an insight into the link between ADHD and excessive video gaming?

In 2009 associate professor of psychiatry Doug Hyun Han and his team at the University of Utah prospectively studied a large number of teenagers, the great majority of whom were male. The subjects all had a history of ADHD, as well as track records of excessive use of video games. The idea was to examine whether video game play and methylphenidate increased dopamine release in a way that could enable them to concentrate better. Han administered *Concerta XL* (similar to Ritalin) and followed up the performance of the subjects after eight weeks. There was a reduction in Internet addiction scores and total time of Internet use, indicating that methylphenidate could reduce the obsessive behaviour in subjects with co-occurring ADHD and excessive video gaming. Although the authors did not clarify how much of the Internet activity was gaming, they came to the fascinating conclusion that, if ADHD and video gaming really are two sides of the same coin, the same brain state, then 'Internet videogame playing might be a means of self-medication for children with ADHD'.[44]

If video games are a kind of self-medication for those suffering from ADHD, the most obvious common factor is excessive dopamine release in the brain, in turn related to addiction, reward and arousal. Paul Howard-Jones at Bristol University has even suggested that this process could be harnessed by allowing children to play video games; they would thereby become more aroused and be cognitively enhanced in the classroom.[45] So, under the right conditions, video games might prove a valuable tool for teachers. Yet, while the amounts of endogenous dopamine released naturally within the brain as a consequence of gaming would probably not lead to the receptor desensitisation that could occur with usual doses of Modafinil or Ritalin, do we really want students to be in a permanent state of high arousal? It would surely not be that different from giving them low doses of amphetamine, a much more familiar and notorious drug that releases excessive dopamine.

Most immediately, it seems there is a clear link between video gaming and attention generally. Although *selective* visual attention for focusing on a screen object or avatar might be improved in the short term with video gaming, it could be to the detriment of the all-important *sustained* type of attention over the longer term, the kind of attention needed to reflect and to understand something in depth. Moreover, the implication of dopamine as a central player in the brain of the video gamer might be providing a truly helpful insight into understanding the appeal of the activity, compared to real life. But could a mind-set used to experiencing reliable if not easy rewards, also be one inclined to aggression and recklessness?

15 VIDEO GAMES, AGGRESSION AND RECKLESSNESS

It seems incredible that the prototype video game *Pong* first appeared as long ago as 1975. But it wasn't until the 1990s when games such as *Double Dragon* and *Mortal Kombat* introduced more violent acts into play. The pictorial resolution of these early games was measured in polygons per second, and can be a good indicator of how fast this technology has developed. For example, the resolution of the first PlayStation model was 3,500 polygons per second, but by 2001 the original Xbox released had a graphics quality of 125 million. Now current electronic games have astonishing graphic resolutions in excess of 1 billion polygons per second! As a result, the screen portrayal of violence in video games has become more detailed and vivid: players are currently exposed to multiple ways of killing and witnessing death in cyberspace more frequently and much more vividly than ever before.

The issue of just how graphic video games might have nasty consequences revisits the now familiar argument that cyber-based activities in general, and gaming in particular, are being disproportionately demonised while older technologies, such as TV, have always been just as detrimental. Not so. Hanneke Polman and her team at Utrecht University explored the difference between playing a video game and a more TV-like experience of passively watching violent video games.[1] After being exposed to the video games, the students had two free-play sessions, after which they completed a questionnaire on aggressive behaviour. Acts were considered aggressive only if the intention was considered hostile. The Dutch team found that, particularly for boys, actively playing a violent video game led to more aggression than just passively watching the same violent video game.

The crucial difference between passively observing media violence and playing a violent video game is, most obviously, the interactivity. In many games, the player is 'embedded' in the game and uses a hand-held controller that enhances the experience and thus could escalate the aggressive feelings. But, then again, violent video games could only affect behaviour in the real world if the player ended up confusing the two. If someone only played *Super Mario Bros.*, would we be concerned they would start to believe in turtle shells that can knock people out and feathers that make you fly?

This is an *ad absurdum* argument. Firstly, no one is claiming that violent video games are the sole and exclusive influence on any individual. Human existence doesn't occur in a vacuum. A bald, irrefutable fact is that even the most avid gamers live a life beyond their consoles: they go to school or college and they learn from their parents and peers. Secondly, comparing cartoon/fictionalised violence to graphic, hyper-real violence is a stretch. People are less likely to be influenced by a game completely devoid of reality such as *Super Mario Bros.* compared to one that mimics reality, such as *Grand Theft Auto V*. Video game violence taps into established mental schemas we already have around aggression and real-world violence. Turtle shells, feathers and being able to fly don't have those established toeholds in our minds, whereas strangers being potential aggressors, and our subsequently feeling hostile and distrustful towards them, do. Additionally, researchers into this subject have questioned the true level of violence in cartoon-style, cute games that are geared towards children, like *Super Mario Bros.*[2] In contrast, the majority of studies have focused on highly graphic and realistic human-on-human character violence, with modern games featuring vividly detailed and gruesome acts such as decapitation. Importantly, this type of realism in the violence depicted in the media *does* appear to impact on levels of subsequent aggression.

Elly Konijn and her group at the University of Amsterdam tested the hypothesis that violent video games are especially likely to increase aggression when players identify with violent game characters.[3] A large group of adolescent boys were randomly assigned to play a realistic violent, fantasy or non-violent video game. Next, they competed with an ostensible partner on a reaction time task in which the winner could blast the loser with loud noise through headphones, which served as the measure of aggression. Participants were told, wrongly, that high noise levels could cause permanent hearing damage. As expected, the most aggressive participants turned out to be those who played a violent game and wished they were like a violent character in the game. These participants used noise levels loud enough to cause 'permanent hearing damage' to their partners, even though their partners had not provoked them. The results suggest that identifying with violent video game characters makes players more proactively aggressive, even after controlling for habitual video game exposure, trait aggressiveness and sensation seeking. Players were especially likely to identify with violent characters in realistic games and with games in which they felt immersed: so it would seem the boys were not simply rehearsing stereotyped 'violent' responses, but were taking on a more generally adversarial mind-set.

Then again, there are those who still question whether video games could ever actually lead to violence. They argue that the video gaming experience cannot actually be harmful because humans have an inherent innate ability to recognise right and wrong. But we've seen time and again in these pages how we are shaped by our individual experiences and how the human brain always adapts to its environment. If that environment for many hours of the day is one of intergalactic warfare or of supernatural heroes with magic powers, then that fiction might increasingly inform the brain's understanding of reality. And this, so it seems, is the case.

Recent evidence suggests that despite a video gamer's awareness that the game world is not real, they still have a real human response to game events. Andrew Weaver and Nicki Lewis at Indiana University designed a project to discover how players make moral choices in video games, and what effects these choices have on emotional responses while playing.[4] Seventy-five participants filled out a 'moral foundations questionnaire' and then played through the first full act of the action video game *Fallout 3*. The majority of players arrived at moral decisions and behaved towards the non-player game characters they encountered as if these were actual interpersonal interactions. The gamers felt guilt when they engaged in an immoral act towards a (non-human) video game character in the game, but, tellingly, this guilt didn't affect their level of enjoyment. It is surely strange that people feel guilt towards a character they know is not a human and doesn't really exist. Moreover, even if for the time being the decisions were 'moral', the enjoyment alongside the culpability suggests that, while feeling guilty may well imply a certain level of empathy, ultimately there is still an interesting decoupling between understanding someone's suffering and caring about it sufficiently to modify your actions.

But you might say that the same argument could be made about books. We can feel an emotional attachment to, and empathy with, characters and pity them, but this in no way lessens our enjoyment of the novel itself. How are video games any different? Well, beyond the opportunity for escapism in both cases, the enjoyment of books could be due to the insight the reader gains from experiencing the lives of others at different times and places, of being able to adjust their views and as a trigger for new ideas of their own. No such claim has been made for video games, where, as we saw previously, much of the pleasure comes from the release of dopamine in a directly interactive and fast-paced experience that does not occur when reading a book. Most significantly, however gripping a novel is during the time of reading, no one would conflate it with the real world around them, as might be possible with video games. Through your avatar, you can live another life. Despite knowing that this world is a fiction, results relating to moral choices indicate that video gamers *do* appear to conflate fantasy with reality in violent video games.[5]

Craig Anderson, professor and chair of psychology at Iowa State University and a leading researcher in the field of video game violence, is concerned that, while violent games do not cause extreme, criminal-level violent behaviour, there is still an enhancement in low-level aggression, and he is convinced that he and others working in this area . . .

> . . . now have a clear picture of how media violence increases aggression in short and long term contexts. Immediately after exposure to media violence, there is an increase in aggressive behaviour tendencies because of several factors. 1. Aggressive thoughts increase, which in turn increase the likelihood that a mild or ambiguous provocation will be interpreted in a hostile fashion. 2. Aggressive affect increases. 3. General arousal (e.g., heart rate) increases, which tends to increase the dominant behavioural tendency. 4. Direct imitation of recently observed aggressive behaviours sometimes occurs.[6]

Anderson's suggestion is that the link between aggression and video gaming is an indirect and generalised association, and that it's quite plausible: subconscious leanings towards violence could be transformed into the overtly conscious via gaming and, through repetition, become automatic, the default mode. It is the rehearsal, the repetition, that is all-important as the player is then immersed in the fantastical narrative played out over and over again. Compared merely to observing a violent scene, in an actual game you have a persona whose aggressive actions are rewarded by the game and trigger a dopamine rush in your own brain; therefore your aggressive mind-set becomes the norm. The individual who has engaged in violent video gaming could lose self-awareness and insight because the tendency to an aggressive disposition has become a strong habit.

We have already seen how visionary psychologist Donald Hebb stated over seven decades ago that 'neurons that fire together wire together'. More recently, video game researcher Douglas Gentile has echoed this theme that 'whatever we practice repeatedly affects the brain and if we practice aggressive ways of thinking, feeling and reacting, then we will get better at those'.[7] The violent content of computer games could have a sensitising effect to violent behaviour towards others, in part by lowering the threshold of response to provocation and through a dwindling in empathy with other people. Now, for example, if someone bumps into you in the corridor, you could over-react with a hostile, 'Who do you think you're shoving!'

In a recent study, Youssef Hasan and his group at the University Pierre Mendès-France showed that violent video gaming does indeed increase expectations that another will act with hostility or aggression, probably as a result of repetitive experience in a game with hostile characters.[8] French college students played either a violent or a non-violent game for just twenty minutes. Afterwards, they read ambiguous story plots about potential interpersonal conflicts, and listed what they thought the main characters would do, say, think or feel as the story continued. Aggression was measured using a competitive computer game in which the winner could apparently blast the loser with loud noise through headphones. Results showed that the violent video game players expected more aggressive responses from the main characters presented in the story. Moreover, they chose significantly louder and longer blasts of noise for their human opponents in the game. As predicted, video game violence increased the hostile expectation bias, which in turn increased actual aggression: violent video games appear to increase aggression because the individual expects others to be hostile. What will be the longer-term implications of this state of affairs?

One suggestion is that there could actually be some positives. For example, violent video games may provide a safe outlet for aggression and frustration.[9] In this spirit, research currently being led by Cheryl Olson and her team at Massachusetts General Hospital's Center for Mental Health and Media at Harvard indicates that violent games actually help students deal with stress and aggression. Apparently, over 45 per cent of boys and 29 per cent of girls use violent games such as *Grand Theft Auto IV* as a safety valve for their anger.[10] But then again, there is little evidence that violence is an internally generated biological imperative akin to hunger or sleep – a drive that builds up in the body come what may, as a natural need that sooner or later must be met. Furthermore, anger is not the same as aggression, although the former might sometimes lead to the latter. In any case, it could be that there are more effective ways for understanding and helping someone cope with their anger than providing an opportunity for violence, however simulated.

The only 'proof' that violent games might have positive effects, according to Olson and many other gaming aficionados, seems to be that the violent crime rate is going down while the popularity of M-rated video games has increased. But then decreases in crime rate are most likely to be caused by a host of complex socio-economic factors. Most importantly, no one has ever actually demonstrated a direct link between violent video games and a decrease in actual violent crime, or indeed suggested the converse, that games directly drive the player to go out on the rampage.

However, the change towards a *more aggressive disposition* as a result of video games does seem to be a definite global phenomenon across different cultures. A recent longitudinal study designed to explore long-term violent game effects on the mentality of American and Japanese school-aged young people has shown that, in as little as three months, high exposure to violent video games increases physical aggression, such as punching or kicking someone or getting into physical fights.[11] Other recent, similar studies in Germany[12] and Finland[13] have revealed similar effects over two years.

Although the systematic study of video games is relatively new, the evidence seems strong in identifying a link between playing video games and an aggressive mind-set. The most comprehensive meta-analysis to date has drawn on 136 papers detailing 381 independent tests of association conducted on a final number of 130,296 research participants to find that violent game play led to significant increases in desensitisation, physiological arousal, aggressive cognition and aggressive behaviour, while prosocial behaviour decreased.[14] As is the way in the peer-reviewed scientific literature, this report was immediately criticised in the same issue of the journal in which it was published, for a number of methodological flaws, in particular a bias in the selection of studies included, and allegedly trivial size effects.[15]

Yet, as we saw at the very beginning, scientists usually disagree, and one paper is never automatically accepted universally as conclusive. In any event, as is the way of scientists' sparring, the refutation, appropriately entitled 'Much Ado about Nothing' was itself rebutted in an article entitled 'Much Ado about Something'.[16] The original authors, Brad Bushman and his colleagues, denied that there was evidence of bias in their selection of data, and countered that the effects observed, far from being trivial in size, were bigger than many effects deemed sufficiently large to warrant action in medical domains. So the main argument against the potentially detrimental effects of violent video gaming comes down to one of detail: namely the real-world implications of those effects, their magnitude and the methodology for evaluating them, but not to whether any exist in the first place.[17]

Violent video games clearly *do* have a demonstrable effect on the inner functioning of the brain and body, beyond aggressive behaviour towards others. Research has linked violent video games to changes in the fight-or-flight system that has evolved to prepare the body for action, by pumping blood around the body more quickly, putting digestion on hold, cooling down the skin with sweat and so on. It seems that players can become habituated to this adrenal rush that living through a realistic violent experience will trigger.[18]

Nicholas Carnagey, a psychologist at Iowa State University, demonstrated that brief exposure to violent video games influences activation of the part of the nervous system that usually gets your heart racing automatically.[19] The subjects played a violent or a non-violent video game for twenty minutes and immediately after playing the game viewed a ten-minute video clip of actual real-world violence (not Hollywood reproductions) - for example a prison fight in which a prisoner was stabbed repeatedly - while heart rate and skin conductance were measured. Those who had played the violent video game demonstrated less change in heart rate and less sweating of the palms while watching the video, compared to those who played the non-violent video game. The violent video game had made the subjects less affected and upset by the real-world aggression.

The consequences of such physiological desensitisation could be quite significant: when individuals are desensitised by violent video games, they are less likely to aid a victim of violence. In one particular study by Brad Bushman and Craig Anderson at Iowa State University, subjects played one of the video games before a fake fight was staged outside a laboratory towards the end of the study.[20] Participants who had played the violent video game were less likely to report hearing the fight, judged the event as less serious and were slower to respond when they did offer help, compared to those participants who had played the non-violent video game.

Perhaps not surprisingly, playing violent video games has corresponding effects that can be observed in the brain itself. Brain activity monitored during game play shows that there are definite neuronal correlates to real-life behaviour. Investigators recorded brain activity of experienced gamers, who normally played an average of fourteen hours per week, while they played a first-person shooter game.[21] Watching violent scenes caused certain areas of their brains to change in activity, specifically one particular area, the rostral anterior cingulate. This area is normally active during detection of discrepancies in incoming information, such as in the Stroop Test, when reaction time is slower because the name of a colour (e.g., blue) is printed in a colour not denoted by the name, such as red. Gaming was also correlated with the deactivation of the amygdala, a brain region normally linked to emotionally charged memory, such that decreased activity in this area would lead to the suppression of fear and an overall drop in emotion. The brains of the gamers were therefore less sensitive and emotionally reactive to discrepant actions, such as sudden violence. Importantly, the activation pattern reflected a sequence of the individual's own brain-environment interaction rather than just merely registering what was going on.

In a second imaging experiment, regular male video gamers played a first-person shooter game and their actions in the game and their corresponding brain scans were analysed.[22] Results showed that areas of the brain linked with emotion and empathy (again the cingulate cortex and the amygdala) were less active during violent video gaming. The authors suggest that these areas must be suppressed during violent video gaming, just as they would be in real life, in order to act violently without hesitation. Furthermore, there was activation of areas associated with aggression and cognition, and this activation resulting from virtual violence paralleled that activation which occurs during real life violence.

Does this mean that the brain can't tell the difference between engaging in a virtual act of violence and a real-world act of violence? This is the same as asking whether an individual (who, after all, *is* their brain) can make such a distinction. We've already seen that gamers can conflate reality and the virtual world. If the opposite were true, that there was some kind of neuronal reality check, it's hard to see where and how it would operate in the physical brain as a mechanism capable of bestowing objectivity independent of all other brain processes. If, as I've been suggesting, the mind is the personalisation of the brain through personalised neuronal connectivity, each of us will, in any case, have unique and very different views of an external reality. It would be foolhardy to assume that the human brain *always* knows the difference between fantasy and reality. Neuroscientist Rodolfo Llinás of NYU Medical Center has gone so far as to argue that our default consciousness is internally generated, modified only to greater or lesser extents by an intermittent input from an external reality.[23] Meanwhile the extreme idea that all reality is illusory and external objects exist only by being perceived goes back centuries to the philosopher George Berkeley. Here is not the place to discuss the nature of physical reality, but suffice it to say that there is no automatic switch in the brain for detecting it, or for assuming that it is a simple concept in the first place, easily distinct from the imagination, that we can take for granted, let alone define.

Although we have focused here on the heavy gamers, those who might be obsessive or even addicted, the picture that is emerging is one of a clear relationship between violent video gaming and increases in aggressive thoughts, feelings and behaviour. But what does this actually mean for life beyond the screen? We know from multiple well-designed laboratory studies that playing violent video games can increase our aggressive view of the world. But how long these effects last, and whether they translate inevitably into real-world situations, remain unclear.

Our exploration of video games started with the idea that, in playing games, we rehearse many of the skills useful for survival in the real world. The possible link between aggression and gaming is still debated even after twenty-five years of research, because terms such as 'aggression', 'aggressive behaviour', 'anger', 'hostility' and even 'aggressive cognition' are often poorly defined, measured indiscriminately and used interchangeably. But above all we need to distinguish 'anger', 'aggression' and 'violence'. There is no evidence that video games lead directly to criminal-level violence, but a large body of data strongly indicates that they do induce an aggressive disposition in everyday life. This is particularly worrying in the light of recent statistics that violent video games account for approximately over 60 per cent of video game sales.[24] Moreover, at the time of writing, the top five most popular video games (*Grand Theft Auto V*, *Batman: Arkham Origins*, *Assassin's Creed IV: Black Flag*, *Call of Duty: Ghosts*, *Battlefield 4*) are all extremely violent in content.

As we've seen throughout these pages, humans are mandated by evolution to adapt to the environment. Children have always learned best by observing behaviour and then trying it out for themselves. The consequences of these experimental forays influence whether they repeat the behaviour, or never do it again. All violent media, of any type, has the potential to teach specific violent behaviours, as well as to colour the circumstances when such behaviours seem appropriate and useful. In this way, violent behavioural scripts are learned and stored in memory. Video games provide an ideal environment in which to learn violence because they place players in the role of the aggressor and often reward them for successful violent behaviour. Games allow players to rehearse an entire behavioural script, from provocation, to choosing to respond violently, to resolution of the conflict. Players are incentivised to re-enact these scenarios repeatedly and for long periods of time in order to improve their scores and advance to higher levels. Inevitably, this repetition increases their effectiveness and the likelihood of such behaviour being repeated. In turn, aggressive behaviours will be adopted. The potential shift to a more aggressive behavioural pattern and attitude over time could affect society and what we expect from each other, possibly lowering our expectations of respect and tolerance and increasing our distrust of others and our need for self-preservation.

Any surge in hostility implies a decrease in normal self-control and an increase in recklessness heedless of the consequences. If a neuroscientist is asked to say something about excessive risk-taking, then they may well start by pointing to neurological syndromes where brain malfunction is characterised by taking too many risks. We saw previously, in the case of Phineas Gage and his damaged prefrontal cortex, how the injury made him, in the words of his physician, Dr Harlow, 'exceedingly capricious and childish, impatient at restraint'.[25]

This is still an accurate description of the common behavioural profile seen in the various examples featured in Table 8.1 (page 99), where an underactive prefrontal cortex can also be characteristic of obese people,[26] gamblers[27] and schizophrenics,[28] as well as of children.[29] These groups are different and distinct, but they all share a preference for the here and now that trumps the long-term consequences. Anyone who over-eats knows what will happen, but for those with a high body mass index (weight relative to height) the thrill of the taste of the food trumps the consequences that it will pile on the calories. Similarly research has shown that obese people are more reckless in gambling tasks, and are comparable to compulsive gamblers for whom the thrill of the horse past the finishing post, or the roll of the dice, trumps the consequences that they may well lose all their money.[30] But then, what of schizophrenics who may be neither obese nor compulsive gamblers?

A detailed excursion into schizophrenia is outside the scope of our current discussion, but the main feature to flag is that schizophrenics place a higher emphasis on the outside sensory world, which they often think is imploding in on them. They think that outsiders can see and hear their thoughts, since there is no firewall between their brains, or rather their minds, and the incoming flood of sensory stimulation impinging on them. We've seen that, as we develop, the sensory world is overtaken by a more cognitive one, where personalised associations, *meaning*, dominates our interpretations of the world. In schizophrenia, this transition is far less emphatic and, as the senses remain overly dominant, those with schizophrenia are more easily distracted by novel stimuli and have shorter attention spans.[31] Those with schizophrenia also struggle with proverbs and metaphorical thinking, which we saw previously with the characteristically literal interpretation of the statement 'People who live in glass houses mustn't throw stones' as signifiying 'If you live in a glass house and I throw a stone at it, then your house will break.' Schizophrenics have trouble understanding one thing in terms of something else because the ability to make such associations is usually based on a robust functional connectivity between networks of neurons – a connectivity that grows and is personalised throughout life.[32]

Another group of people who see the world literally and take it at a sensory face value, are children. A young boy or girl instructed not to cry over spilt milk might look around in surprise at the absence of an overturned glass. Young children can be compared to people with schizophrenia in that they have shorter attention spans, are more readily distracted and, significantly, are also more reckless. They too have an underactive prefrontal cortex, which fully matures only in the late teenage years or even early twenties.[33]

As we saw earlier, the common factor underlying obesity, schizophrenia, gambling recklessness and childhood is how the sensory present trumps the long-term consequences: the press of the here and now environment is unusually paramount. And this suppression of the past and future in favour of the present moment seems to be related to an underactive prefrontal cortex. Does this mean that, despite all the health warnings in the earlier chapters against regarding specific brain regions as independent mini-brains, the prefrontal cortex is indeed some kind of HQ for cognition and loftier thoughts beyond the moment? Not at all. Far from being a kind of autonomous super mini-brain, the prefrontal cortex has more inputs to all other cortical areas than any other region of cortex, and therefore plays a key role in operational brain cohesion. So, if this pivotal area is underactive for whatever reason, there could be a profound effect on holistic brain operations, which are normally functional for accessing memories and planning ahead. One interesting effect of damage to the prefrontal cortex can be 'source amnesia', where memory is still intact but is more generic and is removed from a specific context or episode.[34] The patient is not linked to a continuous narrative of particular events, but is more in an ill-defined, hazy present.

When dopamine is unleashed on the prefrontal cortex, it inhibits the activity of the neurons there,[35] and so recapitulates in some ways the immature brain state of the child, or indeed of the reckless gambler, the distracted schizophrenic or the food junkie. Just as children are highly emotional and excitable, adults in this condition are also more reactive to sensations rather than calmly proactive. Small wonder that this much cited transmitter heightens arousal and arousal is often linked to pleasure whether it be in extreme sports, drugs, sex or rock and roll. It's a brain state dominated by the heightened sensational moment for the passive recipient. As we saw back in Chapter 8, when you 'blow your mind', you temporarily suspend access to the personalisation of neuronal connections developed over an individual lifetime which characterises your proactive uniqueness. Now, for the time being at least, those connections are not being accessed fully, thanks either to psychoactive drugs or to an environment that has little cognitive content because the senses are being rapidly and powerfully stimulated, as in the context of sport or sex or raves.

How might this scenario apply to video games? A character you've just shot in a video game can become obligingly undead the next time around. Perhaps the biggest difference between video games and real life is that actions do not have irreversible consequences in games. You can afford to be reckless in a way that would have dire results in the three-dimensional world. The consequence-free nature of video gaming is a basic part of its ethos (remember that one of Nicole Lazzaro's essential criterion for a successful game, is to 'suspend consequences').[36] Depending on the game, sometimes you'll even be rewarded for behaving recklessly while playing. This parallel world not only facilitates recklessness, but also promotes and rewards it and this cyber-based irresponsibility can have serious effects in the real world. After playing a video game where reckless driving was part of the game such as crashing into other cars, driving on the sidewalk or driving at high speed, gamers were more likely to behave recklessly and take risks in a simulated driving situation.[37] One longitudinal study found that playing violent, risk-encouraging video games, including the driving game *Grand Theft Auto*, was associated with self-reports of risky driving, even after controlling for other variables that influence this type of behaviour.[38] Specifically, video gaming was associated with vehicle accidents, being stopped by the police and unsafe driving habits including speeding, tailgating and the willingness to drink and drive.

With modern video games, the mere experience of recklessness itself can be fun. We've already seen that games could be providing a comparable fast-paced and exciting experience, one that we have discovered is associated with the excessive release of dopamine.[39] So, since dopamine is well known to inhibit the prefrontal cortex, would the brains of video gamers also show up less activity in this crucial brain region? Several studies have indeed linked the cyber lifestyle to decreases in prefrontal cortex activity.[40] A recent report from China found structural abnormalities in the prefrontal cortex in the brains of Internet addicts (and, as we saw in Chapter 14, the majority of Internet addiction studies involve individuals whose main addictive behaviour is video gaming), which suggests that Internet addiction might result in brain structural alterations.[41] The study involved scanning the brains of adolescents who played on average ten hours of online video games per day for nearly three years and compared the results with scans of comparable subjects who played fewer video games. The results showed abnormalities in white matter, the fibres in the brain connecting regions involved in emotional processing, attention, decision-making and cognitive control.

Similar changes have been observed in forms of addiction to substances such as alcohol and cocaine. Microstructure abnormalities were seen in key brain areas, including the very ones that have featured here: the ventral striatum, where dopamine is released, and the prefrontal cortex, where it acts.[42] In addition to reduced activation in the prefrontal cortex, recent research into video game addicts has shown, alarmingly, lower activity in the regions of the brain associated with visual and auditory processes.[43] The authors suggest that extended video gaming can diminish the responsiveness of the visual and auditory regions of the brain. Perhaps too much gaming in a visually and auditorily stimulating world reduces our reaction to the relatively dull real world because our brains have recalibrated to the video game world that now seems the norm.

It is possible that the following cycle of events could unfold, especially for action video games. The experience of a fast-paced, vivid, interactive, screen experience is arousing, hence dopamine is released. As we saw earlier, the level of dopamine released while playing a video game is comparable to that produced by amphetamine or methylphenidate (the generic name for prescription drugs such as Ritalin or Modafinil).[44] Once released, dopamine will inhibit the prefrontal cortex, thereby putting

Figure 15.1 A continuous cycle of stimulation, arousal and reward in addiction that could account for a compulsion to play games. Typical gaming responses are fast and exciting, leading to a higher level of arousal and release of dopamine. Dopamine also underlies rewarding experiences and addiction, so that the behaviour continues and yet more dopamine is released. This excessive dopamine will inhibit the prefrontal cortex, to the degree that the mind-set is now compatible with various other conditions, with the common denominator that actions are performed heedless of their consequences in the drive for sensation at the expense of a wider cognitive take on the world. The gaming experience meets this drive particularly well, and so the cycle continues.

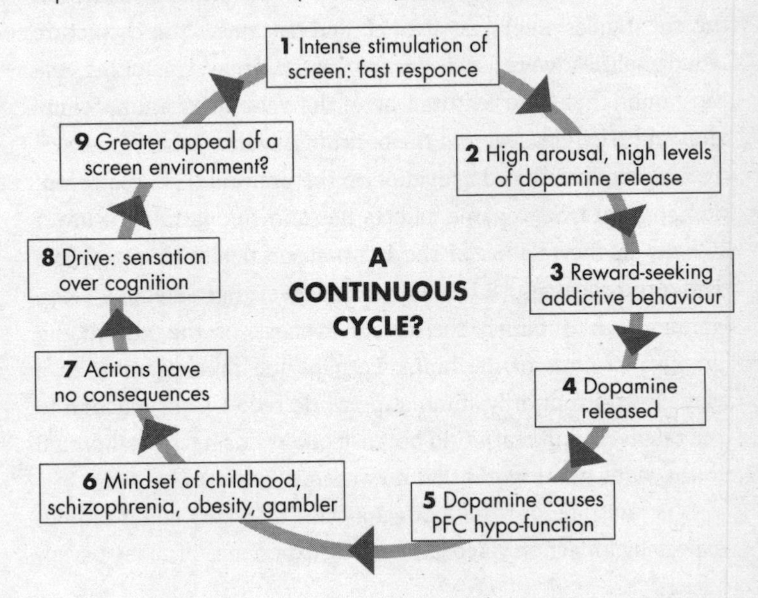

the brain into a mind-set where the here and now trumps the consequences, so the fast-paced sensation of the screen will have still more appeal than the slow, dull real world. As the gamer continues, more dopamine is released and, as with excessive eating, compulsive gambling or drug taking, this continual dopamine will activate reward and addiction pathways, leading to the desensitisation of its receptors. Because more dopamine is needed to create the same original effect, so the same behaviour is perpetuated to greater or lesser extents. In some 10 per cent or so of individuals it will be extreme enough to be regarded as addictive or obsessive behaviour.

We may now be living in an unprecedented era where an increasing number of people are rehearsing and learning a new default mind-set for negotiating the world: one of low-grade aggression, short attention span and a reckless obsession with the here and now. This profile, as a simple minimal list, could amount to the 'mindless' behaviour underlying road rage or the mitigating *crime passionnel* in French law, where the anger is so great it can be excused since the individual has truly 'lost' their mind. But, although excessive video gaming may ramp up arousal levels and feelings of reward, it does so in the cognitive context of the Internet game. And this simulated context can perhaps become the new narrative that, in extreme cases, substitutes for the less simple, less successful, less fun story-line that is the player's real life.

16 THE *SOMETHING* ABOUT SURFING

'I wanted something that expressed the fun I had using the Internet, as well as hit on the skill, and yes, endurance necessary to use it well. I also needed something that would evoke a sense of randomness, chaos, and even danger. I wanted something fishy, net-like, nautical.'[1] These reminiscences from librarian Jean Polly, who claims to have been the first to have used the term 'surfing' in 1992, as she 'cast about for a metaphor' for an article title. But many find this version of events hard to believe. The term is more likely to have evolved from TV channel surfing, as an ironic commentary on how unsporty, safe and inactive flicking a remote at a television is, compared to the actual riding of the real waves. Alternatively, perhaps channel surfing could resemble actual surfing in that both a channel surfer and Internet surfer have little interest at all in what is going on at the deeper levels but just enjoy going along for the ride, wherever it takes them. In any event, the very word 'surfing' conjures up excitement, health, youth and speed as you skim effortlessly across sites, film clips and facts. It is an activity that is unique to cyberculture.

For the first time ever a vast mass of humanity has easy access to an effectively infinite amount of information via search engines and websites: we can see any backyard in the world via sites such as Google Earth and, if need be, gain instantaneous updates of world events unfolding as they happen. Traditional notions of space and time no longer have the same relevance and no longer impose the same constraints on our lives, while most governments trying to monitor their state media no longer have unfettered control over what their citizens can access. Then there is the darker side of surfing: the far less savoury opportunities, for example, to learn how to make an improvised explosive device, determine the most effective way to commit suicide or, unbelievably, find the best method for cooking human flesh. Anyone anywhere can access such sites.

This free-of-charge, casual and rapid acquisition of information even applies to more formal education, with lessons and lectures from all over the world. Since 2001, the Massachusetts Institute of Technology, for example, has made openly available on the Internet the materials for nearly all of its courses, while more recently the Khan Academy has set up 2,700 high-quality micro-tutorials on the web (www.khanacademy.org), and computer games developed by Marcus du Sautoy, a mathematician at Oxford University, are enabling children to engage with complex problems that people would have once said were far too advanced for them.[2]

But surfing is much more than formal learning. 'Without Google and Wikipedia I'm stupid, not just ignorant,'[3] So claimed the journalist and visiting Harvard researcher John Bohannon, who went on to speak of the 'Google effect', the phenomenon where the Internet becomes a personal memory bank, replacing the collective efforts of family members as a primary source of recall. Bohannon even goes so far as to suggest that many had 'made the Internet their husband and wife', a vivid turn of phrase describing how some people now assume Google will complement their memory processes in a way that previously a spouse might have done. Is Bohannon just a one-off weirdo speaking in hyperbole, or has he put his finger on a growing trend? An ever growing part of society might have been lured away from an internalised cognitive framework that has been painstakingly constructed over time in favour of constant access to a vast but unstructured morass of facts.

Bohannon's concerns about the Google effect were based on the results of experiments devised by Betsy Sparrow and her collaborators, Daniel Wegner of Harvard and Jenny Liu of the University of Wisconsin. Their findings illustrating this Google effect on cognitive performance made the headlines in 2012 with a paper in the high-impact journal *Science*.[4] Participants read simple statements such as 'An ostrich's eye is bigger than its brain.' One group of subjects was then tested for their recall of the statements when they believed these had been saved (i.e., they were accessible to them later, as is the case of the Internet), the other when they believed the statements had been erased. Perhaps not surprisingly, subjects didn't learn the facts as well when they believed the information would be readily accessible later. They performed worse on the memory test than the group who believed the information was no longer available, and therefore had had to rely on their own cerebral resources from the get-go.

Before we go any further and talk about the impact of Google on memory, we need to sort out the different types of memory[5] that may or may not be affected: *non-declarative*, *implicit* or *procedural* memory (the terms are interchangeable) involves the remembered skill set that enables you to ride a bicycle or learn to swim: this type of recall wouldn't be affected by a reliance on Google for summoning up facts. The other kind of memory is known as *declarative* or *explicit* memory, where the process of active recall is in turn either episodic or semantic. *Episodic* memories have a specific time-space coordinate and hence can be linked to many other different events and facts that are personal to each individual episode. So, although the September

11 attack on New York's World Trade Center was a clear event that took place at a specific time and location, the actual memory of it will be very different for each of us, depending on our own circumstances and personal history, and the individual contextual framework in which it was embedded. In contrast, Sparrow's experiments were dealing with mainly *semantic* memory: objective, stand-alone facts of the type that many would now argue no longer have to clog up our synapses because they can be accessed more accurately externally. Although only you can access your personal memories, the idea is that Google, or any search engine, could eventually act as an outsource for this type of recall of objective facts.

Sparrow devised a subsequent test to explore whether there might be a difference between memory for the information itself and memory for where the information can be found. When asked to remember the folder names, subjects did so with greater success rates than they recalled the trivial factual content itself. Analysis revealed that people do not necessarily remember *where* to find certain information when they can remember *what* it was, and that, conversely, they tend to remember where to find information when they can't remember the information itself. Sparrow and her colleagues summed this up:

> The advent of the Internet, with sophisticated algorithmic search engines, has made accessing information as easy as lifting a finger. No longer do we have to make costly efforts to find the things we want. We can 'Google' the old classmate, find articles online, or look up the actor who was on the tip of our tongue.[6]

This new strategy will swiftly leave its mark on the brain. Gary Small and his colleagues at UCLA studied twenty-four middle-aged individuals, of whom twelve had minimal Internet search engine experience (the 'Net Naive' group) and twelve had more extensive experience (the 'Net Savvy' group).[7] The scientists scanned the brains of these subjects during a novel Internet search task, or during a control task of reading text on a computer screen that had been formatted to simulate the prototypic layout of a printed book. While the brains of the two groups showed similar patterns of activation during the text reading task, the picture, literally, was different during the Internet search task. The brain scans of the Net Naive group showed an activation pattern similar to that of their text reading task, whereas the Net Savvy group demonstrated significant increases in activity in additional regions that control decision-making, complex reasoning and vision. Yet, amazingly, after only five days of spending a few hours on the Internet, the erstwhile Naive group were showing brain activation patterns similar to their Savvy counterparts. Once again, we can see the powerful adaptability of the human brain. However, it's not clear whether this seemingly efficient change to the new environment of the Internet is such a good thing. The new brain patterns indicated a switch in strategy from actually reading what was displayed to fast searching, in turn suggesting that success in a Google search depends not on detailed scrutiny or in-depth reflection, but instead on fast evaluations at face value.

Of course, using dictionaries, log tables and encyclopaedias also requires quick acts of evaluation but, unlike the Google effect, these more traditional resources have never posed a comparable threat to memory but have always been an adjunct to a large number of more commonly known facts already present in the brain. The potential problem lies in how an increasing reliance on the Internet might erode the line between facts that we can assume almost everyone knows and the kinds of facts that may well not be common knowledge and that you'd always need to look up. For example, if two adults in the developed Western world met each other today, they could take it for granted that they would both know what and where Barcelona was, or who Napoleon or Shakespeare was, without having to look it up on their mobile phone. They would be able to have an interesting conversation on the assumption that they shared a sufficient number of certain basic facts – a general knowledge – which provide a starting point for developing ideas. What we have in common with others already determines the scope of our interaction and conversation, but let's take it to an extreme. Imagine that in the future people become so used to external access for any form of reference that they have not internalised any facts at all, let alone put them into a context to appreciate their significance and to understand them. Any discussion would be punctuated by lengthy pauses while each interlocutor looked up a name or a phrase on their digital device. Of course, some people have always known more than others. There has never been a clear divide as to what we can assume everyone knows, and what is considered arcane and therefore acceptable to admit ignorance of. But if the balance eventually shifts more in one direction, perhaps normal, real-time face-to-face conversation (already imperilled by social networking sites) may be downgraded to the simplest interchanges where minimal general knowledge is assumed, or slowed down to such an extent that offline conversations, via text or email, become even more the norm.

The ease of looking something up on a search engine is already transforming not just memory strategies, but our thought processes themselves. It is hard now to think back to the days of the question-rich, answer-poor environment in which many of us were students, a world where we had to leaf through heavy and cumbersome encyclopaedias, or plan a time-consuming trip to a reference library. Nothing came quickly or easily: there was a constant uphill struggle to obtain the exact information you wanted, and you had to focus on what was really essential. When you try and find an answer to a question, you're on a quest, a journey with a very clear goal: each step is sequentially linked in a linear path that eventually leads to a specific and different destination. As we've seen, this is how a thought process would differ from a raw instantaneous feeling, through the sense of a narrative over time. It is this experience of a goal-directed passage of time that I've suggested gives each of us a unique life story and the events and people within it a unique meaning. As T.S. Eliot so eloquently described it in *Little Gidding*:

> We shall not cease from exploration
> And the end of all our exploring
> Will be to arrive where we started
> And know the place for the first time.[8]

This last line is the whole point, the original place is actually now somewhere different. The very effort we invest in the journey of discovery, in the time spent joining the dots and making connections across networks of neurons, gives an importance, a significance, to what we learn, so that we see things in a new way. Now we are in danger of entering the reverse scenario, an arguably question-poor world where our brains are saturation-bombed with answers but where it is hard not to be distracted nor lose sight of what we wanted to know at the outset.

James Thurber, the American author, cartoonist and celebrated wit who died in 1961, well before surfing ever meant anything other than surmounting looming walls of salty water, once said: 'It is better to ask some of the questions than to know all of the answers.'[9] The experience of endless surfing over an infinite sea of responses might trump the original goal of articulating a question in order to find a defined and definite answer. And in turn this new easy-come, easy-go way of handling incoming information may have new effects on the ever adaptable human brain. In order to investigate this possibility, we need to unpack what the effects of being inundated by so much content may be having on the mind. It's not just the amount of material available but, perhaps more crucially, the speed and therefore ease with which we can all interact and deal with it.

Now, thanks to Google and other search engines, we've gone from articulating questions to weaving and bobbing through answers. The Internet presents an endless stream of facts, but deep and interesting questions remain less obvious. Consider the example in the Sparrow study (see above) that 'An ostrich's eye is bigger than its brain.' It may be that you never set out to learn much about ostriches, but in the course of Googling, say, 'eyes', this fact popped up. In and of itself the fact won't help you understand how eyes work, if indeed that had been your original question, but it will distract you, make you pause for a moment to say 'Wow' and even store it away in your memory as an isolated, disconnected fact for pulling out of the hat when conversation in the bar or at the water cooler lapses. At best it will rupture a linear train of exploration in finding out about eyes, and at worst it would have confused you as to what the most important issues concerning eyes might be.

The problem could now be one not so much of relying too heavily on an external source for facts, but of letting that mentality of collecting isolated bits and pieces of information overtake the erstwhile normal process of making use of these facts, of joining up the dots, as would normally happen in an internalised conceptual framework. In a 2013 investigation by Malinda Desjarlais at Brock University, undergraduate students with high and low levels of sustained attention were tasked with navigating the Internet for twenty minutes to learn about how tropical cyclones form, a topic about which they knew little at the outset; this was then followed by a test.[10] Students with high levels of sustained attention more frequently guided their learning in a linear manner, alternating between search engine results and first links. Rarely did these learners select hyperlinks presented on the links themselves, and it was these students who performed better on the test. Low-attending learners typically took advantage of the opportunity to jump around between sources of information. While they alternated between search engine results and first links, the low-attending learners engaged in far more exploration of the hyperlinks presented than the high-attending learners. However, the hyperlinked sources were typically irrelevant. So, perhaps not surprisingly, those with short attention spans performed more poorly than those who were able to focus for longer.

Such variations in performance can be even more marked when we look across age groups. David Nicholas, director of CIBER Research, has investigated how different generations use the Internet to search for information, and the confidence they have in their search abilities. The Google generation (born after 1993), Generation Y (born after 1973 and before 1994) and Generation X (born 1973 or earlier) were compared for their Internet information-seeking abilities. The younger generations spent a fraction of the time the older generation did looking for an answer to both simple and complex questions. However, by their own admission, they were less confident about the answers they found, as demonstrated by the fact that they viewed fewer pages, visited fewer domains and undertook fewer searches compared to the older generation searchers. Also, tellingly, the answers they provided to the simple and complex problems were much more the product of cut and paste. The younger generation also turned out to have poorer working memories and to be less competent at multi-tasking, despite engaging in it more.

The researchers came to the conclusion that 'the propensity to rush, rely on point-and-click, first-up-on-Google answers, along with growing unwillingness to wrestle with nuances or uncertainties or inability to evaluate information, keeps the young especially stuck on the surface of the "information" age, too often sacrificing depth for breadth.'[11]

These findings have profound implications for the Digital Natives and their ability to research information on the Internet, and more widely still for learning in general and thus overall success in life. Those with more facts at their immediate disposal can build richer constructs of reality and thus have a world view informed by a context that enables deeper understanding, more *wisdom*. Although the number of facts internalised does not automatically guarantee wisdom, facts constitute the all-important dots that you connect, interpret and place within your personal schemas to give them meaning. But if you can only remember the places to look for answers rather than the answers themselves, then even these dots will not be learned and therefore cannot be joined up with other dots to form an individual perspective of the world.

Another unprecedented experience offered by search engines that could impact on how and what we learn is YouTube.[12] Watching YouTube or similar sites is a form of learning in the most general sense, since watching a video involves the processing of an input coming into your brain from the screen. After all, you have acquired a tiny nugget of information; you now know something that you didn't know previously, even if it be that a cycling dog is alive and well and performing in Ohio. But many people watch YouTube videos without any explicit motivation to acquire any new information. The appeal is that YouTube presents visual information, actions rather than spoken words. Actions do indeed speak louder than words and the watching of actions rare, exciting or funny anchors you in the moment, as what you see is what you get. Granted, YouTube also enables commentary, and links are frequently shared between friends, so that social networking can also flourish around a common subject, just as it might over a film or a book. The big difference is that the duration is usually limited to only fifteen minutes so, unlike a film or book, the YouTube video typically has a shorter, and therefore less complex, story to tell.

An action such as a dog cycling or humans dancing the Harlem Shake (where different groups of people dance to a song of the same name) has a face value all of its own; it need not stand for or symbolise anything unless it is placed in an elaborate conceptual framework of a story where the behaviour has associations with previous actions or specific characters that give it a special relevance not intrinsic to the physical features of the event. It is very rare for such elaborate or complex story-lines, which might be more readily seen in a TV programme, to be played out on YouTube. Yet, while there is some evidence of substitution of web viewing for conventional television viewing, the time spent on viewing programming on the web, on average some 6.8 hours per week, far exceeds the reduction in weekly traditional television viewing of only some seven minutes.[13] Perhaps more important still, overall time spent on network-controlled viewing (television plus network websites) has increased by almost four hours a week.

In real life, actions always have consequences and, as we know only too well, cannot be reversed. Unlike in video games, no one can become undead; killing someone is therefore a highly significant and meaningful act. By contrast, as we've discussed, dropping something on the floor and immediately picking it up is meaningless: the action has effectively been completely reversed. Most of life, however, unfolds between these two extremes:

much of what we do seems meaningless at the time, but on reflection it sets in train a chain of cause-and-effect reactions that give rise to a certain outcome. Even the dropping of a coin and its retrieval may lead to a particular outcome, even if only that people watching regard you as a bit weird!

Alternatively, actions may lead not just to a predictable immediate effect, but to one with many indirect ramifications. Surely it is this intricate sequencing of cause and effect, of indirect consequences, that amounts to a good story. The more unpredictable, but in retrospect understandable, the sequence of cause and effect, say in a murder mystery, the more absorbing the narrative. If, on top of that, the characters also have intrinsic significance by virtue of what they've done in the past or simply because of their association with other characters, then the story is even better still: it is just like real life. By contrast, a character in a YouTube clip usually has no complex back-story, no personal relationships, and their actions have no long-term consequences; they are frozen in a tiny time window of a quarter of an hour. What you see doesn't really *mean* anything.

Could such a statement also apply to the freeze-frame of a painting? No, because a painting is showing you the world through the highly subjective and idiosyncratic eyes of the artist. If anything, a better analogy would be a photo, or a series of photos, of people, objects and events with which you have no connection. Given the millions of videos that YouTube hosts, perhaps the competition between them for your attention, and the ease and speed with which they can be circulated, may suggest that quantity trumps quality, where brevity is interlinked with a shorter attention span and a lower level of personal involvement or insight.

Therefore, in itself it may seem baffling, sad or worrying or, for others, perfectly understandable that people wish to spend their time passively watching something that is not necessarily even a story, but that makes you smile, gasp, shake your head or cry, just for a moment. This is perhaps the most minimal activity of all those associated with digital technologies; a few moments where the outside world is replaced by the cyber one, for no purpose, requiring no response, making no point other than capturing your passive attention for a few moments. Then, of course, you can play it back again and again. The 'Harlem Shake' viral video might be a good example. Perhaps it is the time out from real life, the fact that no effort is required, no input and arguably not even any thought, that is the appeal. If so, we have come a long way from both committing facts to memory and learning so that we can translate information into knowledge.

> What I . . . found fascinating [about asking people where they did their best thinking] was that only one person said in the office, and they said very early in the morning . . . in other words, when the building wasn't really functioning as an office at all. Interestingly, not a single person mentioned digital technology . . . Technology, it seems, is good for spreading and developing ideas, but not much use for hatching them.[14]

Once again, futurist Richard Watson is the pessimist. But, as our society spends increasing amounts of time surfing, swimming or drowning in Google or YouTube, perhaps Watson has a point. The magical *something* about surfing is perhaps not its value in offering infinite content, unprecedented speed and ease of access. Perhaps the opportunity for an experience that can be an end in itself and that is impossible to obtain elsewhere is the true appeal. This online ongoing experience could easily trump the longer-term reason for surfing in the first place: to find something out. If so, then we are about to witness a radical change in how the next generation thinks.

17 THE SCREEN IS THE MESSAGE

Back in 1964 Marshall McLuhan argued in his now legendary work, *Understanding Media*, that technology wasn't a neutral conduit but that in and of itself it would have an impact on mental processes: 'The medium is the message.'[1] McLuhan then went on to develop the distinction between 'hot' and 'cold' media. 'Hot' media does most of the work for you; with TV, radio or even a simple photograph, you are nothing but a passive recipient. In contrast, 'cold' media, such as a cartoon or a telephone, require some kind of input from you, in response to a much more minimal offering. Interestingly enough, cyber experiences can be regarded as hot, on the one hand, leaving nothing to the imagination with ever more exotic and startling screen displays; on the other hand, they can qualify as cold since their huge appeal comes from the interactive, participative experience they offer. The very medium of the digital technologies, the screen itself and what lies behind it, might now be driving our thought processes in an unprecedented direction. The physical difference of a screen compared to a book, the availability of hypertext, the opportunity to multi-task or engage in brain-training regimes are all unprecedented in their possible impact on our brain processes.

The first, most obvious physical feature of the screen is that the text is lit up on a hard surface as opposed to print on a fragile page. Back in 2001, Abigail Sellen and Richard Harper argued in *The Myth of the Paperless Office* that good old-fashioned paper would continue to play an important role in office life.[2] The basis of their rationale was the fascinating concept of *affordances*, the idea that the physical properties of an object allow, or afford, certain activities. The reasoning was that paper, which can be thin, light, porous and opaque, affords activities such as grasping, carrying, folding, writing and so on. That being so, the affordances of the laptop and mobile phone will be very different.

Anne Mangen at the Oslo and Akershus University College of Applied Sciences set out to explore the importance of the affordance of actually touching paper, by comparing the performances of readers of paper with those who read on the screen.[3] Her conclusion was that e-reading resulted in poorer comprehension, as a result of the physical limitations of the text that forced readers to scroll up and down, thereby disrupting their reading with a spatial instability.[4] This is an important factor, since having a good spatial mental representation of the physical layout of the text leads to better reading comprehension. Those who understand well, compared to those who comprehend poorly, are significantly better at remembering and relocating the spatial order of information in a text, so there could well be a link between the physical layout of what you're reading and how well you understand it.[5]

A further consideration in reading from a screen is the greater potential for eye strain. Even the appearance of the printed page, compared to the screen itself, can make a vital difference to visual ergonomics. The visuospatial perceptual processes of reading rely on the legibility of the text, which in turn is dependent on letter detection and word identification, light source, ambient luminance, character size, display time, interline spacing and so on. Each of these processes impacts reading performance, visual fatigue and search time. Even between different types of electronic media, lighting is a differentiating factor.[6]

Hanho Jeong, from Chongshin University, Seoul, aimed to assess the usability of electronic and paper books with objective measures such as eye fatigue, along with perception and reading comprehension in sixth-year state school students.[7] The results showed a significant 'book effect' on quiz scores: compared to reading e-books, reading paper books resulted in better reading comprehension. Moreover, the students had significantly greater eye fatigue after reading e-books than after reading the paper counterparts and, although they are 'satisfied' with the e-book, they claimed they actually preferred paper books. Most of them grew tired of reading on the screen. In turn, this fatigue could have an adverse effect on both reading comprehension and the perception of e-books: further analysis of users' responses showed that many of their critical remarks were based on the screen or text size or clarity, rather than on the e-book itself.

A second distinguishing feature of digital technology is the temptation and opportunity that it offers for multi-tasking. In his book *The Shallows*, Nicholas Carr is in no doubt as to the potential detrimental effects: '. . . the Net seizes our attention only to scatter it. We focus intensively on the medium itself, on the flickering screen, but we're distracted by the medium's rapid fire delivery of competing messages and stimuli.'[8] Media multi-tasking can be operationally defined by all too familiar and highly irritating scenarios such as switching from checking emails to having an instant messaging conversation with someone, text messaging while watching television, or jumping from one website to another. In a survey of 2,000 8- to 18-year-olds, the time spent multi-tasking between more than one technology medium in 1999 was 16 per cent but had almost doubled to 29 per cent ten years later in 2009.[9] In a survey of US college students, 38 per cent said they could not go for more than ten minutes while studying without checking their laptop, smartphone, tablet or e-reader.[10]

Since media multi-tasking involves, by definition, shifting attention between multiple sources, much research has focused on how much information can be retained, and how efficiently, when individuals multi-task between media. One study put students through a series of three tests. In each case, the subjects were split into two groups: those who regularly engaged in frequent media multi-tasking and those who didn't. The three tests in the study involved the subjects looking at shapes, numbers or letters, but the task was to remember something about just some of the images on the screen and to ignore the others.

In all three tests, the high multi-taskers seemed unable to ignore the shapes they were told to, and were unable to filter out what wasn't important to that particular task. In all cases the low multi-taskers outperformed their high multi-tasking counterparts. The researchers had originally set out to learn what benefits multi-tasking conferred, but Eyal Ophir, the study's lead author and a researcher at Stanford's Communication between Humans and Multimedia Lab, concluded: 'We kept looking for what they're better at and we didn't find it.' Ophir's explanation was that 'the high multi-taskers are always drawing from all the information in front of them. They can't keep things separate in their minds.'[11] Anthony Wagner, a psychologist, amplified this idea further: 'When they (high multi-taskers) are in situations where there are multiple sources of information coming from the external world or emerging out of memory, they're not able to filter out what's not relevant to their current goal. That failure to filter means they're slowed down by that irrelevant information.'[12]

Multi-tasking has also been cited as a reason for why the reading time for an e-textbook is significantly longer,[13] and research shows that college students multi-task for approximately 42 per cent of class time.[14] An experimental investigation into multi-tasking and lecture comprehension found that comprehension was significantly impaired when students were set simple Google, YouTube and Facebook search tasks that occupied only 33 per cent of class time.[15] Overall, students who multi-tasked for a third of the lecture scored 11 per cent lower on a post-lecture comprehension test. One answer to this apparent sad state of affairs is fairly simple: students who want to learn will do so, and those who become bored or unmotivated during lectures switch off. However, investigators went one step further and found that, for non-multi-tasking students, even the visible presence of other students multi-tasking during a lecture had a significant negative effect on their comprehension. Students who were in direct view of a multi-tasking student perusing Facebook, Google or YouTube had a 17 per cent poorer performance on the subsequent comprehension test, indicating that the distracting effect of personal computer technologies in the classroom had an impact not just on bored students, but also on motivated ones.

Outside of class, is multi-tasking during study also affecting academic performance? Researchers observed middle school, high school and university students engaged in academic work for just fifteen minutes in their homes.[16] They factored in the presence of other technologies and open computer windows in the learning environment prior to studying, and conducted a minute-by-minute assessment of on-task behaviour and off-task technology use. Astonishingly, students averaged *less than six minutes* on task prior to switching, most often as a result of technological distractions including social media, texting and a self-reported preference for task switching. Having a positive attitude towards technology did not affect being on task during studying; however, those who preferred to task-switch had more distracting technologies available and were more likely to be off task than others. It's no real surprise that concentration is the key and that multi-tasking can be counterproductive.

Instant messaging has become one of the most popular forms of computer-mediated communication for college students, through programs such as *Skype* and *Facebook Chat*. Unsurprisingly, in a large-sample web-based survey of college students over half of them reported that instant messaging while studying had a detrimental effect on their academic performance.[17] Similarly, two studies have found that there is a negative relationship between amount of time spent on Facebook and grade point averages, or GPAs.[18] Facebook users also reported spending fewer hours each week studying compared to non-users.[19]

While students may be aware of the detrimental effect of instant message multi-tasking, a more formal investigation set out to measure how well students can perform in a test when they have been multi-tasking during study. In one investigation, the prediction was that students who engaged in instant messaging while reading a psychology passage online would take longer to read the passage and would perform more poorly in a comprehension test.[20] Participants were randomly assigned to one of three conditions: instant messaging before reading, instant messaging during reading or no instant messaging. Students took significantly longer to read the passage when they were instant messaging during reading, not including the time taken actually to send the message. The researchers cautioned that students might feel as though they are achieving more in a shorter period of time while multi-tasking, which was patently not the case.[21]

In summary, although the ability to be engaged in several things at once sounds like it might be wonderful for keeping pace with the speed of twenty-first-century life, the price paid could be high. Evidence is mounting regarding the negative effects of attempting to process different streams of information simultaneously, and results now indicate that multi-tasking leads to increased time needed to achieve the same level of learning, as well as an increase in mistakes while processing information, compared to those who sequentially or serially process the same information.

A third basic feature of the screen that the printed book can never offer is hypertext. Although individual differences between readers, such as their working memory capacity and their background knowledge, all play a part in final reading performance, the increased demands of decision-making and visual processing in hypertext can have a distracting or even detrimental effect on students' efficiency.[22] Hypertext is, after all, a deviation from the path of linear thought, a tangent that may or may not be a red herring, but you only discover which once you've deviated. A detour that might lead to further meandering away from your initial intellectual journey arguably presents more of a deviation/distraction from the path of linear thought than, say, a traditional one-off footnote, which is finite and leads no further. Moreover, a hypertext connection is not one that you have made yourself and that will not necessarily have a place in your own unique line of reasoning and eventual conceptual framework. It will, therefore, not necessarily help you understand and digest what you're reading, at your own appropriate pace.

This notion of reading at your own pace is an important part of what is known as metacognition. 'Metacognition', or the ability to monitor and be aware of your own cognitive performance, matches up closely with good reading comprehension. Rakefet Ackerman and Morris Goldsmith from the Technion-Israel Institute of Technology and University of Haifa compared reading performance from on-screen learning and paper learning, and found that performance did not differ significantly under fixed test conditions. However, when study time was self-regulated, they found a poorer performance in screen reading than in paper reading. The lower test performance of those working from the screen was accompanied by significant overconfidence with regard to predicted performance, whereas subjects learning from paper monitored their performance more accurately. Ackerman and Goldsmith came to the conclusion that people appear to perceive the medium of print as more suitable for effortful learning, whereas the electronic medium, in this case a computer, is better suited for 'fast and shallow reading of short texts such as news, emails, and forum notes . . . The common perception of screen presentation as an information source intended for shallow messages may reduce the mobilization of cognitive resources that is needed for effective self-regulation.'[23]

This brings us to the fourth and most crucial issue of all: the reason for picking up a book or switching on an e-book in the first place. Recent research analysing reading behaviour in the digital environment over the past ten years has revealed that decreases in sustained attention are increasingly characterising people's literacy skills and habits.[24] With a growing amount of time spent reading electronic documents, a profile of screen-based reading behaviour is emerging characterised by more time spent browsing and scanning, keyword spotting, one-time reading, non-linear reading and reading more selectively, while less time is spent on in-depth and concentrated reading. So reading on a screen may take longer than reading a book, as a consequence of potential distractions, for example hypertext links, as well as encouraging a more browsing-oriented strategy. Which of the two, the book or the screen, might be the harder work?

At Johnannes Gutenberg University in Germany, Franziska Kretzschmar's team measured brain waves (EEG) and eye tracking to evaluate the cognitive effort involved in reading in each type of medium.[25] Results replicated previous findings in that participants overwhelmingly chose the paper page over an e-reader or a tablet computer as their preferred reading vehicle. However, actual cognitive effort did not differ between media, indicating that while *subjectively* readers rank digital devices as more of an effort, objective results on comprehension or cognition were indistinguishable. This subjective perception may account for why electronic textbooks specifically are still not very popular with college students. Textbooks will be read for different reasons and with different strategies than, say, novels as e-books.[26]

Certainly skills beyond comprehension and cognition may flourish more readily as a result of reading paper textbooks. For example, one investigation at Sheffield University followed students as they identified woodlice, with one group using a conventional paper-based identification guide, and the other group using the same key on a computer.[27] It turned out that the group using conventional textbooks were more curious and questioning of the information. Perhaps a book has a sense of permanence and immediate structure that enables the student to feel more secure and confident in asking questions. Alternatively, they may feel that they have more time to reflect, that there is no rush to press a key for the next entry on the screen. So perhaps it's this sense of personal exploration at their own pace that underlies the subjective preference of students seen in the other studies.

And yet here's the paradox: despite the appeal of paper books, in the rapidly changing circumstances of our increasingly digital world, reading is becoming an ever more digital experience. E-book sales are rapidly growing, while sales for traditional books have slowed down.[28] In the United States in 2012, e-book sales outpaced hardback book sales for the first time.[29] The slow growth in the sale of paper books will inevitably have knock-on effects for retailers. Independent booksellers in the United Kingdom have been shutting down year after year, and are now down a third since 2005.[30] Over-riding socio-economic and lifestyle factors such as the novelty, cheapness and accessibility of e-books are clearly key factors that are trumping other, more intellectual, considerations. Books and screens offer very different kinds of experiences and consequently will elicit different performances, responses and priorities.

Perhaps the greater appeal of the printed book, but one that will not be at a premium when the more everyday workaday considerations of money and convenience are taken into account, is its cultural symbolism. Paper books are of a fixed time and place, have permanence and therefore offer a reassuring security that an e-book can never deliver. As I look around my study, with bookshelves covering three of the four walls around me, I try to imagine these walls denuded in favour of a small stash of flash drives. Just seeing and touching those hard and paperback coloured objects of different sizes, and in varying degrees of dilapidation, is like being surrounded by old friends. In many cases I remember the time in my life when I acquired a certain book and devoured the facts it contained, or was stunned at the ideas it set out; even though the contents of some of them may long have been obsolete, the prospect of throwing any one, or indeed any book, out with the garbage would seem almost like a kind of murder. Beyond the functional value offered by the particular properties of the printed page, and beyond personal memories, there is also the powerful iconography of physical books. On 10 May 1933, Nazi students burned upwards of 25,000 volumes of 'un-German' books, including the writings of Albert Einstein, as well as non-German authors such as Ernest Hemingway. Now, on that site in Berlin, a large glass-covered opening in the cobbled square reveals an excavated area below of wide walls of empty bookshelves in a simple but chilling testimony . . . to what? Books *stand for* knowledge, new ideas and the inventiveness of the human spirit and imagination. Will the Digital Native in the future appreciate such a non-interactive object with its fixed time and place, its unchangeable story locked away in its fragile pages?

Printed works may always have something special to offer, despite our changing lifestyle, agenda and mind-set. Books and screens may become complementary objects rather than rivals, just as the book and the film, the radio and the TV, or the bicycle and the car play different but complementary roles in many of our lives. And a new part of that life now is the acquisition of facts through digital devices. Will this change in medium change how *effectively* we process those facts; how we learn, remember and think?

Aside from the more general activities of hypertext and multi-tasking, the digital technologies could offer unique, formal pedagogic opportunities. There are many 'brain-training' products that claim to improve cognitive function through the regular use of screen-based exercises, and modest but positive effects have been reported in some studies of older individuals and of preschool children.[31] Adrian Owen and his colleagues in Cambridge and London were, nonetheless, not convinced there was sufficiently hard empirical evidence of their efficacy.[32] They investigated the key question of whether the benefits accrued during training would transfer to other untrained tasks, or indeed lead to any general improvement in the level of cognitive functioning. Over a six-week online study, they monitored some 11,000 participants trained several times each week on cognitive tasks designed to improve reasoning, memory, planning, visuo-spatial skills and attention. Improvements were apparent in every one of the cognitive tasks in question, as might have been expected; but the crucial observation was that there was no evidence for the transfer of these effects to untrained tasks, even when those tasks were closely related in the thought processes required.

But wait. Didn't we just see in the earlier discussion on video games the precise opposite: that there was indeed robust evidence that the skills learned while gaming could be transferred to more generalised contexts? So, simply at face value and without drilling down into the relative merits of specific games and training regimes, where might the crucial distinction lie? One important difference, with all the usual caveats of stereotyping, might be that video games, as we saw, are by definition providing an experience that is more exciting and stimulating than what the dull, three-dimensional world can offer. In contrast, to the best of my knowledge, brain training is rarely marketed as exciting. After all, if we are thinking in terms of the serious acquisition of knowledge, and selling that as a product, it is the long-term acquisition that needs to be emphasised to the customer rather than a short-term moment of frivolous fun. The motivation for buying a brain-training program is self-improvement. On the other hand, the primary reason for choosing to play a video game is not to learn but to enjoy yourself.

The difference between short-term sensation and long-term cognitive improvement in the brain is, at least in part, determined once again by the participation of our faithful old friend, the transmitter dopamine. Could the presence or absence of high dopamine levels make the difference, at least hypothetically, between whether or not you can apply a skill learned from one task to other tasks and activities? Simplistic though it might seem, one possibility springs from the fact that dopamine operates like a fountain in the brain, emanating from the more evolutionarily basic parts to access wide reaches of the 'higher' cerebral regions. Dopamine can also serve as a modulator, acting as an agent that can predispose brain cells to be more sensitive to stimulation when it arrives. Scenarios such as video gaming, where dopamine is released as a result of raised arousal and reward, could enable more brain circuitry to be harnessed, and hence for learning to be more generalised.

We shouldn't ever underestimate the importance of enjoyment. Part of the appeal in studying lies in its potential for social interaction, the feeling that it gives us, that we belong, that we are part of the crowd and are not being left out. Networked interactivity is one of the essential factors that differentiate the most recent online educational games from traditional stand-alone CD-based games. Kwan Min Lee and his colleagues from the University of Southern California measured how networked interactivity influenced game users' learning outcomes in online educational quiz games, offline educational quiz games and traditional classroom lectures.[33] The researchers found that networked interactivity in the online educational quiz game condition enhanced game users' positive evaluation of learning, test performance and feelings of social presence. Further analyses indicated that it was the *feelings* of social presence in an interactive network that was what counted in the various learning outcomes. So, by promoting the feeling of being connected with others, screen technologies act as a positive driver. It is unsurprising that the best environment for learning, it turns out, is one where you are having fun and interacting with others, irrespective of whether these key ingredients are provided through a screen or a more traditional scenario.

While the screen can readily offer a more rigorous rehearsal regime in mental processing than people or paper ever can, does the same apply to how *effectively* we learn? Computer-assisted technologies have, of course, been used for decades in classrooms, and their moderate use continues to enhance the learning experience of students. In particular, the case for screen devices in education seems most conclusive for special needs students, whether they have a visual impairment, dyslexia or some other learning difficulty. So far, the use of 'errorless' software, where there are no right or wrong answers, has proved to be one of the best approaches. Instead, trial and error, as well as exploration, are rewarded with fun noises, humorous animations, vivid graphics, music and natural sounding speech. For children with learning needs, this non-judgemental interactive software, with its fast-paced and colourful displays, is easily more motivational than a simple printed book.[34]

Touch tablet devices certainly seem to be beneficial for a range of cognitive impairments in students with developmental disabilities. One review looked at fifteen studies covering five domains: academic, communication, employment, leisure and transitioning across school settings.[35] The studies in question reported outcomes for participants who ranged from 4 to 27 years of age and had a diagnosis of autism spectrum disorder and/or intellectual disability. Most studies involved the use of iPods or iPads and aimed either to deliver instructional prompts via the iPod Touch or iPad or to teach the individual to operate an iPod Touch or iPad to access preferred stimuli. The latter also included operating an iPod Touch or an iPad as a speech-generating device to request preferred stimuli. Taken together, the results were largely positive, suggesting that iPods, iPod Touch, iPads and related devices are viable technological aids for individuals with developmental disabilities.

The benefits of screen technology are also evident in mainstream learning. For example, one meta-analysis of forty-six different original studies involving a total of 36,793 students showed significant positive effects of computer use on mathematics achievement.[36] Similarly, a recent large-scale analysis reviewed how educational software programs affect reading outcomes, in a total of eighty-four studies based on over 60,000 students.[37] The findings suggested that various reading programs, predominatly computer delivered, generally produced a positive, though small, effect on reading skills. However, any innovative technology applications and integrated literacy interventions showed more positive evidence when there was teachers' support. So the greatest promise of the digital devices lies not so much in the software and screen delivery themselves, but in their use in close connection with teachers' efforts.

For anyone who's read *The Prime of Miss Jean Brodie* or *Goodbye Mr Chips*, this will come as no new insight. Nothing beats an inspirational and exciting teacher. However, direct face-to-face instruction is declining in higher education. Lecturers have also observed another trend in university courses: 55 per cent of academic staff recently reported that lecture attendance had decreased as a result of introducing digital audio recordings of their presentations.[38] Back in 2006, one of the main reasons college students gave for not attending lectures was the availability of materials online.[39] In the same spirit, when asked why they did not attend lectures, almost 70 per cent of students surveyed at an elite Australian university reported that they could learn as effectively using digital audio recordings as they could by attending the corresponding lecture in person.

However, one report found that economics students who learned course material via virtual delivery performed significantly worse compared to those who attended traditional lectures.[40] While the two groups did not differ in regard to their grasp of basic concepts, the group learning virtually fell significantly behind in their grasp of complex material. This indicates that sophisticated ideas cannot be transferred via the screen as effectively as in person. Another study found similar results, favouring person-to-person instruction for academic performance.[41] Indeed, when college students in a large introductory microeconomics course were randomly assigned either face-to-face lectures or video-streamed presentations, the students who attended face-to-face lectures had higher average test scores.

It seems that the benefits of dialogue, of face-to-face discussions of issues and problem-solving still exceed the benefits of virtual communication. Surely, when it comes to education, regardless of the number of screens in a classroom and the time spent in front of them, there is always a strong case for real classrooms with real teachers overseeing real-life conversations. Recent studies suggest that e-books and tablets might be useful educational tools but crucially, once again, only when used alongside adult supervision. Ofra Korat and Adina Shamir at the School of Education, Bar-Ilan University in Israel, examined the effects of e-book reading on 5–6-year-old students' reading skills, with and without an adult.[42] While one group read an e-book independently, a second group read an e-book with adult mediation, a third read the printed book with adult mediation and the fourth read the printed book with no adult intervention. The results showed that the activity of reading the e-book with adult assistance achieved greater progress in the recognition of letter names, emergent word reading and general emergent reading level than all other groups. So, here, the e-book might be superior to a traditional book, *but provided an adult is around.*

Education doesn't take place in a bubble but is an integral part of a person's life and relationships. Different lifestyles will therefore also play their part in determining whether or not, and to what extent, the screen can make a difference to learning. For example, another factor associated with higher test scores in mathematics and reading is having a home computer, even after allowing for family income and for cultural and social capital.[43] However, home computing may generate a 'Sesame Street effect' whereby an innovation that held great promise for poorer children to catch up with more affluent children educationally, in practice, actually widens the educational gap between affluent and poor, between boys and girls and between ethnic minorities and whites. This gap could grow as different must-have (i.e., expensive) digital devices appear at an ever faster rate.

The iPad is now a mainstay source of education and entertainment for many children. While most schools in the United States don't have the purchasing power to provide all their students with iPads, the children who *do* have them are getting them from their families and other adults who, presumably, are using them as well. The iPad plays an increasingly integral part in the American system. In a recent list of the top 100 enterprises with the largest iPad roll-outs worldwide, nearly 70 per cent of the list were US schools.[44] Apple signed a US$30 million deal in 2013 with the Los Angeles School Board of Education, the second largest public school district in the United States, to roll out iPads to every single student by 2014.[45] Other Western countries are also zealously integrating iPad technology into the formal education system.

Known as 'one-to-one classrooms' and fully supported by Apple (for whom the commercial implications shouldn't be ignored), schools around the world are adopting tablet-only classrooms, replacing textbooks and traditional computers with a tablet-only program for classes as young as kindergarten. One elementary school in Arizona outfitted a classroom solely with iPads, dubbing it the 'iMaginarium'.[46] If we're going to try to evaluate how the newly pervasive cyberculture affects how the brain adapts to different styles of learning, the large-scale introduction of iPads into the classroom might be a good place to start.

Consider, for example, an email I received recently from a concerned mother who is also a physician:

> My daughter's school in Australia is aggressively introducing digital learning from Grade 5 . . . They will use nothing but a computer slate from the age of 9 or 10 which is also web enabled. As a health professional, I have done extensive Internet searches myself and am yet to find any evidence for the benefits apart from 'expert opinion' and anecdotes. Do you know of any scientific evidence for the neurophysiological effects of using nothing else but computers for learning?

One typical iPad enthusiast is Lisa Wright, head of a school in Essex in the United Kingdom, who claims the flexibility of the curriculum means that iPads could be used right across the primary school. Mrs Wright is a clear convert:

> Year Four children [8–9-year-olds] have used them in maths lessons and reception children have played some maths and phonics games . . . Year Ones [4–5-year-olds] had them in their religious education lesson and Year Five and Six pupils [9–11-year-olds] have been using iPads in their topics, such as learning about the Titanic by getting on the Internet . . . We bought the iPads because they're so flexible and versatile. We've got a lovely outdoor space here so the children can take them outside and even use them to take pictures. We want learning to be fun for the children. The iPads are in use all the time. If you walk around the school, there's a child somewhere or a group using the iPad, which is what I want to see.[47]

Although Mrs Wright also insists that books and conventional teaching methods, such as pencil and paper, are equally important, in many one-to-one classrooms the tablet computer has replaced all traditional teaching methods.

In contrast to such an overwhelming vote of confidence, a recent report claimed that millions of dollars' worth of tablet computers were sitting in British school cupboards as a result of teachers' over-enthusiasm in purchasing new technology without any evidence that it actually improved educational outcomes.[48] We often assume that any new technology is automatically superior because it is the next step in cutting-edge progress: advances in knowledge and understanding become ascribed to the gadget itself. This view is frequently based on availability and novelty but not on other factors such as the type of supervision being given or the inspirational character, or otherwise, of the teacher. But, more to the point, just what evidence is there that iPads and other digital aids really do make a serious difference?

A critical and potentially confounding factor to bear in mind is the formidable physical appeal of the iPhone and iPad. David Furió and his team at the Polytechnic University of Valencia set out to compare learning outcomes and preferences of 8–10-year-olds who played an educational game either in its traditional form or on an iPhone.[49] Ninety-six per cent of the children indicated that they would like to play the iPhone game again, and 90 per cent indicated that they preferred the experience with the iPhone game over the traditional one. The design of the physical object itself was clearly an important factor.

A similar result emerged in a 2013 study comparing desktop computers and iPads.[50] Students received an online multimedia lesson on a desktop iMac in a lab or on an iPad in a courtyard outside. The students then experienced either a continuous lesson with no headings or an enhanced lesson, where each slide had a helpful heading and where the learner clicked on a button to go on to the next slide. In both cases, perhaps not surprisingly, the enhanced group outperformed the standard group. However, irrespective of type of instruction, the iPad group produced stronger self-reported ratings than the iMac group on their willingness to continue learning. Given that switching to iPad-based classrooms blindly assumes that traditional teaching materials are inferior, this current trend is very worrying. Until we have solid scientific evidence that iPads really do have superior pedagogic powers rather than just being prettier, it seems foolhardy to replace traditional teaching methods, which may actually be more effective, albeit less flashy, with these devices.

Interestingly enough, a backlash against the premature adoption of technology in classrooms is gathering momentum in California, with many schools opting for low-tech teaching methods. 'Engagement is about human contact, the contact with the teacher, the contact with their peers,' says a parent of three children, who is also an employee of a high-tech company. Meanwhile Paul Thomas, a former teacher and an associate professor of education at Furman University, who has written twelve books about public educational methods, stresses that 'Teaching is a human experience. Technology is a distraction when we need literacy, numeracy and critical thinking.'[51]

There are 160 Waldorf schools in the United States which subscribe to a teaching philosophy focused on physical activity and learning through creative, hands-on tasks. All digital devices are actually banned, as the school credo is that computers inhibit creative thinking, movement, human interaction and attention spans. Interestingly, the *New York Times* reported that the Waldorf school in Los Altos was, tellingly, popular with the very Silicon Valley parents who were themselves immersed in the digital industries.[52] This seems like a particularly fascinating trend, not only for education, but for Mind Change as a whole.

If the clever minds behind video games, social networking and tablets are wary about immersing their own children in these technologies, perhaps a general growing scepticism about their educational benefits is warranted.

One very extreme consequence of using high-tech methodologies in classrooms is that it could have a collective effect on literacy. If information is increasingly conveyed through the spoken word and visual images, we might have to face the possibility that literacy will be less and less relevant in our future lifestyle. Why learn to read or write when everyday communication can be so readily accomplished without either of these skills? Already literacy standards are declining: research has shown that many children are more likely to own a mobile phone than a book.[53] Another study by academics at Dundee University found that teenagers now prefer easier reads such as the *Harry Potter* and *Twilight* series.[54] Astonishingly, Eric Carle's classic picture book *The Very Hungry Caterpillar*, which charts a caterpillar's transformation into a butterfly over a week, emerged as the most popular book among girls aged 14 to 16.

The value of pervasive digital technology in education will be hard to appreciate for some time, as the jury will be out until the pre-teens of today take up their first jobs. Currently, it seems that any short- or medium-term impact will depend on the context in which screens feature: on what is being taught, by whom and where. More generally, for all of us, these powerful interactive screen technologies are not just exciting experiences but critical tools that have and will continue to reshape our cognitive processes with both benefits and problems. The difference between silicon and paper, the distractions of multi-tasking and hypertext, and the tendency to browse rather than to think deeply all suggest fundamental shifts in how our brains are now being asked to work.

18 THINKING DIFFERENTLY

When the Nobel Prize-winning physicist Niels Bohr took his colleague to task for not thinking but just being logical, what particular talent in the exclusively human cognitive tool-kit did the great intellectual pioneer feel was being neglected? Nothing less presumably than the quintessential mental activity that has enabled our species to probe into the meaning of our existence, and to express those insights through science and the arts. Yet, perhaps nowadays, there's a danger that growing numbers of us are taking the more straightforward path and thinking increasingly like a computer, the more we interact with and adapt to its algorithmic mode of functioning determined by digital culture;[1] so our brains will function more like suboptimal computers.

Then again, sometimes such logical thinking is just what's required for solving a specified problem. Of course problems come in all shapes and sizes, from simple IQ tests and sudoku right up to solving an economic crisis or trying to reignite the faltering Arab Spring, or seemingly insoluble personal crises. But it's easiest to start with the most straightforward brain teasers where, unlike real life, the problem has a clear and unambiguous pre-existing solution. The skills needed here are the type of agile computational processing that is measured in IQ tests.[2]

Though many admit that intelligence can be defined and expressed in many ways, IT aficionados such as the physicist Ray Kurzweil focus on a narrow definition of intelligence denoted as *g* and assume, therefore, that this multifaceted phenomenon can be expressed as a computational process.[3] Contrary to popular belief, a high or low IQ may not be something you're simply born with. The largest genetic study on children has shown that only between 20 and 40 per cent of *g* is inherited.[4] Leaving aside the question of how accurately IQ scores measure mental prowess, the strong impact of the environment can be evidenced in the significant and long-sustained increase in IQ scores seen in the past 50–60 years.[5] This increase, known as the 'Flynn effect', may be caused by a number of factors, with the eponymous James Flynn himself suggesting that this rise may be due to the more stimulating environment of modern times.[6]

Another possible explanation for the rise in IQ test proficiency may be the increased rehearsal of test-specific skills. Since the beginning of the twentieth century, the rise of films, television, video games and the Internet has exposed us to more visual media, allowing us to become increasingly adept at visual analysis. One variant of the IQ test, the Ravens Progressive Matrices IQ Test, emphasises visuospatial skills and, tellingly, the increase in those scores has been dramatic. Steven Johnson, author of *Everything Bad is Good for You*, elaborates on the idea that video gaming and competence at IQ tests exercise the same mental processes. Digital natives are developing certain skills better than previous generations reared on books as a result of increased interaction with the screen.[7] This suggestion is persuasive when we compare the kinds of skills for performing well in IQ tests with those rehearsed in computer games. Both are abstracted processes, requiring the ability to see connections and anomalies and, above all, to detect rules independent of a wider context or requiring any background knowledge. Johnson also suggests that screen culture is developing minds that are better adapted to greater complexity, and greater proficiency at multi-tasking. This ability to solve problems while keeping in mind multiple rules and contingencies (working memory) is further enhanced with the rehearsal for faster problem-solving, or the ability to juggle problems at a faster rate as, indeed, has been shown to be the case.[8]

This is the most likely *type* of intelligence that our evolving cyberculture is helping to nurture, a computational ability where we are already outstripped by silicon and which impresses Ray Kurzweil so much that he predicts that digital devices will one day supersede the human brain. However, Kurzweil overlooks the fact that computational processing requires a specific end point, a clear solution to a specified problem. The type of intelligence enhanced by prolonged screen interaction involves discerning patterns and processing connections so that the correct solution is reached within a given time. In contrast, other manifestations of intelligence, such as writing *War and Peace* or imagining how the brain might generate consciousness, are infinitely more open-ended. When the problem is finding the solution to a defined puzzle, or searching for a fact, then accessing the screen will help, but if it is parsing the meaning of life, then juggling tasks and audio-visual expertise will be of little use.

'Game players are not soaking up moral counsel, life lessons or rich psychological portraits,' Steven Johnson readily admits.[9] So what ability enables the human mind to progress beyond mere reasoning, to escape the computational mind-set admired by Kurzweil but cautioned against by Bohr?

Although IQ scores have risen, interestingly enough, other abilities have remained constant. There has not been a concomitant increase in insights into the economic situation; no really noticeable increase in the creative arts, nor even on the horizons of neuroscience, compared to previous decades. However it's important to bear in mind that the Flynn effect lies mainly in the middle range of ability, within the group that do not usually win the Nobel Prize or compose symphonies, or even just venture into politics or the outreaches of academic research.

John Newton, head of Taunton School in Somerset, fears that 'We will raise a generation who do not love learning but simply see the screen as a source of opinion or nuggets of information, poorly digested, that will suit their point of view without testing their veracity.' Just as rote memorisation differs from true learning, Newton believes that critical thinking requires 'balance and a firm grasp of facts and context to avoid being led astray'.[10] I have deliberately selected this quote from many similar ones voiced by teachers around the world because Newton highlights two crucial terms, 'facts' and 'context':

> 'Now, what I want is, Facts. Teach these boys and girls nothing but Facts. Facts alone are wanted in life. Plant nothing else, and root out everything else. You can only form the minds of reasoning animals upon Facts: nothing else will ever be of any service to them. This is the principle on which I bring up my own children, and this is the principle on which I bring up these children. Stick to Facts, sir.'[11]

Extreme though it may seem, this view of Thomas Gradgrind's in Charles Dickens's *Hard Times* is perhaps closer to where the current mind-set could be heading than we might care to admit.

> 'Bitzer,' said Thomas Gradgrind. 'Your definition of a horse.'
>
> 'Quadruped. Graminivorous. Forty teeth, namely twenty-four grinders, four eye-teeth, and twelve incisive. Sheds coat in the spring; in marshy countries, sheds hoofs, too. Hoofs hard, but requiring to be shod with iron. Age known by marks in mouth.'

The facts are indeed all there, and accurate. It's just that the dots are not joined up at any level, from the literal to the metaphorical. The Gradgrind approach conflates efficient information processing with real understanding: the insight and the knowledge that characterises a gifted mind is more than the regurgitation of facts. You can train a brain (in certain cases even that of a parrot) to give the right responses to a given input, to recite poetry or to answer factual questions with factual answers. But real intelligence requires a synthesis between facts, context and meaning that encompasses far more than efficient responding.

Although we might access information efficiently and even regurgitate it on demand, success in such activities as Trivial Pursuit or pub quizzes is not regarded by even the most enthusiastic fans as the pinnacle of intellectual endeavour. Facts on their own are not enough! While collecting information is gathering dots, knowledge is joining them up, seeing one thing in terms of another and thereby understanding each component as part of a whole. The more connections you can make across an ever wider and disparate range of knowledge, the more deeply you will understand something. Search engines and video games do not provide that facility: nothing does, other than your own brain.

Even when you read at second hand someone else's idea, whether in a book or in a condensed form on Google, it's only by incorporating it into *your* own personal conceptual framework that you derive your own take of whatever it may be. Hence *your* interpretation, *your* evaluation, *your* understanding will inevitably be individual to you and different from everyone else's. And this *conceptual framework* will have developed since you were small. Your experiences, the stories you hear from others and read yourself, the facts you've been taught all build up into an ever more complex system of cross-referencing.[12] This connectivity, achieved through the plasticity of neuronal connections during development, may then be the key feature that defines real learning, which sets the human brain above and beyond the information processing of a computer. This is why the concept of *context*, beyond mere facts, is so important.

When actual context comes into play, when the question requires a 'crystallised' intelligence that is based within a 'conceptual framework', then it turns out that the Flynn effect is actually reversed.[13] The largest gains appear on IQ tests that measure a more computational type of mental agility, the 'fluid' intelligence discussed earlier (see Chapter 7). The Ravens, the Norwegian matrices, the Belgian Shapes, the Jenkins and the Horn are all examples of tests that are designed to measure fluid intelligence. They emphasise problem-solving and minimise a reliance on specific skills or familiarity with words and symbols, and have shown on average an increase of about 15 points per generation.[14] However, tests like the Wechsler and the Stanford-Binet – which measure verbal abilities as well as more direct problem-solving skills – show fewer IQ gains.

But, then, how do we use this crystallised intelligence to think in our special human way? I've been suggesting that *meaning* is an association between at least two elements, whether they are objects, people or events. A wedding ring has particular significance if it is yours, even though it looks quite generic. The associations that this particular object, and no other, imbue it with a special association for you that is not apparent to anyone else, nor is it intrinsic in the physical qualities of the ring.

So, the greater our ability to forge these links the greater our *understanding*. We bring together two previously disparate and independent elements, and can see one thing in terms of something else; for example, the snuffing out of a candle stands for the extinguishing of a life. As we live our individual existence, the linking of certain objects, people and actions with previous objects, people, actions and emotions will imbue them with a cognitive rather than a mere sensory quality, a meaning shared by no one else, and which is unique to you. When we encounter a person or an object, we create personal meaning, and when we link that person or object to a wider framework our understanding grows richer and deeper. Finally, as we develop a sequence over time that links these meaningful things into a linear causal sequence, the original meaning and understanding changes and adapts. This is the kind of *thought* process that characterises the mature human mind.

The work of the late educational neuroscientist John Geake provides hard evidence for this suggestion. Geake's imaging studies of gifted children revealed that their brains showed greater interconnectivity than the brains of those with average cognitive ability.[15] Specifically, the findings led to the idea that giftedness is linked to 'analogical reasoning' (e.g., the analogy of the candle going out with death), a kind of reasoning that compares similarities between established concepts, and then uses those similarities to gain an understanding of new concepts. This ability to make connections where they didn't exist before, to connect the dots, could account for talents in a number of academic areas, including philosophy, mathematics, science and music.[16]

A similar pattern seems to hold for adults. In Bejing, Professor Ming Song and his colleagues in the Chinese Academy of Sciences showed that brain imaging could demonstrate correlations between high intelligence and the strength of the functional connectivity distributed widely across the cortex.[17] The authors concluded that these observations were further evidence for a 'network view of intelligence', and that, even in the resting state and in the absence of any explicit cognitive tasks, this connectivity was operative.

So, if connections enable deeper understanding, then the process of making these connections can loosely be termed 'thinking'. Earlier, I suggested that the crucial distinction between a raw feeling and a thought was a time-frame. Simply being conscious, as for any infant or non-human animal, always entails some kind of subjective sensation, as revealed by tail-wagging, purring, gurgling, smiling; but never at any time does the animal in question suddenly turn into an automaton or zombie. It is impossible to disentangle consciousness from this subjective state of feeling. In fact, I would argue that they are pretty much synonymous.

By contrast, although all animals have degrees of consciousness, and therefore feeling, not all animals are capable of what we would recognise as thought processes. It is a skill that even humans have to develop as the years unfold. So what do a fantasy, a rational argument, a memory, a hope, a grievance, a business plan and a joke all have in common? Remember that insightful quote, 'Thinking is movement confined to the brain', and how movement is characterised by a fixed sequence of muscle actions? So it is with thought: both processes share a specified, linear sequence where one step leads to the next. You start off in one place and end up somewhere else. And this sequence of linear steps unfolds over time, with a clear beginning, a middle and an end. Unlike a raw feeling, the thought process transcends the here and now; it has to, as it links a past with a future.

In brain terms, the prefrontal cortex is once again pivotal. We've already seen how an underdeveloped prefrontal cortex is linked to an underdeveloped understanding of figurative language, as well as an inability to connect current actions to future consequences. It may not be surprising, therefore, that this part of the brain, when fully functional, plays a part in the human experience of time-frames and time passing. We saw a little earlier that damage to the prefrontal cortex can, in addition to the many other deficits, lead to source amnesia – not so much the loss of a memory as the loss of how and when a memory was created.[18] Memories will now be free-floating, no longer tethered to any personal context. If you have source amnesia, all your memories will blur instead of being compartmentalised into specific incidents. You may remember a fact but not how and when you learned it. Your recollections would be more like the memories of a small child or a non-human animal, hazily aware of the past insofar as it colours the here and now but lacking any kind of order or chronology, and therefore any meaning. Your life story will make no sense, not even to you.

The notion of your life story, any story, is compelling to most people perhaps because it represents an amplification of the basic human thought process. The traditional custom of reading children stories has been the best possible way to develop the cognitive skills of imagination, attention span, empathy and insight into the minds of others. Research from the University at Buffalo, State University of New York, measured the impact on the empathy of undergraduates reading passages from J.K. Rowling's *Harry Potter* and Stephenie Meyer's *Twilight* books. Participants then answered questions designed to measure how they identified with the worlds they had been reading about. Results showed that participants who read the *Harry Potter* chapters self-identified as wizards, whereas participants who read the *Twilight* chapter self-identified as vampires. More fascinating still, membership of these fictional communities actually provided the same mood and life satisfaction people derive from affiliations with real-life groups. The authors, Shira Gabriel and Ariana Young, concluded: 'Books provide the opportunity for social connection and the blissful calm that comes from becoming part of something larger than oneself for a precious, fleeting moment.'[19]

Although this particular study focused on children, the power of stories and story-telling extends equally to adults. Keith

Oatley, a professor in the department of human development and applied psychology at the University of Toronto and a published novelist himself, expands on this point:

> I think the reason fiction but not non-fiction has the effect of improving empathy is because fiction is primarily about selves interacting with other selves in the social world. The subject matter of fiction is constantly about why she did this, or if that's the case what should he do now, and so on . . . In fiction, also, we are able to understand characters' actions from their interior point of view, by entering into their situations and minds, rather than the more exterior view of them that we usually have.[20]

A novel can, unsurprisingly, be as much of a learning tool as a textbook. We need fiction, someone else's story, in order to understand our own facts. The characters in question have a meaning because they can be linked in a conceptual framework, a context, to others and to past events, just like in our own lives. When we read fiction, as opposed to non-fiction, we are transported into the world of the characters and start to connect with them, the experiences they have and the decisions they make. We may feel positive or negative emotions towards them as people and care deeply about what happens to them in a way that would be much less likely with a character in a video game who is little more than an icon. The journalist Ben Macintyre sums it up beautifully:

> From the moment we become aware of others, we demand to be told stories that allow us to make sense of the world, to inhabit the mind of someone else. In old age we tell stories to make small museums of memory. It matters not whether the stories are true or imaginary. The narrative, whether oral or written, is a staple of every culture the world over. But stories demand

> time and concentration; the narrative does not simply transmit information, but invites the reader or listener to witness the unfolding of events.[21]

By observing what happens, by following the linear path of a story, we can convert information into knowledge in a way that exercises emphasising fast response and constant stimulation cannot. As I see it, the key issue is *narrative*. In a narrative there is a sequence, a chain of cause and effect in a non-random, strictly ordered sequence. Any narrative will, in some way, echo a life story. Stories arrange events into a context, a conceptual framework, and this order creates meaning. While narratives are the *sine qua non* of books, they are far from guaranteed on the Internet, where parallel choices, hypertexting and randomised participation is more typical. While empathy may be developed from reading books, it may not be automatically guaranteed in a cyber lifestyle that favours the rushed, the shallow and the disconnected.

But surely search engines could free us up for more challenging questions and deeper thinking than we could ever have imagined possible, just as the printing press once granted more people access to knowledge. Maybe so, but we first need to have some story-lines already in place. Without a personalised conceptual framework that enables us to use the Internet to frame and think about open-ended and difficult questions, we run the risk of being passively driven by isolated facts as we lurch from one disconnected but amazing screen experience to another. It's worth noting that even the chair of Google, Eric Schmidt, believes that sitting down and reading a book 'is the best way to really learn something'.[22] We need time to think about, and understand, the world around us. The sequence of steps, the 'movement confined to the brain' will not happen in an instant but within a time-frame as a 'train' or 'line' of thought. It seems that cyberculture does not encourage the development of the attention spans necessary for deep thought, and thus we fail to construct the adequate conceptual framework that gives the world around us meaning.

The reading of stories has to be the best possible way to develop the cognitive skills of imagination, attention span, empathy and insight into the minds of others, as well as to provide us with a grasp of abstract concepts. After all, how would you convey honour, for instance, as an icon? Yet anyone reading Malory's *Le Morte d'Arthur* would soon get a sense of what honour means. Hence a novel can be as much of a learning tool as a textbook. We need fiction to understand facts. And if all this is so, then search engines are not the best vehicles for gaining understanding or for acquiring knowledge.

This critical issue facing us is how we negotiate a transition from the old question-rich, answer-poor environment of the twentieth century to make sense of, indeed survive in, the current question-poor, answer-rich environment delivered by a fast-paced technology. In my view there are three essential factors often overlooked in current education, and certainly not necessarily inspired by the current cyber lifestyle: firstly, to have a strong sense of one's own individual identity (and to respect it in others); secondly, to have a sense of individual fulfilment; and, thirdly, to be useful to society. How might these somewhat abstract goals be realised?

There is something that ticks all three boxes: creativity. By creativity I don't mean necessarily writing a symphony or revealing some great new insight into science or the human condition, although such activities would of course qualify. On a more basic level, surely the essence of creativity is simply seeing something in a new way, whether it be rearranging the bedroom furniture or interpreting a social situation from a different angle. Let's unpack the idea further.

Creativity is often associated in particular with young children. It is also associated by some, such as the clinical psychologist Louis Sass at Rutgers,[23] with schizophrenia, and by others (usually the individuals themselves) with the taking of recreational drugs. But not all children, schizophrenics or drug takers are overtly creative, nor do creative people have to be young, mentally ill or doped. The clue here might lie in the fact that some of the features exhibited by children, schizophrenics and drug takers could be a necessary, but not sufficient, requisite for creativity. Meanwhile the same condition may well be attained by people who fall into none of these three categories. What could it be?

Young children, as we saw, have sparse brain connectivity, so they cannot readily see one thing in terms of anything else. Schizophrenics resemble children in taking the world literally and not being able to interpret proverbs; in both cases what they get is what they see. Finally, as a consequence of the psychoactive substances impairing their neuronal connectivity, drug takers have impaired associative powers. For them, meaning is fragile and idiosyncratic. So could it be that the crucial first step in the creative process, but only a first step, is the ability to dissociate previously conventionally connected elements? This kind of deconstruction is familiar in art, where the whole trick is to reduce a cognitive take on an image, a vase of flowers say, to an abstract sensory conglomeration of colours, shapes and textures that you then try and reproduce. Similarly in science, the essential first step is to challenge dogma, as for example Barry Marshall did with the notion that ulcers were not caused by stress but by a bacterium.

However, it's important not just to challenge dogma but also to replace it with an alternative, a *new* association that has been never been tried before: words combined in a special way, a certain convergence of colours and shapes, a familiar object or person in an unexpected context or a link between two previously unrelated features of the physical world, such as the parallels between the immune system and the idea of Darwinian survival of the fittest, which was first pointed out by the brilliant Australian immunologist Frank Burnet.[24]

But such deconstruction and reconstruction does not guarantee a creative act, as anyone experimenting with odd ingredients in a new culinary concoction will testify. Another example would be a child's painting, where there may well be unusual colours or shapes depicting an animal or a person but the final work wouldn't qualify for exhibition in an art gallery. What is the third all-important step that is not just necessary but also sets apart true creativity? The crucial final step, as I see it, is that the work or idea should mean something, help you see the world in a new way. Whether through science, art, literature or any other medium, new connections are established in the brain that in turn give the world a new meaning. For connections to have a meaning, as we have seen, they cannot be just random: they need to link to ever wider conceptual frameworks that give a correspondingly ever deeper meaning.

Creative thinking cannot be purchased, downloaded or guaranteed but it can be fostered with the right environment. Developing individual conceptual frameworks for understanding and interpreting the world also means encouraging individuals to have the confidence to question and deconstruct dogma and traditional views, to possess the courage to make new associations without fear of the opinions or cynicism of others. It is not a happy scenario to imagine a world peopled by individuals who have brilliant sensorimotor coordination, can multi-task and perform well in IQ tests, but who are incapable of reflective thought and understanding, let alone original ideas.

In 1964, at the New York World's Fair, the science fiction writer Isaac Asimov came up with this appropriate, enormously prescient prediction for 50 years hence:

> Even so, mankind will suffer badly from the disease of boredom, a disease spreading more widely each year and growing in intensity. This will have serious mental, emotional and sociological consequences, and I dare say that psychiatry will be far and away the most important medical specialty in 2014. The lucky few who can be involved in creative work of any sort will be the true elite of mankind, for they alone will do more than serve a machine.[25]

Then again, perhaps to people in the future, the priorities of the ancient thinkers, of visionaries such as Asimov, and certainly of Digital Immigrants like myself, will seem as obsolete, as risible and as inappropriate for the mid-twenty-first-century agenda as the mind-set of the Victorians was to that of the twentieth century. Still, we cannot ignore the real world. However much digital technologies draw us into their pixelated, frenetic hall of mirrors, this world still serves as a parallel to the ever present, bulky, three-dimensional environment in which even the geekiest technophiles still have to exist.

MIND CHANGE BEYOND THE SCREEN

19

In Shakespeare's time the age of 40 was considered old. In jaw-dropping contrast, a baby born today has a one in three chance of living to be 100 years old, at least in our privileged developed world.[1] Diseases such as polio and diphtheria are now spectres of the past, with new advances in medicine raising our expectations of good health ever higher. Meanwhile whole new branches of medicine, such as gene therapy[2] and regenerative medicine,[3] are opening up wonderful possibilities.

How will the existence of these pioneering medical technologies impact on the twenty-first-century mind-set? Upcoming generations will probably take these advances for granted, just as we baby boomers never regarded polio or TB as serious health threats in the way that our parents had done. And further back, in the early decades of the twentieth century, most people would have accepted discomfort at best and pain at worst as the norm, whether from a rotting tooth, cataracts, joint pain or infection. Nagging minor ailments would have been a way of life, and the brain would have adapted, as is its evolutionary mandate, to whatever ongoing situation presented itself. But then again, if it was the default to be physically uncomfortable, people would not have been able to reflect so readily on themselves and their lives in the way that is possible today. Moreover the highly plausible likelihood of some capricious and indiscriminate illness suddenly wrecking your life, or that of someone close to you, would have overshadowed your daily existence. Nowadays, such fears are receding, and in the future biomedical technologies might further encourage the belief that good health is the birthright of the human species.

However, there is one disease, or rather range of diseases encompassing one particular dreaded symptom, which is more devastating than any other. If we are concerned about Mind Change, then we also need to think about mind loss not just through mindless screen activities, but more permanently through brain disease, *dementia*, literally a 'loss of mind'. As we've already seen, if the mind can be regarded as the personalisation of neuronal connections, then the gradual dismantling of those connections would be the physical process that underlies the confusion and loss of memory that characterises diseases such as Alzheimer's. By the middle of the twenty-first century, 2 million people in the United Kingdom alone will be suffering from Alzheimer's disease, which accounts for about 70 per cent of the instances of dementia.[4] Think about how many people love you in the world. For the ease of the ensuing maths, let's say ten; that means there will be 20 million lives turned upside down, about a third of the British population. It was estimated that, in 2010, 35.6 million people were living with dementia worldwide, with numbers expected to almost double every twenty years, to 65.7 million in 2030 and 115.4 million in 2050.[5] In a 2013 US study, dementia emerged as a more expensive economic burden to society than heart disease or cancer.[6]

Dementia is a singularly cruel affliction in its devastation of such a large number of lives: although heart disease, say, or cancer can be life-threatening diseases, the patient is still the person they ever were, still aware that they are your husband, wife, mother, father, brother, sister, and therefore still have a meaningful relationship with you even though they may be seriously ill. Not so with dementia.[7] As the disease takes its remorseless toll with the slow yet continuous loss of brain cells, so the carer can undergo indescribable distress, as an afflicted parent or spouse may deny any relationship with them, as well as a great sense of loss every bit as sharp as if their loved one had actually died or been killed. Carers often undergo all the signs and stages of bereavement but without the consideration and allowances society normally affords those suffering a personal loss. There is currently no effective treatment for the spectrum of neurodegenerative disorders characterised by dementia.[8]

But let's assume, and indeed hope, that sooner or later someone can come up with a breakthrough. Imagine going to your GP for a routine blood test, just as you might to check your cholesterol levels, and the doctor calmly looks you straight in the eye and says, 'Well there's good news and bad news. The bad news is that you have an elevated biomarker for neurodegeneration in your blood. This means, according to the chart here, that in your case, in about two years, certain symptoms will appear - short-term memory difficulties or problems finding the right word for an everyday object. However, the good news is that we now have an oral medication that will stop any more of your brain cells dying. So start taking these tablets today, and you'll need to take them every day from now on, but as long as you do you'll never experience any symptoms because we'll have stopped the neurodegenerative process in its tracks.' This scenario of a routine blood test and daily medication is a serious reality rather than a fantasy. The crucial bit of knowledge still needed is what makes specific cells in the brain embark on the remorseless cycle of cell death that we call neurodegeneration.[9] The identification of this basic mechanism underlying Alzheimer's and related diseases is the Holy Grail that will then lead to early, ideally presymptomatic diagnosis, and the all-important medication for stopping any more cells dying.

So let's assume that this wonderful prospect is realised and that dementia eventually joins those other diseases of the past that once were, or seemed to be, death sentences but are now containable thanks to new biomedical strategies. By the second half of this century, many of us will be looking forward to a long and healthy life. We will also look younger as a result of being healthier, and we will be able to reproduce for much longer, perhaps eventually for our entire lives. As the technology improves, it could even become the norm for a woman to have her eggs frozen when she is in her reproductive prime, to be thawed, perhaps even when she is post-menopausal, so that she can have a child, albeit by IVF. Let's take the scenario further to an extreme. Unpalatable and far-fetched though it might sound, it is not beyond reasonable scientific expectation that in the future anyone, regardless of gender, age or sexual orientation, could have a child with anyone else. If it were possible to extract the genetic material from any cell in the body and combine half of it with someone else's, there would be no further need of sperm or egg.[10] What would be required would be an evacuated egg and a womb, which could be supplied by different people. Therefore, in principle, a child could eventually have six parents: the genetic donors, the donor of the egg, the donor of the womb, and the two parents who raise the child. The main point is that, one way or another, you could be a new parent, caring for a small baby, throughout adulthood.

Finally, there's work. Traditionally, paid work was outside of the home and often entailed physical fitness. Now that the knowledge economy and the cyber world have made working from home possible, and physical strength and mobility no longer essential, there is a growing argument against having a fixed retirement age; indeed, this is now becoming the case in many organisations and societies. If we weight the case further with the idea that stimulation of the brain is much better for you than passive disengagement from the outside world, then work might even be sold to society as being good for the brain. Suffice it to say that if we have an increasingly ageing sector that is mentally agile and healthy, retiring on a pension to play golf or sudoku will be the exception rather than the norm.[11]

When you first meet someone, you most probably, perhaps subconsciously, allocate them to a particular generation on the grounds of (1) how healthy they seem, which will impact on (2) what they look like, (3) their reproductive status, and (4) whether or not they are still working. If the biotechnology-driven trends now in train play out to the logical conclusions outlined above in all these four crucial areas of our lives, such compartmentalisation into one generation or another will not be so easy.

So much for a changing outside world – but one grounded in a good old-fashioned 3-D physical reality as opposed to the 2-D cyber life. Yet now imagine if the two were to merge. What if the digital technologies previously confined to the screen could now affect the way you experience the real world? Nobody nowadays wants to just sit still, sheet-anchored to a clunky keyboard and a cumbersome separate screen. Already, smartphones are hand-held computers that happen to have a phone facility, and there is a burgeoning preference for mobile devices rather than laptops which offer all manner of apps and video games. The next generation of smartphones will be *context-aware*, exploiting the growing availability of embedded physical sensors and data exchange abilities. As a result, phones will start keeping track of your personal data, and will adapt to anticipate the information you need based on your intentions and location.[12] As well as monitoring you, the phone will monitor your surroundings: an x-ray device will reveal information about any place at which you point your phone.

Now imagine what life might be like if only the much valued, protective feature of texting was oral as the universal, default mode rather than written after all. You'd avoid the difficulty and embarrassment of interacting directly with someone, even on the phone, by recording messages which are then accessed as swiftly and easily as written text messages are today. You wouldn't even have to be literate. This new invention would create a firewall between you and the squalor of real, immediate human contact, along with the growing disaffection with laborious reading and writing skills. Welcome to the world of Google Glass.[13]

In appearance, Google Glass looks just like a pair of normal spectacles with a small black oblong at the top on one side, which shows you information and through which you can access the Internet via simple voice commands. Soon you will be able to record whatever you see, hands-free, and share it in real time with others. Moreover, you'll be able to get directions and find out anything about your current location, have your words translated and receive information about wherever you are, without even asking explicitly.

Until now, sessions of video gaming, social networking and surfing all come to an end at some stage. You can always turn the device off and walk back into the real world. Google Glass and other such technologies will make most of these activities possible every waking moment. Just as it's now commonplace to see passers-by with wires snaking into their ears talking loudly to themselves - people who would once have seemed plain loony - there's now the prospect that these same people will have morphed into a species with minimally notable rimless specs, living in the Google Glass 'augmented reality'.[14] The technology functions by *enhancing* one's current perception of reality and therefore should not be confused with virtual reality, which replaces the real world with a simulated one. Instead, augmented reality is an ongoing view of a physical real-world environment whose elements are 'augmented' by computer-generated sensory input such as sound, video, graphics or GPS data.[15] In this way, 'artificial' information about the environment and what it contains will be constantly overlaid on the real world.

The plan is for Google Glass to be launched in 2014, so you might even be reading these words right now with your own glasses ready to hand, and longing to put them back on. In any event, the implications of mass adoption of this, literally, new way of seeing the world are as diverse as they are profound. Predictions for wearable computing devices like Google Glass, or Apple's proposed iWatch, are that they will become the norm for most of us within five years, with 485 million annual device shipments by 2018.[16]

Once you're all wired up to an augmented reality, just imagine how terrible it will be to be on your own, how hard it would be to abandon this new dimension and just to switch everything off. Already, the majority of phone owners are emotionally attached to their smartphones. In one 2012 study of US phone users, 73 per cent said they felt 'panicked' when they misplaced their phones; 14 per cent said they felt 'desperate', while 7 per cent felt 'sick'.[17] In the United Kingdom, 66 per cent of phone users reported a fear of losing their phones, which now even has a name, 'nomophobia'.[18] If this type of attitude already exists, then it's breathtaking to contemplate the type of emotional attachment we might have to intensively integrated devices that provide more entertainment, faster answers and even more sanitised socialisation, all seamlessly.

It is hard to understand how the human brain will absorb such a tsunami after tsunami of information. With Google Glass, you will have the facts in your face without the need to try to work out the answer yourself. If search engines are already offering a faster and easier option than taking your brain through its otherwise necessary work-out, you'll now run the risk of becoming mentally flabby in a way that isn't even possible at the moment, with the proactive typing or touching still required for surfing on mobile phone or laptop. You will no longer be driving what you look at: the display will be driving you. The most immediate feature of Google Glass is its interactivity, with the emphasis on the constantly updated present moment. This constantly ongoing literal world will permanently trap users in an endless hyper-connected present. There will be nothing private to remember, nor anticipate.

Google Glass could also sound the final death knell, once and for all, for privacy. Andrew Keen, who describes himself as 'a British-American entrepreneur, professional sceptic and the author of *The Cult of the Amateur* and *Digital Vertigo*', has been quick to flag this issue: 'these glasses, a kind of digital surrogate for our eyes, are strange in a creepy, Hitchcockian, *Rear Window* sort of way. Or the same way that Big Brother's ubiquitous cameras were strange in George Orwell's *Nineteen Eighty-Four*. And in the same way that a future in which "promethean" data companies like Google rule the world now appears strange.' He continues:

> But *Google Glass* opens an entirely new front in the digital war against privacy. These spectacles, which have been specifically designed to record everything we see, represent a developmental leap in the history of data that is comparable to moving from the bicycle to the automobile. It is the sort of radical transformation that may actually end up completely destroying our individual privacy in the digital 21st century. When we put on these surveillance devices, we all become spies, or scrooglers, of everything and everyone around us. [19]

So here is a truly new type of future straight out of science fiction, where the currently nascent obsessions with monitoring the lives of others and broadcasting every moment of your own existence are now finally liberated completely from keyboard and touch screen. Instead you're truly interfaced directly with a digital device: it is an extension of your body. My concern is not only, as it is for Keen, with the ethics and legality of the possible loss of privacy, but also with what such a loss will mean to us as the independent individual entities we've all been until now.

The Google Glass wearer may well feel pressurised to opt into the hyper-connected cyber world all the time for fear of otherwise missing out or of being left behind. The trade-off for the resulting disclosure in what they are doing every minute of the day is, as it always has been, loss of privacy. Until now, privacy has been precious because it has been the other side of the coin to our identity. We see ourselves as individual entities, in contact with the outside world for sure, but at the same time always distinct from it. A sense of privacy keeps the two distinct. We don't disclose certain facts about ourselves, not because we're ashamed or embarrassed by them, but quite simply because we feel that not everyone should know what we are feeling or thinking. *By holding back, we are preserving a sense of self distinct from the outside.* Privacy provides the boundary: it stops us being transparent. This is why most of us draw the curtains at night to prevent strangers looking into our homes. We interact with the outside world, yes, but always in dialogue with our brain. You have secrets, memories and hopes to which no one else has automatic access, a *private* life as distinct from a professional *public* one, and multifaceted one-on-one friendships where you vary what and how much you confide in someone else. But, above all, you have that third type of life, an inner narrative, an ongoing thought process that is yours alone, a *secret* life – until now.

If you're now trapped in the present, constantly catering for and to the demands of the outside world, that inner narrative might be harder to sustain. Your secret sense of identity might become less and less important, less meaningful because it no longer has the all-important context, the inner conceptual framework where one event, object or person relates to another according to your own unique framework of connectivity. The *you* now externally constructed by Google Glass may not allow much time and opportunity for those internal memories, the secret reflections, to develop and blossom fully. But if privacy were needed only to protect this inner awareness, if there were no longer a secret life anyway, then privacy is meaningless. In contrast, if you define yourself by the degree of attention you receive from others, the loss of privacy is to be welcomed in order to permit a new type of identity: a connected one.

Let's go one step further. What if you were integrated with the outside world all the time? Perhaps this would lead to a kind of life where the second-hand thrill of self-reporting, posting and receiving feedback completely trumps the experience itself. Your identity is now paradoxically *online* moment to moment but essentially *offline* in that its importance lies in its reporting. The excitement you feel is generated not by the raw first-hand experience, but by the slightly delayed, indirect and continuous reaction of others.

If we live in a world where face-to-face interaction becomes uncomfortable, and where personal identity is increasingly defined by the approbation of a virtual audience, the most personal relationships might change as well. It will be a hard transition for an individual accustomed to an audience of 500 'friends' who share a collective flood of consciousness to switch to a one-on-one long-term relationship that is exclusive and completely private. Interestingly, two of the most technologically advanced collective/socially minded countries today (Japan and South Korea) are facing huge problems in declining birth rates.[20] Of course, any decline in interpersonal skills for conducting deep and meaningful partnerships doesn't imply a comparable decline in sex. It may be a relatively straightforward process to extrapolate from the sensory-laden sexual adventures of a video game to similar experiences in real life. Sex would now be more casual, less meaningful and highly transient.[21] On the other hand, perhaps even sex itself, involving as it does even at the level of the basic act, issues of self-confidence, trust and vulnerability, may also develop into an aversion. Once again, evidence from Japan and Korea indicates a lack of sex, or even of interest in dating, among the younger generations. Tellingly, nearly half of all Japanese women aged 16–24 are 'not interested in or despise sexual contact' and nearly a quarter of men feel the same way.[22]

Another ramification of the technologies on the move will be the abandonment of the sedentary cyber lifestyle. A trend we are already seeing is that a screen life may be leading to an under-stimulation not only of the sense of touch, but also of taste and smell, which in turn could be a factor leading to ever more indulgence in eating and drinking. The prevalence of obesity in England has more than tripled in the last 25 years. The latest Health Survey for England data show that, in England in 2010, 62.8 per cent of adults (aged 16 or over) were overweight or obese and 30.3 per cent of children (aged 2–15) were overweight or obese, with 26.1 per cent of all adults and 16 per cent of all children crossing the line into obesity.[23] While there are many and complex reasons to account for this alarming rise, including a poor diet of high sugar and high calories, and the availability and popularity of cheap but unhealthy junk food, another definite factor is insufficient physical exercise, which can be linked to a life spent sitting in front of a screen. Surely here the mobile technologies will offer at least the obvious advantage of a reduction in obesity through increased movement. But an alternative perspective is that the drive for stimulation of the senses of touch, taste and smell, for which the screen does not cater and which may be too risky to achieve in a close physical relationship, may be met by further eating which would then offset any potential reduction in obesity.

So, there you are weaving among the crowds but oblivious to them. At least one of your hands is holding something easily edible and in your ear there's an incessant stream, perhaps of music but more likely previously recorded oral text messages, or perhaps information as to where you can buy the latest goods that your personal traffic history has revealed are just right for you. Cyberspace is no longer limited to the two-dimensional screen, but extends to the three dimensions, thereby transforming reality. Your world is more like a bubble. Outside other people are passing by, but you are protected from them by the transparent shield encompassing your virtual space, your new dimension. You can touch and smell things, as well as hear and see them, but you are never alone, never independent. Always there's the voice in your ear, your best friend acting as intermediary and therefore distancing you from everyone and everything else as the same time as it paradoxically connects you.

Bear in mind that you will have no strong sense of who you are, no past or future, just the atomised moment. You'll be in a continuous state of high arousal, craving novelty and stimulation as each input is evaluated on purely (literally) sensational terms and thus soon palls. You will be very vulnerable to manipulation, both in how you see the world and how you react to it. Like a small child, you'll readily obey and conform, since you have adapted to expect the constant approval of others. So you'll be grateful for the voice since you may be a little confused. After all, you'll no longer have a conceptual framework for understanding what is happening around you. Added to this blurring of self with the outside world will be a blurring of fact and fiction. Since you are no longer just using your senses, but everything is aided and abetted by your cyber best friend, the boundary between reality and fantasy will be increasingly smudged, as is your now ambivalent generational status, thanks to advances in biotech. The three age-old distinctions that formed the basic constructs of our lives – the private inner self versus external others; fact versus fantasy; child versus parent versus grandparent – may for the first time start to erode.

An extreme and far-fetched scenario? Of course. Yet none of these future developments is a sci-fi fantasy on a par with time travel, say, or perpetual motion machines. *They are all starting to happen right now*. These and similar technologies will have enormous and far reaching implications for the long and healthy lives opening up to the next generations on how they will behave and, most importantly, how they will think. The critical issue facing us is one of transition: how do we not only make sense of, but flourish in, the current question-poor, answer-rich technological blizzard? For those born in the second half of the twentieth century, extraordinary advances in resources, health and culture have increased our life expectancy compared to those born a generation or so earlier. As a result, larger swathes of the developed world have more options, more privileges and more time in which to explore their full potential. So how can we ensure a future where our technology does not frustrate, but actively fosters, deep thinking, creativity and real fulfilment?

20 MAKING CONNECTIONS

Just think back to a decade ago, when there was neither Facebook nor Twitter, and when Wikipedia had fewer than 50,000 articles instead of the 4,500,000+ available today. And could anyone have predicted in the early 1980s that within just a few decades, 6 billion of the 7 billion people in the world would have access to a mobile phone, while only 4.5 billion have access to a working lavatory?[1] The past was indeed a foreign country, as L.P. Hartley observed: they did things differently there. So what will the new country of the mid-twenty-first century look like? More significantly, how would we like it to look?

Some sneer at any attempt to predict the future. The seeming arrogance of previous generations can appear ridiculous and naive with the glory of hindsight. One often quoted and apocryphal example is that of Thomas J. Watson, former head of IBM, who foretold that, at best, there might be a market for five computers in the world.[2] While this shows that accurate predictions of the long-term outreach and mass adoption of an invention is uncertain, carrying the basic scientific *concepts* envisioned a step further can raise interesting questions about the world we are creating. While we may not be able to predict consumer enthusiasm, we can contemplate where new technologies could lead if taken to the extreme. For example, George Orwell's *Nineteen Eighty-Four* envisaged a world of surveillance and manipulation of thought, where an omnipresent Big Brother ruled absolutely. This book remains a classic because it suggests eerie parallels to our world today.

'Might man become a mere parasite of machinery, an appendage of the reproductive system of huge and complicated engines which will successively usurp his activities.' You might think that this is a quote from Richard Watson, Nicholas Carr, Larry Rosen or any of the current thinkers cited in these pages. In fact, the quote is from a paper in 1923 by the brilliant biologist J.B.S. Haldane delivered to the Heretics Society at Cambridge University.[3] Haldane entitled his paper *Daedalus* after the father of Icarus in Greek mythology, referencing him as the creator of the labyrinth, home to the Minotaur. Haldane's purpose was to focus on the terrible consequences of our own cleverness.

Still reeling from the horrors of the mechanised butchery of the First World War, he explored the future of science, which he described as 'the free activity of man's divine faculties of reason and imagination'. Many of the predictions in *Daedalus* are not only spookily prescient but articulate fears that resonate with the worries we've explored in the previous chapters. Although he envisaged that chemistry would continue to transform life with explosives, dyes and drugs, it was in the application of biology that Haldane foresaw the big transformations. Looking hard at the nascent eugenics movement of the time, he wondered if this might result in 'eugenics officials' and 'marriage by numbers'.[4] These are prospects that may have come to pass with the advent of genetic screening and online dating, respectively.

Along with foreseeing our ability to cure many infectious diseases, Haldane predicted the development of a 'nitrogen-fixing' plant, which anticipated genetically modified food. Perhaps even more impressively, he actually prophesied the development of IVF and the complete dissociation of sex and reproduction with his concept of 'ectogenesis'. So troubling and fascinating were these ideas that they inspired Aldous Huxley to write his famous dystopian novel, *Brave New World*, which anticipated a

Central London Hatchery for babies and the worst consequences of genetic manipulation. Haldane was also uncannily on target in predicting hormone replacement therapy: 'This change seems to be due to a sudden failure of a definite chemical substance produced by the ovary. When we can isolate and synthesise this body we shall be able to prolong a woman's youth, and allow her to age as gradually as the average man.' Even mood-bending drugs were on his horizon: 'to control our passions by some more direct method than fasting or flagellation'. This idea was also appropriated by Huxley: the citizens of his dystopia routinely take 'soma' (Greek for 'body') pills and become immediately and unconditionally ecstatic.

Haldane listed in *Daedalus* the big questions of science that are still with us today: 'first of space and time', in our terminology the Big Bang; 'then of matter as such', for us the persistent quirkiness of quantum theory and the dream of nanoscience; 'then of (man's) own body and those of other living beings', surely the synthesis of different branches of biomedical science, along with the greatest question of how a brain can generate the subjective experience of consciousness; 'and finally the subjugation of the dark and evil elements in (mankind's) own soul': at a stretch, the big question of how we shall use this knowledge to work out the degree of biological determinism, the ultimate question of free will in the digital age.

Granted, we may not be able to predict the precise technologies and consumer products of the future, but it *is* possible, as Haldane, Huxley and Orwell have shown, to articulate the underlying scientific idea, observe its current manifestation and predict where such technology might be headed in its possible impact on human existence, society and mind-set. The preceding chapters have given snapshots of where we are at the moment, but the most important question of all is where these new developments could lead us if they continue unabated and unfocused. Sleep-walking into the unknown proudly unprepared and unreflective, and hoping for the best, is surely the most perilous option. By letting our imaginations unfold and by looking towards more distant horizons, we admittedly run the risk of straying into mere speculation, but proactive thinking allows us to take critical stock of our world today and puts us in the best possible position to devise a game plan for an optimal future.

Most typically, humanity has always had a love–hate relationship with 'progress', in equal measure delighted by the convenience a new invention brings and worried that it might just rob us of some quintessential quality. Some 400 years before the birth of Christ, Socrates was concerned that writing would destroy mental prowess, with eerily similar arguments to those we've explored here with respect to the Internet. He argued that writing

> will create forgetfulness in the learners' souls, because they will not use their memories; they will trust to the external written characters and not remember of themselves. The specific which you have discovered is an aid not to memory, but to reminiscence, and you give your disciples not truth, but only the semblance of truth; they will be hearers of many things and will have learned nothing; they will appear to be omniscient and will generally know nothing; they will be tiresome company, having the show of wisdom without the reality.[5]

These perennial worries were dramatically inflamed at the beginning of the twentieth century, when the mass adoption of automation became a recognisable force in our lives, along with the electricity that powered it. The underlying plot is perhaps obvious and readily seen as 'romantic': despite the benefits it brings, mechanisation will somehow rob us of all the less tangible but most basic features that we hold dear about our species, our emotions.

An early illustration of suspicion of the pitiless robot is captured in the 1927 German expressionistic film by Fritz Lang, *Metropolis*, which plays to the fear that technology will dehumanise us. In the film (a visual masterpiece combining Art Deco and industrial imagery) we see the horrors of mechanisation through the eyes of Freder, the spoilt son of the owner of the large industrial city, as he discovers how the workers are effectively treated as machines.

Another dim vision of the future is evoked in Edwin Muir's 1952 poem *The Horses*, which describes the immediate aftermath of a world destroyed by technology and how the survivors embrace the old traditional way of life. The speakers refuse to return to:

> That old bad world that swallowed its children quick
> At one great gulp . . .
> The tractors lie about our fields; at evening
> They look like dank sea-monsters couched and waiting.
> We leave them where they are and let them rust:
> 'They'll moulder away and be like other loam.'[6]

A third, and perhaps most familiar, fictional scenario where technology poses a threat to humanity is that of the robot HAL in Stanley Kubrick's 1968 classic, *2001: A Space Odyssey*. HAL is capable of speech, speech recognition, facial recognition, natural language processing, lip reading, art appreciation, reasoning, chess playing and, most unsettling of all, interpreting and reproducing emotions. When, eventually, the astronaut Dave gradually removes his modules one by one, HAL's consciousness slowly disintegrates in a way that seems painfully human, going all the way back to childhood songs:

> 'I'm afraid. I'm afraid, Dave. Dave, my mind is going. I can feel it. I can feel it. My mind is going. There is no question about it. I can feel it. I can feel it. I can feel it. I'm a . . . fraid. Good afternoon, gentlemen. I am a HAL 9000 computer. I became operational at the H.A.L. plant in Urbana, Illinois on the 12th of January 1992. My instructor was Mr. Langley, and he taught me to sing a song. If you'd like to hear it I can sing it for you.'

And in real life the reverse can also send a chill: not so much machines trying and failing to be human, but humans trying to escape the ravages of emotion by trying to be machines. In 1959 the child psychologist Bruno Bettelheim published an account of 'Joey: The Mechanical Boy', a case history of a very disturbed little boy who converted himself into a robotic-type entity as a defence against the world. At the end of the article, after successful treatment, Joey makes a banner for the Memorial Day parade with the words 'Feelings are more important than anything under the sun.' 'With this knowledge,' concludes Bettelheim, 'Joey entered the human condition.'[7]

But could this now be the very way we are headed into a mechanised future devoid of all the human qualities we cherish? If enthusiasm for technology has usually been tempered in previous generations with worries that it could be dehumanising, it seems that Digital Natives typically do not have such qualms. To summarise the preceding chapters: social networking sites could worsen communication skills and reduce interpersonal empathy; personal identities might be constructed externally and refined to perfection with the approbation of an audience as priority, an approach more suggestive of performance art than of robust personal growth; obsessive gaming could lead to greater recklessness, a shorter attention span and an increasingly aggressive disposition; heavy reliance on search engines and a preference for surfing, rather than researching, could result in agile mental processing at the expense of deep knowledge and understanding.

These snapshots may seem a bit unfair in that their brevity boils down complex differences across cultures, generations and individuals to simplistic caricatures, but they can be useful for us to reflect on where they might lead. Interestingly enough, the profile emerging from this list is *not* of a ruthless robot but of an all too human mind-set amplified in all its frailty and vulnerability, craving attention as unique individuals and, at the same time, paradoxically, needing desperately to belong and to be embraced within a collective identity and mind-set. No wonder Digital Natives don't have the age-old concerns about mechanisation robbing them of their humanity, when feelings and emotions are amplified and constantly held at a premium. So what exactly is problematic about a culture that taps into such deep-seated biological needs?

The difficulty arises when, thanks to the unprecedented nature of the digital lifestyle, these natural tendencies become exaggerated as never before. The first basic human need is to be acknowledged as special. We've seen how narcissism is increasing thanks to social networking sites. Indeed, only recently a word was reported as increasing in frequency 17,000 per cent since it was first used in 2002: 'selfie', the taking of your own picture.[8] Without the handbrake of body language that usually constrains interpersonal communication, and with access to a community larger than any group of real-life friends could ever be, the drive to be someone special could get out of hand, even become obsessive.

The cyber life obligingly offers an unprecedented level of status, measured for the first time ever not by possessions, talent or job. Without question, the excessive flaunting of such culturally acknowledged traditional signs of status can be pernicious and detrimental, as argued persuasively by Oliver James in *Affluenza*,[9] but status is now simply measured by how 'cool' one is, how many followers and friends one can attract in cyberspace, and not by one's talents or achievements. Add to the mix the unprecedented opportunity for concealing the real self, and the possibilities for an individual never to feel at ease in meaningful face-to-face relationships are even greater: the answer is to retreat instead into the safe world of the screen in the quest for approval, having done little to earn it, and indeed not even existing in the same way that people do in the real world.

The second natural human desire is to be accepted as one of the tribe, to be a small part of a larger collective identity. Once again, the screen world can cater to this need on an unprecedented scale in that you can join with others without the real-world effort or skills normally required to be in a choir or a football team, and even without the physical effort of going to a football match as a supporter. But while football teams and choirs generate an objective end product, and even purely fun hen or stag nights have a specific ending, an Internet community has the boundless time, numbers and lack of accountability to turn in on itself and develop a collective identity that may or may not be for the good. Bertrand Russell remarked in his reply to Haldane, *Icarus*, that 'men's collective passions are mainly evil',[10] while behaviour on 4chan has been likened by one of the site's devotees to that of the schoolboys turned savages in William Golding's *Lord of the Flies*. A recent example of a collectively negative cyber mind-set is the case of the woman threatened with rape on Twitter, not just by one deranged man, but by a whole following. Her crime? Suggesting that, since no woman is currently featured on any British banknote, the universally acclaimed author Jane Austen should grace the latest edition of the £10 note. Once the hue and cry was raised, a mob mentality took over.[11]

A final and third aspect of being human, which is nonetheless exaggerated in cyberspace, is our impulsivity, the desire for instant gratification. We've seen that a key attraction of video games is that actions do not have long-term consequences in that participants can, for example, obligingly become undead, but this is just the tip of the hedonistic iceberg. The sheer pleasure not just of playing games, but of watching YouTube or of disclosing everything about yourself on Facebook trumps any long-term implications. Pandering to this, indeed providing an excuse at the end of any account of reckless and often thoughtless actions, is the simple term 'YOLO' (You Only Live Once) appended to a description, for example, of outrageous or excessive behaviour as justification or explanation.[12] By focusing on the moment, by being the passive recipient of a sensational time, you've 'let yourself go'. The big difference between now and the recreational abandonment of previous generations is that now you can do it much more often, on demand – almost all of the time if you want to.

It just might be that the cyberculture enables you to satisfy all three basic drives more fully and more easily in combination than at any other time in human history.[13] Think back to the imagined scenario in Chapter 19 in relation to mobile technologies. Firstly, there is the strong sensory stimulation of the exciting audio-visual inputs that distracts you from thinking ahead or reflecting on the past (YOLO). Secondly, at the same time, you're going to be connected, increasingly hyper-connected, say by Google Glass, and therefore are always one of the tribe. Thirdly, you are constantly acting and reacting as a single player before your audience: you require constant feedback from them, paradoxically living a life indirectly, at second hand and offline, but in an online mode of constant read-out, which, if you're 'cool', brings you recognised status as someone special.

So, instead of the digital age being just like earlier technologies in posing the age-old threat of dehumanising us, of pandering to the perennial fear that scientific and technological progress will turn us all into zombie-like cyborgs, I suggest that the *exact opposite* is the case. Some of the very worst aspects of being all too human - the desire for status irrespective of talent, mob mentality and uncaring recklessness - are now being given free rein throughout the unchartered territory of cyberspace. What can or should we do?

In Douglas Adams's *Hitchhiker's Guide to the Galaxy*, a group of hyper-intelligent pan-dimensional beings demand to learn the 'Answer to the Ultimate Question of Life, the Universe, and Everything' from the supercomputer, Deep Thought. Deep Thought then needs 7.5 million years to compute and verify the answer, which turns out to be: 42. But note that even here the Ultimate Question itself is unspecified. Even though many have articulated comparably ambitious thoughts on the meaning of life through the centuries, they still amount to a tiny minority privileged with the leisure to continue to contemplate the significance of who they were and what they were doing, while still fewer have had the opportunity to express their reflection in literature, music, art or science. But we are now entering a time, potentially, of real opportunity to stretch ourselves *en masse* to our true potential, to ask big questions and to develop original and exciting solutions.

Before we get too carried away with the prospect of such a rosy future, we need first to decide what our priorities are, what kind of society we want and what kind of individual traits we value. To this end, the traditional print and broadcast media could get the ball rolling. After all, they can access the broadest range of different types of people, not just the overheated blogosphere; moreover, unlike those ranting in cyberspace, they have the legal obligation to be accurate. Debates and in-depth interviews with a range of specialists would ensure that everyone has access to as many views and insights as possible. Perhaps someone might even think of making a film. After all it was *An Inconvenient Truth* that woke up the silent majority of us to climate change.

Step 2 would be to take the pulse of societies around the world. It would be really helpful to have formal surveys of the views of stakeholders such as parents and teachers, psychiatrists and neuroscientists, as well as the Digital Natives themselves. As we saw back in Chapter 1, the kinds of surveys published so far have been mainly simple numbers, statistics and demographics. Now we need surveys that go beyond raw statistics to canvass the *opinions* of all sectors of society. Mind Change encompasses questions that could be every bit as complex and varied as climate change. But a big difference is that, while most people would prefer the planet not to overheat, the possible and desired outcomes from Mind Change may vary widely according to different tastes and predilections, so we need to look at the full spectrum of views out there.

The next key issue is the thorny one of evidence. While specific experiments in the lab can and have been designed to answer specific questions, further funds and resources are still needed from both the private and the public sectors for more basic lab-based research, epidemiology and psychological and sociological studies: this constitutes Step 3. As we've seen in the previous chapters, the scientific method can be tricky, with more questions being raised than answered by the findings. Much more clarification and detail, as well as simply more data, is needed. It is only by investigating on all levels, from the molecular to the societal, how the human brain is developing over months and years that we can assess the real long-term impact of the new technologies on how an individual thinks and feels. So the longer we wait before commissioning this type of work, the fewer the options and the narrower the scope we may have in the future. We need to start right now.

Further, there is no reason why the technologies discussed here shouldn't be part of the solution. Step 4 would be the invention of completely novel software that attempts to compensate and offset any possible deficiencies arising from excessive screen-based existence. [14] Of course, these four steps are not really steps at all, in that one is not consequent on the other. Rather, these very different strategies could all be deployed simultaneously.

We come back to H.L. Mencken's famous quote: 'For every complex question, there is a simple answer, and it's wrong.' Never has that been more true than for the complex situation generated by the all-pervasive cyberculture of the early twenty-first century. The snapshots captured in these pages which, taken together, constitute Mind Change, amount to a phenomenon whose enormity and impact is comparable to climate change. Both climate change and Mind Change are in our hands: in both cases, it's up to us to be proactive and to do something.

Yet there's a further, utterly crucial difference. For Mind Change there is no answer as such, because there is no clear question or goal. Unlike the unambiguous agenda set by climate change, Mind Change depends on what each of us wants and where we want to go as individuals. Moreover, while climate change involves at best damage limitation, the same is not true for Mind Change. With Mind Change, we have the opportunity to harness the powerful technologies it encompasses to positive and unprecedented, albeit as yet unspecified, ends. If we do indeed wish, in the late futurologist Jim Martin's words, not to ask what will happen in the future, but to proactively 'shape the future', then we should expect no quick Manichaean answers, no catchphrase nor sound bite, no easy collective doctrine. We cannot predict what wondrous new technologies will appear, nor even the developments and rate of advance of those already in train, such as mobile technologies. But we *can* emulate Haldane, Russell, Huxley and Orwell in discerning trends in how we humans adapt to that technology, and how it transforms the way we see the world.

The theme of connectivity might provide a good ending point for this current journey. We have seen that, by connecting neurons in a unique configuration, the physical brain is personalised and shaped into an individual mind. It is these connections, the personal association between specific objects and people, that give them a special significance. Our experiences over time give each and every one of us meaningful episodes that in turn contribute to a linear narrative, a personal story whose very unfolding echoes the thought process itself. But, as we become increasingly hyper-connected in the cyberspace dimension, might not our global environment begin to mirror the networking in our individual physical brain? Just as neuronal connectivity allows for the generation and evolving expression of a unique human mind, the hyper-connectivity of cyberspace could become a powerful agent for changing that mind both for good and for ill. Working out what this connectivity may mean, and what we decide to do about it, is surely the most far reaching and exciting challenge of our time.

NOTES

Chapter 1 A GLOBAL PHENOMENON

1 *Mind Change* poses and answers questions using empirical, epidemiological, testimonial and anecdotal evidence. While all of these styles of evidence are included in the book, the latter three are used mostly to develop questions, whereas significant weight is given to empirical research to answer them. It is not claimed that the research collated here is either a systematic or an exhaustive review of the literature. Studies published up to July 2013 were eligible for inclusion. Preference was given to meta-analyses and peer-reviewed journal publications in instances where the research field of the topic was established. Preference was given to higher-ranking journals where applicable. For areas of research that are brand new, and where few peer-reviewed publications yet exist, less robust literature such as conference proceedings and technical reports were consulted. It is important to remember that the scientific field lags behind technological advances, and that the speed at which the cyber world changes creates significant challenges for this area of research. Where possible, preference was given to studies that used the most current forms of technology. Throughout *Mind Change*, notes contain additional references and comments on various topics. Readers are strongly encouraged to source the papers discussed here and beyond, as *Mind Change* is designed as a current snapshot of the literature only.

2 An Australian digital publisher, Sound Alliance, recently commissioned a national survey of some 2,000 16- to 30-year-olds (Mahony, M. (2013, April 22). Sound Alliance reveals results of national youth research project [Weblog post]. Retrieved from http://thesoundalliance.net/blog/sound-alliance-reveals-results-of-national-youth-research-project). Among the participants, who typically had an undergraduate degree or at least secondary education to 18 years, 53% looked to social media, rather than TV or newspapers for their news, while 93% used Facebook daily even though 22% of them thought it a 'waste of time'. Meanwhile 89% of respondents said they had not yet found a passion or purpose in life but were still searching for it. Of course this continuing quest may well apply to most of humanity, but perhaps more telling is that it is 'FOMO' (the fear of missing out) and 'FONK' (the fear of

not knowing) that drives them constantly to check their phones for Facebook, Instagram, Twitter feeds, and new emails and texts. Stig Richards, the creative director at Sound Alliance, summed it up: 'They have so much information coming in through aggregation, principally Facebook, that they are working very hard to keep up with the constant flow . . . So they aren't able to attribute time and energy into specific passions, to the extent that maybe people could before social media was so pervasive . . . The youth of today are living their lives one mile wide and one inch deep' (Munro, K. (2013, April 20). Youth skim surface of life with constant use of social media. Retrieved from http://www.smh.com.au/digital-life/digital-life-news/youth-skim-surface-of-life-with-constant-use-of-social-media-20130419-2i5lr.html).

3 World Economic Forum (2013). *Global risks report 2013* (8th edn). Retrieved from http://reports.weforum.org/global-risks-2013/

4 Department for Work and Pensions (2011). *Differences in life expectancy between those aged 20, 50 and 80 - in 2011 and at birth*. Retrieved from http://statistics.dwp.gov.uk/asd/asd1/adhoc_analysis/2011/diffs_life_expectancy_20_50_80.pdf

5 World Health Organization (2008). *WHO report on the global tobacco epidemic, 2008: The MPOWER package*. Retrieved from www.who.int/tobacco/mpower/mpower_report_full_2008.pdf

6 Schwartz, M. (2008, August 3). The trolls among us. Retrieved from http://www.nytimes.com/2008/08/03/magazine/03trolls-t.html?pagewanted=all&_r=0

7 Nisbett, R.E., & Wilson, T.D. (1977). Telling more than we can know: Verbal reports on mental processes. *Psychological Review, 84*, 231–259. Reprinted in D.L. Hamilton (Ed.) (2005). *Social cognition: Key readings*. New York: Psychology.

8 Prensky, M. (2001). Digital Natives, Digital Immigrants: Part 1. *On the Horizon, 9*, 1–6. doi:10.1108/10748120110424816

9 Keen, A. (2007). *The cult of the amateur*. London: Nicholas Brealey, pp. xiii-xiv.

10 Selwyn, N. (2009). The Digital Native - myth and reality. *Aslib Proceedings: New Information Perspectives, 61*(4), 364–379. doi:10.1108/00012530910973776

11 Kidscape (2011). *Young people's cyber life survey*. Retrieved from http://www.kidscape.org.uk/media/79349/kidscape_cyber_life_survey_results_2011.pdf, p. 1.

12 Kang, C. (2013, December 10). Infant iPad seats raise concerns about screen time for babies. *Washington Post*. Retrieved from http://www.washingtonpost.com/business/economy/fisher-prices-infant-ipad-seat-

raises-concerns-about-baby-screen-time/2013/12/10/6ebba48e-61bb-11e3-94ad-004fefa61ee6_story.html

13 Grubb, B. (2013, December 16). iPad holder seat for babies sparks outcry. Retrieved from http://www.nydailynews.com/life-style/baby-seat-ipad-holder-sparks-outcry-article-1.1544673

14 The full debate on the impact of technology on the mind can be found at http://www.publications.parliament.uk/pa/ld201011/ldhansrd/text/111205-0002.htm

15 Rideout, V.J., Foehr, U.G., & Roberts, D.F. (2010). *Generation M*^{2}*: Media in the lives of 8- to 18-year-olds*. Retrieved from http://kaiserfamilyfoundation.wordpress.com/uncategorized/report/generation-m2-media-in-the-lives-of-8-to-18-year-olds/

16 Teilhard de Chardin, P. (1964). *The future of man*. London: Collins, p. 159.

17 Badoo (2012). Generation lonely? 39 percent of Americans spend more time socializing online than face-to-face. Retrieved from http://corp.badoo.com/he/entry/press/54/

Chapter 2 UNPRECEDENTED TIMES

1 Watson, R. (2010, October 21). Lecture to the Royal Society of Arts [Weblog post]. Retrieved from http://toptrends.nowandnext.com/2010/10/21/lecture-to-the-royal-society-of-arts/

2 By mid-2013, 56% of US adults owned a smartphone and 34% owned a tablet computer (Smith, A. (2013). *Smartphone ownership: 2013 update*. Retrieved from http://pewinternet.org/Reports/2013/Smartphone-Ownership-2013.aspx). In the same year 51% of US households possessed a dedicated video gaming console (Entertainment Software Association (2013). *The 2013 essential facts about the computer and video game industry*. Retrieved from www.theesa.com/facts/pdfs/ESA_EF_2013.pdf), while 39% of US adults in 2012 reported spending more time socialising online than they do in face-to-face time (Badoo (2012). Generation lonely? 39 percent of Americans spend more time socializing online than face-to-face. Retrieved from http://corp.badoo.com/he/entry/press/54/). The growth in screen use among youth is comparable. In 2012, 37% of all US youths aged 12–17 owned smartphones, up from just 23% in 2011 (Madden, M., Lenhart, A., Duggan, M., Cortesi, S., & Gasser, U. (2013). *Teens and technology 2013*. Retrieved from http://www.pewinternet.org/Reports/2013/Teens-and-Tech.aspx). Twenty-three per cent of the same group owned a tablet computer. As of 2013, the average US household with Internet connection now contains 5.7 Internet-connected devices, and they are often being used simultaneously (Internet

connected devices surpass half a billion in U.S. homes, according to the NPD group (2013). Retrieved from http://www.prweb.com/releases/2013/3/prweb10542447.htm). A survey from 2013 found that Digital Natives switch between digital devices in non-working hours every other minute (27 switches per hour) whereas Digital Immigrants switch 17 times per hour (Moses, L. (2013, March 31). What does that second screen mean for viewers and advertisers? Retrieved from http://www.adweek.com/news/technology/what-does-second-screen-mean-viewers-and-advertisers-148240).

3 In 2010 US youths aged 8–18 reported spending more than 7.5 hours a day in front of a screen watching TV, listening to music, surfing the Web, social networking and playing video games (Rideout, V.J., Foehr, U.G., & Roberts, D.F. (2010). *Generation M^2: Media in the lives of 8- to 18-year-olds*. Retrieved from http://kaiserfamilyfoundation.wordpress.com/uncategorized/report/generation-m2-media-in-the-lives-of-8-to-18-year-olds/). There was a significant jump from the group of 8–10-year-olds who spend an average of 7.51 hours in the cyber world to the older 11–14-year-olds, with an astonishing 11.53 hours, and 15–18-year-olds, with a similar 11.23 hours. While TV watching still outstrips Internet use on average in adults (Pew Internet (2012). *Trend data (adults)*. Retrieved from http://pewinternet.org/Trend-Data-%28Adults%29/Online-Activites-Total.aspx), in youths the rate of TV to Internet use for UK 12–15-year-olds in 2012 was evenly matched (17 hours on each activity per week) (Ofcom (2012). *Children and parents: Media use and attitudes report*. Retrieved from http://stakeholders.ofcom.org.uk/binaries/research/media-literacy/oct2012/main.pdf), whereas 2013 data for US youths and adults shows that TV use is declining, with the biggest differences seen in 12–24-year-olds, with their TV watching down three hours per week compared to 2011 data (Marketing Charts (2013). Are young people watching less TV?. Retrieved from http://www.marketingcharts.com/wp/television/are-young-people-watching-less-tv-24817/). Furthermore, in 2012, for the first time in twenty years, the number of homes in the US with TVs decreased (Stelter, B. (2011, May 3). Ownership of TV sets falls in U.S. *New York Times*. Retrieved from http://www.nytimes.com/2011/05/03/business/media/03television.html?_r=0&adxnnl=1&ref=business&adxnnlx=1396530217-uFZGwm27zoGqpRHf4pOFog). Poverty is one reason given for this effect, in addition to the increasing number of youths who have been raised on laptops becoming young adults and starting their own households, for whom the computer offers all that a TV can, and more.

4 IDC (2013). *Always connected: How smartphones and social keep us engaged*. Retrieved from https://fb-public.box.com/s/3iq5x6uwnqtq7ki4q8wk

5 Rapoza, K. (2013, February 18). One in five Americans work from home, numbers seen rising over 60%. *Forbes*. Retrieved from http://www.forbes.com/sites/kenrapoza/2013/02/18/one-in-five-americans-work-from-home-numbers-seen-rising-over-60/

6 Pew Internet, 2012 (see n. 3).

7 Office for National Statistics (2013). *Internet access – Households and individuals, 2012 part 2*. Retrieved from http://www.ons.gov.uk/ons/dcp171778_301822.pdf

8 Entertainment Software Association, 2013 (see n. 2).

9 Nielsen (2011). *State of the media: The social media report*. Retrieved from http://cn.nielsen.com/documents/Nielsen-Social-Media-Report_FINAL_090911.pdf

10 Bohannon, J. (2013, June 6). Online marriage is a happy marriage. Retrieved from http://www.smh.com.au/comment/online-marriage-is-a-happy-marriage-20130606-2ns0b.html

11 Moss, S. (2010). *Natural childhood*. Retrieved from http://www.nationaltrust.org.uk/document-1355766991839/

12 Frost, J.L. (2010). *A history of children's play and play environments: Toward a contemporary child-saving movement*. New York: Routledge, p. 2.

13 Palmer, S. (2007). *Toxic childhood: How the modern world is damaging our children and what we can do about it*. London: Orion. The list is: Climb a tree; 2. Roll down a really big hill; 3. Camp out in the wild; 4. Build a den; 5. Skim a stone; 6. Run around in the rain; 7. Fly a kite; 8. Catch a fish with a net; 9. Eat an apple straight from a tree; 10. Play conkers; 11. Throw some snow; 12. Hunt for treasure on the beach; 13. Make a mud pie; 14. Dam a stream; 15. Go sledging; 16. Bury someone in the sand; 17. Set up a snail race; 18. Balance on a fallen tree; 19. Swing on a rope swing; 20. Make a mud slide; 21. Eat blackberries growing in the wild; 22. Take a look inside a tree; 23. Visit an island; 24. Feel like you're flying in the wind; 25. Make a grass trumpet; 26. Hunt for fossils and bones; 27. Watch the sun wake up; 28. Climb a huge hill; 29. Get behind a waterfall; 30. Feed a bird from your hand; 31. Hunt for bugs; 32. Find some frogspawn; 33. Catch a butterfly in a net; 34. Track wild animals; 35. Discover what's in a pond; 36. Call an owl; 37. Check out the crazy creatures in a rock pool; 38. Bring up a butterfly; 39. Catch a crab; 40. Go on a nature walk at night; 41. Plant it, grow it, eat it; 42. Go wild swimming; 43. Go rafting; 44. Light a fire without matches; 45. Find your way with a map and compass; 46. Try bouldering; 47. Cook on a campfire; 48. Try abseiling; 49. Find a geocache; 50. Canoe down a river.

14 Moss, 2010 (see n.11).

15 Moss, 2010 (see n. 11), p. 6. Cited in Byron, T. (2008). Safer children in a digital world: the report of the Byron Review. Retrieved from http://media.education.gov.uk/assets/files/pdf/s/safer%20children%20in%20a%20digital%20world%20the%202008%20byron%20review.pdf?

Chapter 3 A CONTROVERSIAL ISSUE

1 Mencken, H. L. (1917, Nov 16). The Divine Afflatus, *New York Evening Mail*. Retrieved from: http://www.archive.org/stream/prejudices030184mbp/prejudices030184mbp_djvu.txt

2 Byron, T. (2008). *Safer children in a digital world: The report of the Byron Review*. Retrieved from http://media.education.gov.uk/assets/files/pdf/s/safer%20children%20in%20a%20digital%20world%20the%202008%20byron%20review.pdf

3 Howard-Jones, P. (2011). *The impact of digital technologies on human wellbeing: Evidence from the sciences of mind and brain*. Retrieved from http://www.nominettrust.org.uk/sites/default/files/NT%20SoA%20-%20The%20impact%20of%20digital%20technologies%20on%20human%20wellbeing.pdf, p. 5.

4 Rosen, L.D. (2012). *iDisorder: Understanding our obsession with technology and overcoming its hold on us*. New York: Macmillan.

5 Turkle, S. (2011). *Alone together: Why we expect more from technology and less from each other*. New York: Basic Books.

6 Batty, D. (2012, February 24). Twitter co-founder says users shouldn't spend hours tweeting. Retrieved from http://www.theguardian.com/technology/2012/feb/23/twitter-cofounder-biz-stone-tweeting-unhealthy

7 Scohnfeld, E. (2009, March 7). Eric Schmidt tells Charlie Rose Google is 'unlikely' to buy Twitter and wants to turn phones into TVs. Retrieved from http://techcrunch.com/2009/03/07/eric-schmidt-tells-charlie-rose-google-is-unlikely-to-buy-twitter-and-wants-to-turn-phones-into-tvs/

8 Michael Rich, associate professor at Harvard Medical School warns: 'Their [Digital Natives'] brains are rewarded not for staying on task but for jumping to the next thing. The worry is we're raising a generation of kids in front of screens whose brains are going to be wired differently' (Richtel, M. (2010, November 21). Growing up digital, wired for distraction. Retrieved from http://www.nytimes.com/2010/11/21/technology/21brain.html? pagewanted=all).

Jordan Grafman, chief of cognitive science at the National Institute of Neurological Disorders and Stroke, says: 'In general, technology can be good (for children's cognitive development) if it is used judiciously. But if it is used in a non-judicious fashion, it will shape the brain in what I think will actually be a negative way . . . a lot of what is appealing about all these types of instant communications is that they are fast. Fast is not equated with deliberation. So I think they can produce a tendency toward shallow thinking. It's not going to turn off the brain to thinking deeply and thoughtfully about things, but it is going to make that a little bit more difficult to do' (Whitman, A., & Goldberg, J. (2008). *Brain development in a hyper-tech world*. Retrieved from http://www.dana.org/media/detail.aspx?id=13126).

The American Academy of Pediatrics has suggested that two hours a day's computer use or more increases the probability of emotional, social and attention problems, a view borne out in findings reported recently by Angie Page and colleagues at Bristol University who concluded that children's screen viewing is related to psychological difficulties irrespective of physical activity. Participants were 1,013 children with an average age of almost 11 years, who self-reported average daily television hours and computer use on a questionnaire. Page found that greater television and computer use were related to higher psychological difficulty scores. Children who spent more than two hours per day watching television or using a computer – which would appear to be the majority of UK and US children – were at increased risk of high levels of psychological difficulties, and this risk increased if the children also failed to meet physical activity guidelines (Page, A.S., Cooper, A.R., Griew, P., & Jago, R. (2010). Children's screen viewing is related to psychological difficulties irrespective of physical activity. *Pediatrics, 126*(5), e1011–e1017. doi:10.1542/peds.2010-1154).

Michael Friedlander, head of neuroscience at Baylor College of Medicine has said: 'If a child is doing homework while on the computer engaged in chat rooms, or listening to iTunes and so forth, I do think there is a risk that there will never be enough depth and time spent on any one component to go as deep or as far as you might have. You might satisfactorily get all these things done, but the quality of the work or of the communication may not reach the level that it could have had it been given one's full attention. There's a risk of being a mile wide and an inch deep' (Whitman & Goldberg, 2008: see above).

9 Bavelier, D., Green, C.S., Han, D.H., Renshaw, P.F., Merzenich, M.M., & Gentile, D.A. (2011). Brains on video games. *Nature Reviews Neuroscience, 12*(12), 763–768. doi:10.1038/nrn3135, p. 766.

10 Pearson UK (2012). New 'Enjoy Reading' campaign and support materials launched to help parents and teachers switch children on to reading for life. Retrieved from http://uk.pearson.com/home/news/2012/october/new-_enjoy-reading-campaign-and-support-materials-launched-to-he.html

11 Purcell, K., Rainie, L., Heaps, A., Buchanan, J., Friedrich, L., Jacklin, A., . . . Zickuhr, K. (2012). *How teens do research in the digital world*. Retrieved from http://www.pewinternet.org/Reports/2012/Student-Research.aspx, p. 2.

12 Those signing this statement were a diverse bunch, from household names like best-selling children's author Philip Pullman, to influential psychologist Oliver James, as well as the founder of Kids Company, the charity for the homeless young, Camila Batmanghelidjh. The diversity of sectors represented certainly revealed the sweep of issues involved – after all, lifestyle is hardly a single activity or issue that is the monopoly of any one narrow field of expertise (Erosion of childhood: Letter with full list of signatories (2011, September 23). Retrieved from http://www.telegraph.co.uk/education/educationnews/8784996/Erosion-of-childhood-letter-with-full-list-of-signatories.html).

13 Anderson, J.Q., & Rainie, L. (2012). *Millennials will benefit and suffer due to their hyperconnected lives.* Retrieved from http://www.elon.edu/docs/e-web/predictions/expertsurveys/2012survey/PIP_Future_of_Internet_2012_Gen_Always_ON.pdf

14 Vinter, P. (2012, September 1). Zadie Smith pays tribute to computer software that BLOCKS internet sites allowing her to write new book without distractions. Retrieved from http://www.dailymail.co.uk/news/article-2196718/Zadie-Smith-pays-tribute-software-BLOCKS-internet-sites-allowing-write-new-book-distractions.htm

15 World Economic Forum (2013). *Global risks report 2013* (8th ed.). Retrieved from http://reports.weforum.org/global-risks-2013/, pp. 23–24. The report states: 'The Internet remains an uncharted, fast-evolving territory. Current generations are able to communicate and share information instantaneously and at a scale larger than ever before. Social media increasingly allows information to spread around the world at breakneck speed. While the benefits of this are obvious and well documented, our hyperconnected world could also enable the rapid viral spread of information that is either intentionally or unintentionally misleading or provocative, with serious consequences . . . It is just as conceivable that the offending content's original author might not even be aware of its misuse or misrepresentation by others on the Internet, or that it was triggered by an error in translation from one language to another. We can think of such a scenario as an example of a digital wildfire.' Such an example occurred in 2012, when someone impersonating a Russian parliamentarian tweeted that Syrian president Bashar al-Assad had been killed or injured. Crude oil prices rose in response before the tweet was revealed to be a hoax (Howell, L. (2013, January 8). Only you can prevent digital wildfires. Retrieved from http://www.nytimes.com/2013/01/09/opinion/only-you-can-prevent-digital-wildfires.html?_r=0).

16 Greenfield, S. (2009, February 12). Children: Social networking sites. UK

Parliament, House of Lords. Retrieved from http://www.publications.parliament.uk/pa/ld200809/ldhansrd/text/90212-0010.htm

17 Ivo Quartiroli in *The Digitally Divided Self* (http://www.amazon.com/The-Digitally-Divided-Self-Relinquishing/dp/8897233007) claims that 'statements such as "it is not scientific" or "we don't have enough data" are typical defences that technologically orientated people use to counteract criticism or expressions of concern' (Chapter 1 Section on 'Technology can't be challenged')

18 A paradigm is, in Kuhn's own words, 'what members of a scientific community, and they alone, share'. According to Kuhn, a paradigm is more than just a single simple theory but the entire world-view within which it exists. Needless to say, such a view may encompass uncomfortable anomalies, facts and findings that just don't fit, but that are for a while brushed aside because of the intellectual discomfort they bring and also because of the explanatory void that might consequently yawn open. But as such anomalies, inevitably those from experimental data, start to accumulate, so some scientists may begin to doubt the whole perspective, not least because they have a more attractive new alternative that can encompass and account for all the erstwhile uncomfortable findings. A 'crisis' ensues in the respective discipline so that eventually, as in France in 1789 and in Russia a little over a century later, a revolution takes place, a struggle between the old order and a new. Comparing such sweeping ideological struggles with academic wrangling might seem far-fetched, but it actually isn't that way off the mark. Bear in mind that what Kuhn was describing were completely different ways of seeing things, so radical that they would influence the way scientists, and therefore eventually everyone, saw the world for generations to come (Kuhn, T.S. (1977). *The essential tension: Selected studies in scientific tradition and change*. Chicago and London: University of Chicago Press, p. 294).

19 Beattie-Moss, M. (2008, February 4). Gut instincts: A profile of Nobel laureate Barry Marshall. Retrieved from http://news.psu.edu/story/140921/2008/02/04/research/gut-instincts-profile-nobel-laureate-barry-marshall

20 The difficulty with the attitude that we cannot even talk about the prospects and implications for humanity of cyberculture until there is conclusive 'scientific evidence' that it is either 'good' or 'bad' is well articulated by Dr Aric Sigman, of the Royal Society of Medicine: 'It strikes me as a terrible shame that our society requires photos of brains shrinking in order to take seriously the common-sense assumption that long hours in front of screens is not good for our children's health' (Harris, S. (2011, July 18). Too much Internet use 'can damage teenagers' brains'. Retrieved from http://www.

dailymail.co.uk/sciencetech/article-2015196/Too-internet-use-damage-teenagers-brains.html).

21 Statistical analysis is conducted on research findings to determine whether the results of the study are likely to apply to the whole population in which the researchers are interested, beyond just the sample obtained for the study. When results of a study are statistically significant, it means that the findings, often in the form of a relationship between variables or a difference between groups of participants, are not likely to be due to chance. The conclusions drawn from statistical methods are sensitive to the particulars of the study design, including the selection of variables and the size of the sample examined. For example, a large sample yields high statistical power, which means that relatively small differences may be detected as statistically significant. Researchers must use their understanding of statistics and the subject matter to determine which of these findings are important as opposed to spurious. There is no magic rule regarding what size sample or number of participants is 'large enough', and this choice in experimental design is somewhat arbitrary. Statistics do not provide an answer and researchers must make a choice based on their understanding of the variables of interest and the effect sizes they might anticipate, i.e. whether or not potential differences will be very dramatic or just marginal. Additionally, statistical analysis cannot account for poor study design, such as how the participants were recruited or how the data collection process occurred. This means that if aspects of the study design were biased, this will increase the likelihood of finding a significant result. Moreover, researchers themselves can manipulate statistical analysis and the subsequent interpretation of results, as publication in a journal can often depend on finding a statistically significant result. Where appropriate, *Mind Change* will comment on significant study findings that may be biased in some way. However, it is beyond the scope of this book to go into this in too extensive detail.

Chapter 4 A MULTIFACETED PHENOMENON

1 Baede, A.P.M. (n.d.). Working Group I: The scientific basis. *Intergovernmental panel on climate change*. Retrieved from http://www.ipcc.ch/ipccreports/tar/wg1/518.htm

2 Witness the popularity of sites like Klout, which gives you a score for your importance in the cyber world. Interestingly enough 'coolness' is now democratised: wealth, gender and age are no longer relevant, but then neither is anything special that you may have done. So the interesting and unprecedented feature of being cool and famous on social networking sites

is that such content need have nothing to do with your particular prowess in any area, and indeed nothing to do with the 'real' you at all. It is important to bear in mind that the interaction between the brain and the environment is a two-way dialogue: just as vital to how we view and use the latest technology is the impact that an environment dominated by compulsive engagement with social networking sites will have on shaping our relationships and our view of our own identity.

3 Lenhart, A., Madden, M., Smith, A., Purcell, K., Zickuhr, K., & Rainie, L. (2011). *Teens, kindness and cruelty on social network sites*. Retrieved from http://pewinternet.org/Reports/2011/Teens-and-social-media.aspx, p. 28.

4 Konrath, S.H., O'Brien, E.H., & Hsing, C. (2011). Changes in dispositional empathy in American college students over time: A meta-analysis. *Personality and Social Psychology Review, 15*(2), 180–198. doi:10.1177/1088868310377395

5 PR Newswire (2013). Facebook reports first quarter 2013 result. Retrieved from http://www.prnewswire.com/news-releases/205652631.html

6 Internet World Stats (2012). Facebook users in the world: Facebook usage and Facebook growth statistics by world geographic regions. Retrieved from http://www.internetworldstats.com/facebook.htm

7 Twitter (2012, December 18). There are now more than 200M monthly active @twitter users. You are the pulse of the planet. We're grateful for your ongoing support! [Twitter post]. Retrieved from https://twitter.com/twitter/status/281051652235087872

8 Ofcom (2013). *Adults' media use and attitudes report*. Retrieved from http://stakeholders.ofcom.org.uk/binaries/research/media-literacy/adult-media-lit-13/2013_Adult_ML_Tracker.pdf

9 Madden, M., Lenhart, A., Duggan, M., Cortesi, S., & Gasser, U. (2013). *Teens and technology 2013*. Retrieved from http://pewinternet.org/~/media//Files/Reports/2013/PIP_TeensandTechnology2013.pdf

10 Arbitron Inc. and Edison Research (2013). *The infinite dial 2013: Navigating digital platforms*. Retrieved from http://www.edisonresearch.com/wp-content/uploads/2013/04/Edison_Research_Arbitron_Infinite_Dial_2013.pdf

11 Smith, C. (2013). By the numbers: 32 amazing Facebook stats [Weblog post, updated June 2013]. Retrieved from http://expandedramblings.com/index.php/by-the-numbers-17-amazing-facebook-stats/

12 Arbitron Inc. and Edison Research, 2013 (see n. 10).

13 Hampton, K.N., Goulet, L.S., Rainie, L., & Purcell, K. (2011). *Social networking sites and our lives*. Retrieved from http://pewinternet.org/Reports/2011/Technology-and-social-networks.aspx

14 Hampton et al., 2011 (see n. 13).

15 McAfee (2010). *The secret online lives of teens*. Retrieved from http://us.mcafee.com/en-us/local/docs/lives_of_teens.pdf

16 Government Office for Science, London (2013). *Foresight future identities: Final project report*. Retrieved from http://www.bis.gov.uk/foresight/our-work/policy-futures/identity

17 Gentile, D.A., & Anderson, C.A. (2003). Violent video games: The newest media violence hazard. In D.A. Gentile (Ed.), *Media violence and children: A complete guide for parents and professionals* (Vol. 22). Retrieved from www.psychology.iastate.edu/faculty/caa/abstracts/2000-2004/03GA.pdf

18 By 2005, a national study commissioned by UK Games Research of individuals aged between 6 and 65 showed a clear age factor slanted towards youth: over 80% of those under the age of 24 years were playing video games (Pratchett, R. (2005). *Gamers in the UK: Digital play, digital lifestyles*. Retrieved from http://crystaltips.typepad.com/wonderland/files/bbc_uk_games_research_2005.pdf). In 2008, 97% of American teens were playing video games (Lenhart, A., Jones, S., & Macgill, A.R. (2008). *Adults and video games*. Retrieved from http://www.pewinternet.org/Reports/2008/Adults-and-Video-Games/1-Data-Memo.aspx), while within a few years (2011) in Australia the number was similar, 94% (Digital Australia (2011). *Key findings*. Retrieved from http://www.igea.net/wp-content/uploads/2011/10/DA12KeyFindings.pdf). Although these statistics come from different countries, the English-speaking developed world cultures are surely similar enough for a comparable trend and trajectory to be discerned.

19 Homer, B.D., Hayward, E.O., Frye, J., & Plass, J.L. (2012). Gender and player characteristics in video game play of preadolescents. *Computers in Human Behavior, 28*(5), 1782–1789. doi:10.1016/j.chb.2012.04.018

20 Rideout, V.J., Foehr, U.G., & Roberts, D.F. (2010). *Generation M^2: Media in the lives of 8- to 18-year-olds*. Retrieved from http://kaiserfamilyfoundation.wordpress.com/uncategorized/report/generation-m2-media-in-the-lives-of-8-to-18-year-olds/

21 Cummings, H.M., & Vandewater, E.A. (2007). Relation of adolescent video game play to time spent in other activities. *Archives of Pediatrics & Adolescent Medicine, 161*(7), 684. doi:10.1001/archpedi.161.7.684

22 Cooper, R. (2012, February 3). Gamer lies dead in internet café for 9 hours before anyone notices. Retrieved from http://www.dailymail.co.uk/news/article-2096128/Gamer-lies-dead-Taiwan-internet-cafe-9-HOURS-notices.html

23 Diablo 3 death: Teen dies after playing game for 40 hours straight. (2012, July 18). Retrieved from http://www.huffingtonpost.com/2012/07/18/diablo-3-death-chuang-taiwan-_n_1683036.html

[24] Tran, M. (2010, March 6). Girl starved to death while parents raised virtual child in online game. Retrieved from http://www.theguardian.com/world/2010/mar/05/korean-girl-starved-online-game

[25] Carter, H. (2010, November 19). Man jailed for murder of girlfriend's toddler. Retrieved from http://www.theguardian.com/uk/2010/nov/18/man-jailed-murder-girlfriends-toddler

[26] Video game fanatic hunts down and stabs rival player who killed character online. (2010, May 27). Retrieved from http://www.telegraph.co.uk/news/worldnews/europe/france/7771505/Video-game-fanatic-hunts-down-and-stabs-rival-player-who-killed-character-online.html

[27] Anderson, C.A., Shibuya, A., Ihori, N., Swing, E.L., Bushman, B.J., Sakamoto, A., . . . & Saleem, M. (2010). Violent video game effects on aggression, empathy, and prosocial behavior in Eastern and Western countries: A meta-analytic review. *Psychological Bulletin, 136*(2), 151. doi:10.1037/a0018251

[28] Kühn, S., Romanowski, A., Schilling, C., Lorenz, R., Mörsen, C., Seiferth, N., . . . & Gallinat, J. (2011). The neural basis of video gaming. *Translational Psychiatry, 1*(11), e53. doi:10.1038/tp.2011.53

[29] Sullivan, D. (2013, February 11). Google still world's most popular search engine by far, but share of unique searchers dips slightly. Retrieved from http://searchengineland.com/google-worlds-most-popular-search-engine-148089

[30] Mangen, A., Walgermo, B.R., & Brønnick, K. (2013). Reading linear texts on paper versus computer screen: Effects on reading comprehension. *International Journal of Educational Research, 58*, 61–68. doi:10.1016/j.ijer.2012.12.002

Chapter 5 HOW THE BRAIN WORKS

[1] The brainstem: the extension of the spinal cord that forms the inner core of the brain around which other structures are elaborated. This is functionally the most basic part of the brain, shared even with reptiles, which mediates respiration, sleep-wake cycles and arousal. Of many possible reviews, see: Siegel, J. (2004). Brain mechanisms that control sleep and waking. *Naturwissenschaften, 91*(8), 355-65; Jones, B.E. (2003). Arousal systems. *Front Biosci, 8*, 438-51.

[2] The cerebellum: nicknamed the 'autopilot' of the brain and mediating fine-tuned sensorimotor coordination. For a recent review, see Reeber, S.L., Otis, T.S., Sillitoe, R.V. (2013). New roles for the cerebellum in health and disease. *Front Syst Neurosci*, 7:83.

3 The cortex: unlike the brainstem and the cerebellum, this is a newer, indeed the newest, brain region in terms of evolution. It is organised in repeating modular circuits like a cookie cutter. Some areas are related to a single sense, while others serve more 'cognitive' functions like learning and memory and are referred to by the umbrella term 'association cortex'. (Shipp, S. (2007). Structure and function of the cerebral cortex. *Curr Biol*, 17, 443-9.)

4 An 'action potential': there is a sharp change in the potential difference (voltage) across the cell membrane caused by positively charged sodium ions rushing into the cell, making it 'depolarised' – a situation that then triggers the efflux of erstwhile internal, positively charged potassium ions, that then makes the potential difference more negative again. For more detailed descriptions see Purves et al. (see n. 6 below).

5 The 'nerve terminal': this is the end of the 'axon', the long process emanating from the cell body along which the action potential is propagated at several hundred miles per hour. Once the 'blip' invades the terminal, the change in voltage triggers the emptying of the contents of small packets (vesicles), namely the transmitter into the synaptic cleft. For more detailed descriptions see Purves et al. (see n. 6 below).

6 See Purves, D., Augustine, G.J., Fitzpatrick, D., Hall, W.C., LaMantia, A.S., & White, L.E. (Eds.) (2012). *Neuroscience* (5th ed.). Sunderland, MA: Sinauer.

7 For example, it could be the case that the input from one neuron 'A' caused a small depolarisation, but not large enough to bring the voltage of the cell to the threshold for being able to generate a full-blown action potential. Now imagine that, during this time period whilst the voltage was raised, another input 'B' arrived that also on its own would normally have caused only a subthreshold depolarisation: because A + B could summate to threshold within this time window, i.e. the combined excitation produced by A and B will now be sufficient for an action potential to be generated, whilst either on their own would have been too weak.

8 'Modulation': a term used when a transmitter or other bioactive compound has no effect on its own but enhances or diminishes the action of another signalling molecule.

9 The most familiar and easiest way of thinking about brain organisation is as a hierarchy, similar to a chain of command with the boss at the top of a pyramid-like structure. Indeed this concept fitted well with scientific findings in the 1960s when two physiologists, David Hubel and Torsten Weisel, made a breakthrough, Nobel Prize-winning discovery. Hubel and Weisel were working on the visual system and monitoring the activity of single brain cells in the different brain regions which processed inputs from the retina, and then further on into the depths of the brain. Their remarkable finding was that, as they went deeper into the brain, further away from

the initial processing of the retina, the cells seemed to become fussier in terms of what turned them on, literally. Initially, the sight of any old blob would excite a neuron, but further up the chain of command it might have to be a line, and then only a line in a certain orientation, and then a line in a certain orientation but only moving in a specific direction (Hubel, D.H., & Wiesel, T.N. (1962). Receptive fields, binocular interaction and functional architecture in the cat's visual cortex. *Journal of Physiology, 160*(1), 106–154. Retrieved from http://www.ncbi.nlm.nih.gov/pmc/articles/PMC1359523/pdf/jphysiol01247-0121.pdf). It was certainly an amazing discovery that a single brain cell could have such an individual signature, but it led to some strange extrapolations. You can see how Hubel and Weisel's discovery easily led to the notion that the further up the hierarchy of the brain you went, the fussier the cell would become, eventually responding only to very sophisticated images, such as a face or even a specific face. The terminology of the time liked to refer to a hypothetical 'grandmother cell' which, as its name suggested, would only respond to the sight of your grandmother as the ultimate stage in the organisation. Although, much more recently, Christof Koch and his team of researchers at Caltech recorded cells in the brains of conscious neurosurgical patients specifically responding, for example, to pictures of Halle Berry (Quiroga, R.Q., Reddy, L., Kreiman, G., Koch, C., & Fried, I. (2005). Invariant visual representation by single neurons in the human brain. *Nature, 435*(7045), 1102–1107. doi:10.1038/nature03687), the idea that a single 'Berry cell' or a grandmother cell could effectively be 'the boss' has been largely discredited, if only by simple logic. If you never had a grandmother, a cell would be wasted; or if you did have a grandmother but your grandmother cell died, as many neurons do daily, then you'd never recognise your grandmother ever again! Just as a brain region can't be an independent 'centre', it is even less likely that a single brain cell can be a final destination – and it certainly can't be the ultimate boss. What would 'the boss' do subsequently? After all, there would be no one further to instruct.

10 Kolb, B. (2009). Brain and behavioural plasticity in the developing brain: Neuroscience and public policy. *Paediatrics & Child Health, 14*(10), 651–652. Retrieved from http://www.ncbi.nlm.nih.gov/pmc/articles/PMC2807801/

Chapter 6 HOW THE BRAIN CHANGES

1 Maguire, E.A., Gadian, D.G., Johnsrude, I.S., Good, C.D., Ashburner, J., Frackowiak, R.S., & Frith, C.D. (2000). Navigation-related structural change in the hippocampi of taxi drivers. *Proceedings of the National Academy of Sciences, 97*(8), 4398–4403. doi:10.1073/pnas.070039597

2 The octopus, who featured in classic memory experiments in the 1960s, more recently received much attention when one of their number, 'Paul', showed apparently prescient powers in being able to predict the outcomes of various matches in the 2011 Football World Cup! See also Young, J. Z. (1983). The distributed tactile memory system of Octopus. *Proceedings of the Royal Society of London. Series B, Biological Sciences,* 135–176.

3 Abrams, T.W., & Kandel, E.R. (1988). Is contiguity detection in classical conditioning a system or a cellular property? Learning in *Aplysia* suggests a possible molecular site. *Trends in Neurosciences, 11*(4), 128–135. doi: 10.1016/0166-2236(88)90137-3

4 Doidge, N. (2007). *The brain that changes itself: Stories of personal triumph from the frontiers of brain science.* Penguin: New York, p. 315.

5 Rosenzweig, M.R. (1996). Aspects of the search for neural mechanisms of memory. *Annual Review of Psychology, 47*(1), 1–32. doi:10.1146/annurev.psych.47.1.1

6 White House, Office of the Press Secretary (1997, April 17). Remarks from the Conference. Retrieved from http://clinton4.nara.gov/WH/New/ECDC/Remarks.html

7 Bavelier, D., & Neville, H. J. (2002). Cross-modal plasticity: Where and how? *Nature Reviews Neuroscience, 3*(6), 443–452. doi:10.1038/nrn848

8 Derbyshire, D. (2011, March 6). The boy whose damaged brain 'rewired' itself. Retrieved from http://www.telegraph.co.uk/news/uknews/1325183/The-boy-whose-damaged-brain-rewired-itself.html

9 Lewis, T. L., & Maurer, D. (2005). Multiple sensitive periods in human visual development: Evidence from visually deprived children. *Developmental Psychobiology, 46*(3), 163–183. doi:10.1002/dev.20055

10 Neville, H.J., & Lawson, D. (1987). Attention to central and peripheral visual space in a movement detection task: An event-related potential and behavioral study. II. Congenitally deaf adults. *Brain Research, 405*(2), 268–283. doi:10.1016/0006-8993(87)90296-4

11 Kleim, J.A. (2011). Neural plasticity and neurorehabilitation: Teaching the new brain old tricks. *Journal of Communication Disorders, 44*(5), 521–528. doi:10.1016/j.jcomdis.2011.04.006

12 Schlaug, G., Marchina, S., & Norton, A. (2009). Evidence for plasticity in white-matter tracts of patients with chronic Broca's aphasia undergoing intense intonation-based speech therapy. *Annals of the New York Academy of Sciences, 1169*(1), 385–394. doi:10.1111/j.1749-6632.2009.04587.x

13 Nudo, R.J. (2011). Neural bases of recovery after brain injury. *Journal of Communication Disorders, 44*(5), 515–520. doi:10.1016/j.jcomdis.2011.04.004

14 Where did such a bizarre idea come from? One suggestion is that the great psychologist William James was working with an accelerated programme of learning for a child prodigy in the 1890s, and generalised from this exceptional case that most people only realised a fraction of their true potential. Maybe so, but it's not because 90% of our brains are not working. This strangely precise figure has been attributed to the American writer Lowell Thomas who, in 1936, tried to summarise James's work. Perhaps he based the estimate on the percentage of brain functions that could be mapped at the time in terms of brain location. While Thomas may not have been party to our current knowledge of the brain, 90/10 is a ratio that coincidentally still features. For example, the key nerve cells of the brain, neurons, are outnumbered ten to one by 'glial' cells (from the Greek for 'glue'), which take care of the basic cerebral housekeeping and ensure a healthy and nurturing brain environment. Moreover, at any one time, only about 10% of neurons are spontaneously active. However, this isn't to say that the remainder are dead or inactive, any more than a football player standing alert but briefly stationary on the pitch would be regarded as not participating in the game.

15 Jenkins, W.M., Merzenich, M.M., Ochs, M.T., Allard, T., & Guic-Robles, E. (1990). Functional reorganization of primary somatosensory cortex in adult owl monkeys after behaviorally controlled tactile stimulation. *Journal of Neurophysiology, 63*(1), 82–104. Retrieved from http://jn.physiology.org/content/63/1/82.full.pdf+html

16 Elbert, T., Pantev, C., Wienbruch, C., Rockstroh, B., & Taub, E. (1995). Increased cortical representation of the fingers of the left hand in string players. *Science, 270*(5234), 305–307. doi:10.1126/science.270.5234.305

17 Gaser, C., & Schlaug, G. (2003). Brain structures differ between musicians and non-musicians. *Journal of Neuroscience, 23*(27), 9240–9245. Retrieved from http://www.jneurosci.org/content/23/27/9240.full.pdf+html

18 Aydin, K., Ucar, A., Oguz, K.K., Okur, O.O., Agayev, A., Unal, Z., . . . & Ozturk, C. (2007). Increased gray matter density in the parietal cortex of mathematicians: A voxel-based morphometry study. *American Journal of Neuroradiology, 28*(10), 1859–1864. doi:10.3174/ajnr.A0696

19 Park, I.S., Lee, K.J., Han, J.W., Lee, N.J., Lee, W.T., & Park, K.A. (2009). Experience-dependent plasticity of cerebellar vermis in basketball players. *The Cerebellum, 8*(3), 334–339. doi:10.1007/s12311-009-0100-1

20 Jäncke, L., Koeneke, S., Hoppe, A., Rominger, C., & Hänggi, J. (2009). The architecture of the golfer's brain. *PLOS ONE, 4*(3), e4785. doi:10.1371/journal.pone.0004785

21 Draganski, B., Gaser, C., Busch, V., Schuierer, G., Bogdahn, U., & May, A. (2004). Neuroplasticity: Changes in grey matter induced by training.

Nature, 427(6972), 311–312. doi:10.1038/427311a. Driemeyer, J., Boyke, J., Gaser, C., Büchel, C., & May, A. (2008). Changes in gray matter induced by learning: Revisited. *PLOS ONE, 3*(7), e2669. doi:10.1371/journal.pone.0002669

22 Boyke, J., Driemeyer, J., Gaser, C., Büchel, C., & May, A. (2008). Training-induced brain structure changes in the elderly. *Journal of Neuroscience, 28*(28), 7031–7035. doi:10.1523/JNEUROSCI.0742-08.2008

23 Engvig, A., Fjell, A.M., Westlye, L.T., Moberget, T., Sundseth, Ø., Larsen, V.A., & Walhovd, K.B. (2010). Effects of memory training on cortical thickness in the elderly. *Neuroimage, 52*(4), 1667–1676. doi:10.1016/j.neuroimage.2010.05.041

24 Draganski, B., Gaser, C., Kempermann, G., Kuhn, H.G., Winkler, J., Büchel, C., & May, A. (2006). Temporal and spatial dynamics of brain structure changes during extensive learning. *Journal of Neuroscience, 26*(23), 6314–6317. doi:10.1523/JNEUROSCI.4628-05.2006

25 May, A. (2011). Experience-dependent structural plasticity in the adult human brain. *Trends in Cognitive Sciences, 15*(10), 475-482. doi:10.1016/j.tics.2011.08.002. p. 4.

26 Mechelli, A., Crinion, J.T., Noppeney, U., O'Doherty, J., Ashburner, J., Frackowiak, R.S., & Price, C.J. (2004). Neurolinguistics: Structural plasticity in the bilingual brain. *Nature, 431*(7010), 757–757. doi:10.1038/431757a. Stein, M., Federspiel, A., Koenig, T., Wirth, M., Strik, W., Wiest, R., . . . & Dierks, T. (2012). Structural plasticity in the language system related to increased second language proficiency. *Cortex, 48*(4), 458–465. doi:10.1016/j.cortex.2010.10.007

27 Begley, S. (2008). *The plastic mind*. London: Constable & Robinson.

28 Pickren, W., & Rutherford, A. (2010). *A history of modern psychology in context*. Hoboken, NJ: Wiley.

29 Diamond, M. C., Krech, D., & Rosenzweig, M. R. (1964). The effects of an enriched environment on the histology of the rat cerebral cortex. *Journal of Comparative Neurology, 123*(1), 111–119. doi:10.1002/cne.901230110

30 Van Dellen, A., Blakemore, C., Deacon, R., York, D., & Hannan, A.J. (2000). Delaying the onset of Huntington's in mice. *Nature, 404*(6779), 721–722. doi:10.1038/35008142

31 Amaral, O.B., Vargas, R.S., Hansel, G., Izquierdo, I., & Souza, D.O. (2008). Duration of environmental enrichment influences the magnitude and persistence of its behavioral effects on mice. *Physiology & Behavior, 93*(1), 388–394. doi:10.1016/j.physbeh.2007.09.009

32 Johansson, B.B. (1996). Functional outcome in rats transferred to an enriched environment 15 days after focal brain ischemia. *Stroke, 27*(2), 324–326. doi:10.1161/01.STR.27.2.324

[33] Young, D., Lawlor, P.A., Leone, P., Dragunow, M., & During, M.J. (1999). Environmental enrichment inhibits spontaneous apoptosis, prevents seizures and is neuroprotective. *Nature Medicine, 5*(4), 448–453. doi: 10.1038/7449

[34] Mohammed, A.H., Zhu, S.W., Darmopil, S., Hjerling-Leffler, J., Ernfors, P., Winblad, B., . . . & Bogdanovic, N. (2002). Environmental enrichment and the brain. *Progress in Brain Research, 138*, 109–133. doi:10.1016/S0079-6123(02)38074-9, p. 127.

[35] Hebb, D.O. (1949). *The organization of behavior: A neuropsychological theory*. New York: Wiley.

[36] Bennett, M.R. (2000, Feb). The concept of long term potentiation of transmission at synapses. *Prog Neurobiol.*, 60(2):109–37.

[37] But this simple chain of electrical and chemical events will not explain how synapses can become 'stronger' (more efficient and effective) the more they are used: something additional must be happening to cause such 'plasticity'. Bliss and Lomo's great discovery was to show that some of the target molecules (receptors) on the receiving cell can be quite fussy about the conditions in which they will work well, and this fussiness can be turned to advantage and form the basis for the adaptability of brain cells. For the fussy type of receptor a simple handshake is not enough, even when interlocking with a transmitter, X; it is just not sufficient to actually cause a change in voltage in the cell. Or, to use another analogy, the boat may be in dock but no car is yet available. Something else must happen next; there must be a further change while transmitter X is already present. The handshake will be effective not just because two hands interlock, but because one of them now squeezes the other. Accordingly, if a second transmitter, Y, now arrives on the scene and also docks into the cell, the contingency of X and Y will at last fulfil the demands of the fussy receptor (a car will appear). An electrical signal will now be generated, but with longer-term consequences. When the fussy receptor starts to work, it will trigger the opening of little channels in the cell so that calcium can flood in. In turn, the calcium will release a chemical that returns back across the synapse to the original incoming cell and makes it release yet still more transmitter than usual. Meanwhile, within the target cell, a cascade of events is set in train that will make the cell more sensitive in terms of how effectively it will respond to the standard amount of input. The same signal will have a much more powerful effect. The synapse now works more powerfully, but things don't just stop there. The calcium that has entered the cell during this process (long-term potentiation) has still longer-term actions: more specialist chemicals are produced inside the cell that stabilise the synapse still further by acting like

sticky badges (cell adhesion molecules). Meanwhile, different proteins kick in to enhance the appearance of yet more neuronal contacts. All this has happened because of the initial requirement of the fussy receptor where two things had to happen within a certain time-frame, and for a sustained period of time, in order for calcium to infiltrate the neuron. In this way, the more a behaviour is repeated or rehearsed, such as a repetitious response to a certain experience, the greater the effect and the stronger the respective synapses will become over time, and hence that experience will literally leave its mark on the brain.

38 Scarmeas, N., & Stern, Y. (2003). Cognitive reserve and lifestyle. *Journal of Clinical and Experimental Neuropsychology, 25*(5), 625–633. doi:10.1076/jcen.25.5.625.14576

39 Frasca, D., Tomaszczyk, J., McFadyen, B.J., & Green, R.E. (2013). Traumatic brain injury and post-acute decline: What role does environmental enrichment play? A scoping review. *Frontiers in Human Neuroscience, 7*, 31. doi:10.3389/fnhum.2013.00031

40 Scarmeas & Stern, 2003 (see n. 38).

41 Frasca et al., 2013 (see n. 39).

42 Winocur, G., & Moscovitch, M. (1990). A comparison of cognitive function in community-dwelling and institutionalized old people of normal intelligence. *Canadian Journal of Psychology/Revue Canadienne de Psychologie, 44*(4), 435–444. doi:10.1037/h0084270

43 Olson, A.K., Eadie, B.D., Ernst, C., & Christie, B.R. (2006). Environmental enrichment and voluntary exercise massively increase neurogenesis in the adult hippocampus via dissociable pathways. *Hippocampus, 16*(3), 250–260. doi:10.1002/hipo.20157

44 Nottebohm, F. (2002). Neuronal replacement in adult brain. *Brain Research Bulletin, 57*(6), 737–749. doi:10.1016/S0361-9230(02)00750-5

45 Nyberg, L., Lövdén, M., Riklund, K., Lindenberger, U., & Bäckman, L. (2012). Memory aging and brain maintenance. *Trends in Cognitive Sciences, 16*(5), 292–305. doi:10.1016/j.tics.2012.04.005

46 Mu, Y., & Gage, F.H. (2011). Adult hippocampal neurogenesis and its role in Alzheimer's disease. *Molecular Neurodegeneration, 6*(1), 85. doi:10.1186/1750-1326-6-85

47 Pascual-Leone, A., Nguyet, D., Cohen, L.G., Brasil-Neto, J.P., Cammarota, A., & Hallett, M. (1995). Modulation of muscle responses evoked by transcranial magnetic stimulation during the acquisition of new fine motor skills. *Journal of Neurophysiology, 74*(3), 1037–1045. Retrieved from http://psycnet.apa.org/psycinfo/1996-25629-001

48 Van Praag, H., Kempermann, G., & Gage, F.H. (1999). Running increases

cell proliferation and neurogenesis in the adult mouse dentate gyrus. *Nature Neuroscience*, 2(3), 266–270. doi:10.1038/6368

[49] Greenberg, R.P. (2005). Endogenous opiates and the placebo effect: a meta-analytic review. *J. Psychosom Res.*, *58*, 115-20.

[50] Tanti, A., & Belzung, C. (2013). Hippocampal neurogenesis: A biomarker for depression or antidepressant effects? Methodological considerations and perspectives for future research. *Cell and Tissue Research*, 1-17. doi:10.1007/s00441-013-1612-z

[51] Begley, 2008 (see n. 27).

Chapter 7 HOW THE BRAIN BECOMES A MIND

[1] Penfield, W., & Boldrey, E. (1937). Somatic motor and sensory representation in the cerebralcortex of man as studied by electrical stimulation. *Brain: A Journal of Neurology*, *60*(4), 389–443. doi:10.1093/brain/60.4.389

[2] Chalmers, D.J. (1995). Facing up to the problem of consciousness. *Journal of Consciousness Studies*, 2(3), 200–219. Retrieved from http://cogprints.org/316/1/consciousness.html

[3] Koch, C., & Tononi, G. (2008). Can machines be conscious? *Spectrum, IEEE*, *45*(6), 55–59. Retrieved from http://ieeexplore.ieee.org/xpls/abs_all.jsp?arnumber=4531463

[4] However, we do know that neurons can interface very well with silicon systems. The pioneering work of Peter Fromherz, for example, has shown the beauty of a 'neurochip' whereby connections are readily made on a circuit board between neurons and silicon nodes. Similarly, if brain cells are able to function in a hybrid device in this way, then the reverse may not be surprising: artificial implants in the brain are already possible and are achieving astonishing effects. For example, Miguel Nicolelis of Duke University has developed a system whereby quadriplegic patients can, through devices implanted in their brain, generate electronic signatures that would normally precede various movements. These electronic signals are then recognized by a computer that can operate an artificial limb, so that a person paralysed from the neck down can 'will' a movement. However these 'neuronal prostheses' are far from the silicon take-over of the brain envisaged in the thought experiment. While silicon-carbon interfacing is possible, at least for the final execution of a movement, namely brain output simulating brain muscle, it should not be conflated with the neuron-neuron interactions that underlie cognitive processes, or confused with AI.

[5] Damasio, A.R., Everitt, B.J., & Bishop, D. (1996). The somatic marker hypothesis and the possible functions of the prefrontal cortex. *Philosophical*

Transactions of the Royal Society of London. Series B: Biological Sciences, 351(1346), 1413–1420. doi:10.1098/rstb.1996.0125

6 Turing, A.M. (1950). Computing machinery and intelligence. *Mind, 59*(236), 433–460. Retrieved from http://cogprints.org/499/1/turing.html

7 For example, Rees, G., Kreiman, G., & Koch, C. (2002). Neural correlates of consciousness in humans. *Nature Reviews Neuroscience, 3*(4), 261–270. Tononi, G., & Koch, C. (2008). The neural correlates of consciousness. *Annals of the New York Academy of Sciences, 1124*(1), 239–261.

8 Koch, C., & Greenfield, S. (2007). How does consciousness happen? *Scientific American*, 297(4), 76–83. Retrieved from http://www.sciamdigital.com/index.cfm?fa=ExtServices.GspDownloadIssueView&ARTICLEID_CHAR=E0E902FE-3048-8A5E-1061447DA58B3813

9 Greenfield, S.A. (2001). *The private life of the brain: Emotions, consciousness, and the secret of the self.* New York: Wiley.

10 James, W. (1890). *The principles of psychology*. Retrieved from http://psychclassics.yorku.ca/James/Principles/prin10.htm

11 René Descartes (1596–1650), often dubbed 'the father of modern philosophy', argued the case that humans are distinctly different from other animals and the rest of the natural world: our unique mind can be attributed to language and reason, features that set our species apart from the rest of the animal kingdom. Descartes suggested that the demonstrative behaviours of all non-human creatures can be explained without having to bother ascribing minds and consciousness to them. He concluded that non-human animals can be regarded as no more than machines, with parts assembled in intricate ways. However, although humans might have minds and consciousness, these phenomena would be separate from the mechanistic working of the body: 'To explain these functions, then, it is not necessary to conceive of any vegetative or sensitive soul, or any other principle of movement or life, other than its blood and its spirits which are agitated by the heat of the fire that burns continuously in its heart, and which is of the same nature as those fires that occur in inanimate bodies.' This notion of a mechanistic physical body extended to the mechanics of the physical brain. For Descartes, the prototype 'dualist', it would mean that the physical brain was distinct from the mind and consciousness, which was left largely undefined and unexplored. More recently, in the twentieth century the advent of the computer brought with it the opportunity to jettison the notion of some airy-fairy parallel consciousness, and instead to ascribe everything to mechanistic processes. (Descartes, R. (1994). The treatise on man. In S. Gaukroger (Ed.), *The world and other writings* (pp. 119-169). Retrieved from http://www2.dsu.nodak.edu/users/dmeier/31243550-Descartes-The-World-and-Other-Writings.pdf, p. 169.)

12 The definition of intelligence is no mere semantic quibble, but would extend to wider moral questions. For example, Hume was at odds with Kant in assuming that intelligence does not necessarily imply moral values and vice versa. However, surely this dilemma once again depends on how we define intelligence. If we take the simple computational concept of g, prowess in IQ tests, then Hume would be correct: after all, why should a simple linear process be predicated on anything other than the rules of the game? But if we take the wider view of intelligence, as I would argue, to imply understanding, then perhaps Kant would be more accurate in viewing intelligence as an understanding that would imply an awareness of the link to particular values.

13 See Frisch, O.R. (1980). *What Little I Remember*. Cambridge University Press, p. 95.

14 Horn, J.L., & Cattell, R.B. (1967). Age differences in fluid and crystallized intelligence. *Acta Psychologica*, 26, 107-129. Retrieved from http://www.sciencedirect.com/science/article/pii/000169186790011X

15 This idea of true, deep mental abilities arising from neuronal connections would fit with the finding mentioned earlier that gifted children do indeed display greater neuronal connectivity.

16 Chalmers, 1995 (see n. 2).

17 Blake, W. (c.1803). 'Auguries of Innocence'. Retrieved from http://www.bartleby.com/41/356.html

Chapter 8 OUT OF YOUR MIND

1 In the mid-twentieth century an American physician, Paul MacLean, developed a theory to explain the inexplicable collective behaviour of the crowds at the Nuremburg rallies during the Nazi era. MacLean's reasoning was that, anatomically, the brain could be compartmentalised into three evolutionary stages: the *reptilian* brain, consisting of the inner core, the basic part of the brain; layered on to that would be the *mammalian* brain, including areas such as the amygdala and hippocampus; and finally, constituting the most sophisticated level of all, would be the cortex, the outer layer of the brain, which is the monopoly of the *neo-mammalian* species. MacLean argued that these three layers represented increasing degrees of sophistication in mental processes. The reptilian brain underpinned very primitive urges, these being channelled into the appropriate context by virtue of the mammalian brain, while the neo-mammalian brain imposed further refinements, even rules, on how one might behave. This hierarchy of three levels corresponds quite neatly to Freud's notion of the atavistic id, the mediating ego and the moralistic super-ego. According to MacLean, emotions were suppressed by logic and reason for most of the time; but within the intermediate limbic system, which

he saw as 'centres for' emotions normally held in check by a logical cortex, regions can also play a key role in that most sensible of activities, memory. Conversely, disruptions to the cortex, especially the prefrontal cortex can be linked to emotional disturbances, such as those seen in addiction, obesity and schizophrenia. Sadly, however, such simple compartmentalisation doesn't stand up to the anatomical and physiological practicalities of what we now know the brain, and indeed the mind, to be capable. Nonetheless, this theory is useful at a more metaphorical level. According to MacLean, the seemingly blind aggression of the Nuremberg crowds could therefore be accounted for by the breakdown in the anatomical hierarchy of the 'triune brain' (MacLean, P.D. (1985). Evolutionary psychiatry and the triune brain. *Psychological Medicine, 15*(2), 219–221. doi:10.1017/S0033291700023485).

2 Greenfield, S.A. (2008). *I.D.: The quest for meaning in the 21st century.* London: Hodder & Stoughton.

3 Olds, J., & Milner, P. (1954). Positive reinforcement produced by electrical stimulation of septal area and other regions of rat brain. *Journal of Comparative and Physiological Psychology, 47*(6), 419–27. Retrieved from http://www.wadsworth.com/psychology_d/templates/student_resources/0155060678_rathus/ps/ps02.html

4 O'Driscoll, K., & Leach, J.P. (1998). 'No longer Gage': An iron bar through the head: Early observations of personality change after injury to the prefrontal cortex. *BMJ, 317*(7174), 1673–1674. Retrieved from http://www.ncbi.nlm.nih.gov/pmc/articles/PMC1114479/#__ffn_sectitle

5 O'Driscoll & Leach, 1998 (see n. 4), p. 1673.

6 Tsujimoto, S. (2008). The prefrontal cortex: Functional neural development during early childhood. *The Neuroscientist, 14*(4), 345–358. doi: 10.1177/107385840831600

7 Sturman, D.A., & Moghaddam, B. (2011). The neurobiology of adolescence: Changes in brain architecture, functional dynamics, and behavioral tendencies. *Neuroscience & Biobehavioral Reviews, 35*(8), 1704–1712. doi: 10.1016/j.neubiorev.2011.04.003

8 Casey, B.J., Getz, S., & Galvan, A. (2008). The adolescent brain. *Developmental Review, 28*(1), 62–77. doi: 10.1016/j.dr.2007.08.003

9 Casey, Getz, & Galvan, 2008 (see n. 8).

10 Steinberg, L. (2008). A social neuroscience perspective on adolescent risk-taking. *Developmental Review, 28*(1), 78–106. doi: 10.1016/j.dr.2007.08.002

11 Callicott, J.H., Bertolino, A., Mattay, V.S., Langheim, F.J., Duyn, J., Coppola, R., . . . & Weinberger, D.R. (2000). Physiological dysfunction of the dorsolateral prefrontal cortex in schizophrenia revisited. *Cerebral Cortex, 10*(11), 1078–1092. doi:10.1093/cercor/10.11.1078

[12] Volkow, N.D., Wang, G.J., Telang, F., Fowler, J.S., Goldstein, R.Z., Alia-Klein, N., . . . & Pradhan, K. (2008). Inverse association between BMI and prefrontal metabolic activity in healthy adults. *Obesity, 17*(1), 60–65. doi:10.1038/oby.2008.469

[13] Pignatti, R., Bertella, L., Albani, G., Mauro, A., Molinari, E., & Semenza, C. (2006). Decision-making in obesity: A study using the Gambling Task. *Eating and Weight Disorders: EWD, 11*(3), 126. Retrieved from http://www.ncbi.nlm.nih.gov/pubmed/17075239

[14] Dang-Vu, T.T., Schabus, M., Desseilles, M., Sterpenich, V., Bonjean, M., & Maquet, P. (2010). Functional neuroimaging insights into the physiology of human sleep. *Sleep, 33*(12), 1589–1603. Retrieved from http://www.ncbi.nlm.nih.gov/pmc/articles/PMC2982729/#__ffn_sectitle

[15] Greenfield, S. (2011). *You and me: the neuroscience of identity*. London: Notting Hill.

Chapter 9 THE *SOMETHING* ABOUT SOCIAL NETWORKING

[1] O'Connell, R. (2011, May 12). The pros and cons of deleting your Facebook [Weblog post]. Retrieved from http://thoughtcatalog.com/2011/the-pros-and-cons-to-deleting-your-facebook/

[2] Hampton, K.N., Goulet, L.S., Rainie, L., & Purcell, K. (2011). *Social networking sites and our lives*. Retrieved from http://pewinternet.org/Reports/2011/Technology-and-social-networks.aspx

[3] Badoo (2012, April 25). Generation lonely? 39 percent of Americans spend more time socializing online than face-to-face. Retrieved from http://corp.badoo.com/he/entry/press/54/

[4] Quoted in McCullagh, D. (2010, March 12). Why no one cares about privacy anymore. Retrieved from http://www.cnet.com/uk/news/why-no-one-cares-about-privacy-anymore/

[5] Protalinski, E. (2013, May 1). Facebook passes 1.11 billion monthly active users, 751 million mobile users, and 665 million daily users. Retrieved from http://thenextweb.com/facebook/2013/05/01/facebook-passes-1-11-billion-monthly-active-users-751-million-mobile-users-and-665-million-daily-users/

[6] Anderson, B., Fagan, P., Woodnutt, T., & Chamorro-Prezumic, T. (2012). Facebook psychology: Popular questions answered by research. *Psychology of Popular Media Culture, 1*(1), 23–37. doi:10.1037/a0026452

[7] Manago, A.M., Taylor, T., & Greenfield, P.M. (2012). Me and my 400 friends: The anatomy of college students' Facebook networks, their communication patterns, and well-being. *Developmental Psychology, 48*(2), 369–380. doi:10.1037/a0026338

8 Grieve, R., Indian, M., Witteveen, K., Tolan, G.A., & Marrington, J. (2013). Face-to-face or Facebook: Can social connectedness be derived online? *Computers in Human Behavior, 29*(3), 604–609. doi:10.1016/j.chb.2012.11.017

9 Quoted in Cohen, J. (2012, Feb 1). Facebook officially files SEC documents for $5B offer [Weblog post]. Retrieved from http://allfacebook.com/facebook-files-ipo_b76165

10 Teilhard de Chardin, P. (1964). *The future of man*. London: Collins.

11 Rutledge, T., et al. (2008). Social networks and incident stroke among women with suspected myocardial ischemia. *Psychosomatic Medicine, 70*(3), 282–287. doi:10.1097/PSY.0b013e3181656e09

12 Cole, S.W., Hawkley, L.C., Arevalo, J.M.G., & Cacioppo, J.T. (2011). Transcript origin analysis identifies antigen-presenting cells as primary targets of socially regulated gene expression in leukocytes. *PNAS, 108*(7), 3080–3085. doi:10.1073/pnas.1014218108

13 Norman, G.J., Cacioppo, J.T., Morris, J.S., Malarkey, W.B., Berntson, G.G., & DeVries, A.C. (2011). Oxytocin increases autonomic cardiac control: Moderation by loneliness. *Biological Psychology, 86*(3), 174–180.

14 Klinenberg, E. (2012, March 30). I want to be alone: The rise and rise of solo living. Retrieved from http://www.theguardian.com/lifeandstyle/2012/mar/30/the-rise-of-solo-living

15 Sigman, A. (2009). Well connected? The biological implications of 'social networking'. *Biologist, 56*(1), 14–20. Retrieved from http://www.aricsigman.com/IMAGES/Sigman_lo.pdf

16 Penenberg, A.L. (2010, July 1). Social networking affects brains like falling in love [Weblog post]. Retrieved from http://www.fastcompany.com/1659062/social-networking-affects-brains-falling-loved

17 Wilson, R.E., Gosling, S.D., & Graham, L.T. (2012). A review of Facebook research in the social sciences. *Perspectives on Psychological Science, 7*(3), 203–220. doi:10.1177/1745691612442904

18 Burke, M., Marlow, C., & Lento, T. (2010). Social network activity and social well-being. *Proceedings of the SIGCHI Conference on Human Factors in Computing System*, 1909–1912. doi:10.1145/1753326.1753613

19 Clayton, R.B., Osborne, R.E., Miller, B.K., & Oberle, C.D. (2013). Loneliness, anxiousness, and substance use as predictors of Facebook use. *Computers in Human Behavior, 29*(3), 687–693. doi:10.1016/j.chb.2012.12.002

20 Skues, J.L., Williams, B., & Wise, L. (2012). The effects of personality traits, self-esteem, loneliness, and narcissism on Facebook use amongst university students. *Computers in Human Behavior, 28*(6), 2414–2419. doi:10.1016/j.chb.2012.07.012

21 Watson, R. (2010). *Future files: A brief history of the next 50 years*. London: Nicholas Brealey.

22 Anderson et al., 2012 (see n. 6).

23 Oldmeadow, J.A., Quinn, S., & Kowert, R. (2013). Attachment style, social skills, and Facebook use amongst adults. *Computers in Human Behavior, 29*(3), 1142–1149. doi:10.1016/j.chb.2012.10.006

24 Bowlby J. (1969). *Attachment and loss*, Vol. 1: *Loss*. New York: Basic Books, p. 194.

25 Oldmeadow, Quinn, & Kowert, 2013 (see n. 23).

26 Skues, Williams, & Wise, 2012 (see n. 20).

27 Tamir, D.I., & Mitchell, J.P. (2012). Disclosing information about the self is intrinsically rewarding. *PNAS, 109*(21), 8038-8043. doi:10.1073/pnas.1202129109

28 Arbitron and Edison Research (2013, April). *The infinite dial 2013: Navigating digital platforms*. Retrieved from http://www.edisonresearch.com/wp-content/uploads/2013/04/Edison_Research_Arbitron_Infinite_Dial_2013.pdf

29 Jiang, L.C., Bazarova, N.N., & Hancock, J.T. (2011). The disclosure-intimacy link in computer-mediated communication: An attributional extension of the hyperpersonal model. *Human Communication Research, 37*(1), 58–77. doi:10.1111/j.1468-2958.2010.01393.x. boyd, d.m., & Ellison, N.B. (2007). Social networking sites: Definition, history, and scholarship. *Journal of Computer-Mediated Communication, 13*(1), 210–230. doi: 10.1111/j.1083-6101.2007.00393.x

30 Trepte, S., & Reinecke, L. (2013). The reciprocal effects of social network site use and the disposition for self-disclosure: A longitudinal study. *Computers in Human Behavior, 29*(3), 1102–1112. doi:10.1016/j.chb.2012.10.002

31 Tamir & Mitchell, 2012 (see n. 27).

32 Mauri, M., Cipresso, P., Balgera, A., Villamira, M., & Riva, G. (2011). Why is Facebook so successful? Psychophysiological measures describe a core flow state while using Facebook. *Cyberpsychology, Behavior, and Social Networking, 14*(12), 723–731. doi:10.1089/cyber.2010.0377, p. 1.

33 Weinschenk, S. (2009, November 7). 100 things you should know about people. #8 Dopamine makes you addicted to seeking information [Weblog post]. Retrieved from http://www.blog.theteamw.com/2009/11/07/100-things-you-should-know-about-people-8-dopamine-makes-us-addicted-to-seeking-information/

34 O'Doherty, J., Deichmann, R., Critchley, H., & Dolan, R.J. (2002). Neural responses during anticipation of a primary taste reward. *Neuron, 33*(5), 815–826. doi:10.1016/S0896-6273(02)00603-7

35 Does Facebook 'addiction' really exist? American psychologist Michael Fenichel has suggested that, like gambling or alcohol, Facebook might have its very own version of addiction. He describes the all too familiar situation in which Facebook usage can trump daily activities like waking up, getting dressed, using the telephone or checking e-mail. Fenichel has accordingly introduced a new term to describe such a state: Facebook addiction disorder, or FAD. He defines FAD as a condition where hours are spent on Facebook, to the extent that the healthy balance of the individual's life is affected. Fenichel claims that approximately 350 million people are suffering from the condition, which can be detected through a simple set of six criteria. People who are victims of the disorder must have at least two or three of the criteria during a six- to eight-month period. For the family members and friends who think they are dealing with an addict, a sign to look out for is, apparently, multiple Facebook windows open. Three or more windows, bizarrely, confirms that they are indeed suffering from this condition. There remains no empirical evidence that Facebook addiction disorder exists (Fenichel, M. (n.d.). Facebook addiction disorder (FAD). Retrieved from http://www.fenichel.com/facebook/).

36 Johnson, D.E., Guthrie, D., Smyke, A.T., Koga, S.F., Fox, N.A., Zeanah, C.H., & Nelson, C.A. (2010). Growth and associations between auxology, caregiving environment, and cognition in socially deprived Romanian children randomized to foster vs ongoing institutional care. *Archives of Paediatrics & Adolescent Medicine, 164*(6), 507–516. doi:10.1001/archpediatrics.2010.56

37 Oldmeadow, Quinn, & Kowert, 2013 (see n. 23).

38 Dumon, M. (2011, October 18). Meet George Clooney's new girl: Stacy Keibler. Retrieved from http://www.examiner.com/article/meet-george-clooney-s-new-girl-stacy-keibler

39 Harkaway, N. (2012). *The blind giant: Being human in a digital world.* London: Vintage.

40 McCullagh, 2010 (see n. 4).

41 McAfee (2010). *The secret online lives of teens.* Retrieved from http://us.mcafee.com/en-us/local/docs/lives_of_teens.pdf

42 Arbitron and Edison Research (2013, April). *The infinite dial 2013: Navigating digital platforms.* Retrieved from http://www.edisonresearch.com/wp-content/uploads/2013/04/Edison_Research_Arbitron_Infinite_Dial_2013.pdf

Chapter 10 SOCIAL NETWORKING AND IDENTITY

1 Government Office for Science (2013). *Future identities: Changing identities in the UK: The next 10 years*. Retrieved from https://www.gov.uk/government/uploads/system/uploads/attachment_data/file/273966/13-523-future-identities-changing-identities-report.pdf

2 Amichai-Hamburger, Y., Wainapel, G., & Fox, S. (2002). 'On the Internet no one knows I'm an introvert': Extroversion, neuroticism, and Internet interaction. *CyberPsychology & Behavior, 5*(2), 125–128. Retrieved from http://www.ncbi.nlm.nih.gov/pubmed/12025878

3 Suler, J. (2004). The online disinhibition effect. *CyberPsychology & Behavior, 7*(3), 321–326. doi:10.1089/1094931041291295. Christopherson, K.M. (2007). The positive and negative implications of anonymity in Internet social interactions: 'On the Internet, nobody knows you're a dog'. *Computers in Human Behavior, 23*(6), 3038–3056. doi:10.1016/j.chb.2006.09.001

4 Zhao, S., Grasmuck, S., & Martin, J. (2008). Identity construction on Facebook: Digital empowerment in anchored relationships. *Computers in Human Behavior, 24*, 1816–1836. doi:10.1016/j.chb.2008.02.012

5 boyd, d.m., & Ellison, N.B. (2007). Social networking sites: Definition, history, and scholarship. *Journal of Computer-Mediated Communication, 13*(1), 210–230. doi:10.1111/j.1083-6101.2007.00393.x

6 boyd & Ellison, 2007 (see n. 5), p. 211.

7 What names are allowed on Facebook? (n.d.). Retrieved from https://www.facebook.com/help/112146705538576?q=name&sid=09QL15Kz6090K35pZ

8 Rogers, C. (1951). *Client-centered therapy*. Boston: Houghton-Mifflin.

9 Bargh, J.A., McKenna, K.Y.A., & Fitzsimons, G.M. (2002). Can you see the real me? Activation and expression of the 'true self' on the Internet. *Journal of Social Issues, 58*(1), 33–48. doi:10.1111/1540-4560.00247

10 McKenna, K.Y.A., Green, A.S., & Gleason, M.E.J. (2002). Relationship formation on the Internet: What's the big attraction? *Journal of Social Issues, 58*(1), 9–31. doi:10.1111/1540-4560.00246

11 McKenna, Green, & Gleason, 2002 (see n. 10).

12 Tosun L.P. (2012). Motives for Facebook use and expressing 'true self' on the Internet. *Computers in Human Behavior, 28*, 1510–1517. doi:10.1016/j.chb.2012.03.018

13 Tosun, L.P., & Lajunen, T. (2009). Why do young adults develop a passion for Internet activities? The associations among personality, revealing 'true self' on the Internet, and passion for the Internet. *CyberPsychology & Behavior, 12*(4), 401–406. doi:10.1089/cpb.2009.0006

14 Zhao, Grasmuck, & Martin, 2008 (see n. 4).

15 Siibak, A. (2009). Constructing the self through the photo selection: Visual impression management on social networking websites. *Cyberpsychology: Journal of Psychosocial Research on Cyberspace, 3*(1), article 1. Retrieved from: http://cyberpsychology.eu/view.php?cisloclanku=2009061501&article=1

16 Goffman, E. (1959). *The presentation of self in everyday life*. New York: Overlook.

17 d.m. boyd interviewed in Rosen, L.D. (2012). *iDisorder: Understanding our obsession with technology and overcoming its hold on us*. Harmondsworth, UK: Palgrave Macmillan, p. 34.

18 Zhao, Grasmuck, & Martin, 2008 (see n. 4).

19 While the majority of social networking research has focused on identity specifically on Facebook, there has been a proposal that, as different social networking platforms offer different types of social networking to users, so different identities might be managed on different social networking sites. For example, LinkedIn may be used to develop the hoped-for professional self, whereas Facebook is the platform to display the hoped-for social self (van Dijck, J. (2013). 'You have one identity': Performing the self on Facebook and LinkedIn. *Media, Culture & Society, 35*(2), 199–215. doi:10.1177/0163443712468605).

20 Zhao, Grasmuck, & Martin, 2008 (see n. 4).

21 Back, M.D., Stopfer, J.M., Vazire, S., Gaddis, S., Schmukle, S.C., Egloff, B., & Gosling, S.D. (2010). Facebook profiles reflect actual personality, not self-idealization. *Psychological Science, 21*(3), 372–374. doi: 10.1177/0956797609360756

22 Rosen, 2012 (see n. 17).

23 Buffardi, L.E., & Campbell, W.K. (2008). Narcissism and social networking web sites. *Personality and Social Psychology Bulletin, 34*, 1303–1314. doi: 10.1177/0146167208320061. Mehdizadeh, S. (2010). Self-Presentation 2.0: Narcissism and self-esteem on Facebook. *Cyberpsychology, Behavior, and Social Networking, 13*(4), 357–364. doi:10.1089/cyber.2009.0257. Ryan, T., & Xenos, S. (2011). Who uses Facebook? An investigation into the relationship between the Big Five, shyness, narcissism, loneliness, and Facebook usage. *Computers in Human Behavior, 27*, 1658–1664. doi:10.1016/j.chb.2011.02.004. Twenge, J.M., Konrath, S., Foster, J.D., Campbell, W.K., & Bushman, B.J. (2008). Egos inflating over time: A cross-temporal meta-analysis of the narcissistic personality inventory. *Journal of Personality, 76*(4), 875–902. doi:10.1111/j.1467-6494.2008.00507.x

24 Twenge et al., 2008 (see n. 23).

25 In a study of Twitter users by Mor Naaman and his team from Rutgers, the

subjects fell into two categories: 'meformers' and 'informers'. As their name suggests, the meformers posted endless updates on their own thoughts and feelings while informers lived up to their particular name by sharing information and interacting more with followers. Of those studied, 80% of the subjects were classified as meformers, fitting well into the profile of our current narcissistic era (Naaman, M., Boase, J., & Lai, C.H. (2010). Is it really about me? Message content in social awareness streams. *Proceedings of the 2010 ACM Conference on Computer Supported Cooperative Work*, 189–192. doi:10.1145/1718918.1718953).

26 Buffardi & Campbell, 2008 (see n. 23). Mehdizadeh, 2010 (see n. 23). Ryan & Xenos, 2011 (see n. 23). Naaman, Boase, & Lai, 2010 (see n. 25). McKinney, B.C., Kelly, L., & Duran, R.L. (2012). Narcissism or openness? College students' use of Facebook and Twitter. *Communication Research Reports, 29*(2), 108–118. doi:10.1080/08824096.2012.666919. Bergman, M., Fearrington, M.E., Davenport, S.W., & Bergman, J.Z. (2011). Millennials, narcissism, and social networking: What narcissists do on social networking sites and why. *Personality and Individual Differences, 50*, 706–711. doi:10.1016/j.paid.2010.12.022. Carpenter, C.J. (2012). Narcissism on Facebook: Self-promotional and anti-social behavior. *Personality and Individual Differences, 52*(4), 482–486. doi:10.1016/j.paid.2011.11.011. Panek, E.T., Nardis, Y., & Konrath, S. (2013). Defining social networking sites and measuring their use: How narcissists differ in their use of Facebook and Twitter. *Computers in Human Behavior, 29*(5), 2004–2012. doi:10.1016/j.chb.2013.04.012

27 Raskin, R., & Terry, H. (1988). A principal-components analysis of the Narcissistic Personality Inventory and further evidence of its construct validity. *Journal of Personality and Social Psychology, 54*(5), 890–902. doi:10.1037/0022-3514.54.5.890

28 Panek, Nardis, & Konrath, 2013 (see n. 26).

29 A potential upside from regularly viewing and modifying your social networking identity may be increased self-esteem. However, earlier research has shown that inducing self-awareness via a mirror can induce a negative mood, particularly for women (Fejfar, M.C., & Hoyle, R.H. (2000). Effect of private self-awareness on negative affect and self-referent attribution: A quantitative review. *Personality and Social Psychology Review, 4*(2), 132–142. doi:10.1207/S15327957PSPR0402_02), so, for some, viewing one's social networking profile may be the equivalent of an online mirror, and may have negative effects on self-esteem. But Facebook is not a true mirror, displaying an unedited image of ourselves; it is a modified and managed mirror that reflects back our self-edited best version of ourselves, and thus

has the potential to be a rose-tinted distortion. Subsequently, research has found that viewing one's own Facebook profile results in higher self-esteem levels compared to those who looked in a mirror, with those who edited their profiles during a short testing period possessing the highest levels of self-esteem (Tazghini, S., & Siedlecki, K.L. (2013). A mixed method approach to examining Facebook use and its relationship to self-esteem. *Computers in Human Behavior*, 29(3), 827–832. doi:10.1016/j.chb.2012.11.010). Unsurprisingly, it seems that the ability to create and present the ideal version of yourself has positive effects on self-esteem. While older forms of media such as glossy fashion magazines and TV shows increase body image issues, particularly in women, research has shown that the strongest media-related predictor of these issues is now social network site use (Tiggemann, M., & Miller, J. (2010). The Internet and adolescent girls' weight satisfaction and drive for thinness. *Sex Roles*, *63*, 79–90. doi:10.1007/s11199-010-9789-z). Girls who spent more time on Facebook and Myspace displayed higher scores of 'drive for thinness', a subscale of an eating disorder diagnostic tool. Facebook use was also linked to girls being less satisfied with their current weight and having higher levels of an internalised thin ideal. These associations were stronger for social networking sites than for traditional culprits of body image disorder in women, such as magazines and TV. Most of the research has been equivocal as to whether social networking can actually promote healthy types of self-esteem. At Canada's York University, psychology student Soraya Mehdizadeh (2010: see n. 23) examined the online habits and personalities of Facebook users at the university, ranging from 18–25 years old. Mehdizadeh explored how narcissism and self-esteem related to the various self-promotional contents of a Facebook profile, and found that individuals higher in narcissism and lower in self-esteem spent more time on the site and filled their pages with more self-promotional content. So filling a Facebook page with positive versions of oneself does not appear to do much for an individual's self-esteem. Perhaps it's because, for real reassurance, we all need real-world feedback, the literal and metaphorical pat on the back that comes with voice tone, eye contact, body language and physical contact. A crucial factor may be the type of online activity involved. One study examined the relationship between self-esteem and Facebook use in a sample of some 200 college students (Manago, A.M., Taylor, T., & Greenfield, P.M. (2012). Me and my 400 friends: The anatomy of college students' Facebook networks, their communication patterns, and well-being. *Developmental Psychology*, *48*(2), 369–380. doi:10.1037/a0026338). Results indicated that self-esteem level was related to engaging in different online behaviours. For example, lower self-esteem was associated with feelings of connectedness to Facebook (that is, to the site itself), more frequently untagging of oneself in photos and accepting friend requests from acquaintances or strangers. In contrast, individuals with higher self-esteem were more likely to report that a positive aspect of Facebook was the ability to share pictures, thoughts and ideas, and that other people's posts could become annoying or bothersome. The conclusion was that individuals with low self-esteem use Facebook to accrue more friends and manage their profiles. Then again, perhaps large audiences inflate self-esteem, and if so those who use Facebook to accrue large networks are potentially at risk of developing unhealthy estimates of their own worth (Gonzales, A.L., & Hancock, J.T. (2011). Mirror, mirror on my Facebook wall: Effects of exposure to Facebook on self-esteem. *Cyberpsychology, Behavior, and Social Networking, 14*(1–2), 79–83. doi: 10.1089/cyber.2009.0411). Meanwhile, participants who also view others' profile pages do not have as high self-esteem as those who focus solely on their own profiles (Gonzales & Hancock, 2011: see above). Accordingly, another study found that those who focused on their own Facebook page had higher levels of self-esteem than a control group (Gentile, B., Twenge, J.M., Freeman, E.C., & Campbell, W.K. (2012). The effect of social networking websites on positive self-views: An experimental investigation. *Computers in Human Behavior, 28*(5), 1929–1933. doi:10.1016/j.chb.2012.05.012). Again, perhaps predictably, individualistic, self-focused social networking has the strongest association with rating yourself highly. However, these studies may only be highlighting correlations between those who most enjoy Facebook and high self-esteem. Does social networking simply reinforce the high opinion of individuals who already have robust self-esteem, or can it actually increase the levels of self-esteem in those who are not so confident in themselves? A critical determinant of any positive effects of social network use is the type of feedback users receive from their Facebook audience (Valkenburg, P.M., Peter, J., & Schouten, M.A. (2006). Friend networking sites and their relationship to adolescents' well-being and social self-esteem. *CyberPsychology & Behavior, 9*(5), 584–590. doi:10.1089/cpb.2006.9.584).

30 Valkenburg, Peter, & Schouten, 2006 (see n. 29).

31 Valkenburg, Peter, & Schouten, 2006 (see n. 29).

32 Facebook cull: Top reasons to unfriend someone. (2013, July 3). Retrieved from http://www.huffingtonpost.co.uk/2013/07/03/facebook-reasons-to-unfriend-someone_n_3541249.html

33 Forest, A.L., & Wood, J.V. (2012). When social networking is not working: Individuals with low self-esteem recognise but do not reap the benefits

of self-disclosure on Facebook. *Psychological Science, 23*(3), 295–302. doi:10.1177/0956797611429709

34 Manago, Taylor, & Greenfield, 2012 (see n. 29).

35 Manago, Taylor, & Greenfield, 2012 (see n. 29).

36 Qiu, L., Lin, H., Leung, A.K., & Tov, W. (2012). Putting their best foot forward: Emotional disclosure on Facebook. *Cyberpsychology, Behavior, and Social Networking, 15*(10), 569–572. doi:10.1089/cyber.2012.0200

37 Sigman, A. (2009). Well connected? The biological implications of 'social networking'. *Biologist, 56*(1), 14–20. Retrieved from http://www.aricsigman.com/IMAGES/Sigman_lo.pdf

38 Kidscape (2011). *Young people's cyber life survey*. Retrieved from http://www.kidscape.org.uk/resources/surveys/

39 Kanai, R., Bahrami, B., Roylance, & Rees, G. (2011). Online social network size is reflected in human brain structure. *Proceedings of the Royal Society Biological Sciences, 279*(1732), 1327–1334. doi:10.1098/rspb.2011.1959

40 Turkle, S. (2012). *Alone together: Why we expect more from technology and less from each other*. New York: Basic Books.

41 James, O. (2008). *Affluenza*. London: Vermilion.

42 Krasnova, H., Wenninger, H., Widjaja, T., & Buxmann, P. (2013). Envy on Facebook: A hidden threat to users' life satisfaction? In *11th International Conference on Wirtschaftsinformatik*. Leipzig, Germany.

43 Marshall, T.C. (2012). Facebook surveillance of former romantic partners: Associations with post-breakup recovery and personal growth. *Cyberpsychology, Behavior, and Social Networking, 15*(10), 521–526. doi:10.1089/cyber.2012.0125

44 Tong, S.T., Van Der Heide, B., Langwell, L., & Walther, J.B. (2008). Too much of a good thing? The relationship between number of friends and interpersonal impressions on Facebook. *Journal of Computer-Mediated Communication, 13*, 531–549. doi:10.1111/j.1083-6101.2008.00409.x

45 Klout scores are then supplemented with three nominally more specific measures, which Klout calls 'true reach', 'amplification' and 'network impact'. True reach is based on the amount of influence, determined by the number of followers and friends who actively listen and react to one's online messages; the amplification score relates to the likelihood that one's messages will generate actions (retweets, @messages, likes and comments); the network score reflects the influence that a person's engaged audience has.

46 Llenas, B. (2011, November 3). Klout CEO Fernandez responds to critics, gives insider tips and thinks ahead. Retrieved from http://latino.foxnews.

com/latino/community/2011/11/03/klout-ceo-fernandez-responds-to-critics-gives-tips-and-talks-future/

[47] Bates, D. (2011, June 17). Leaving Facebook? You can try . . . but 'evil genius' social network won't make it easy. Retrieved from http://www.dailymail.co.uk/sciencetech/article-2004610/Leaving-Facebook-You-try--evil-genius-social-network-wont-make-easy.html

[48] Stieger, S., Burger, C., Bohn, M., & Voracek, M. (in press). Who commits virtual identity suicide? Differences in privacy concerns, Internet addiction, and personality between Facebook users and quitters. *Cyberpsychology, Behavior, and Social Networking*. doi:10.1089/cyber.2012.0323

Chapter 11 SOCIAL NETWORKING AND RELATIONSHIPS

[1] Plato (1925). *Plato in Twelve Volumes*. (H.N. Fowler, Trans.). Cambridge, MA: Harvard University Press; London: William Heinemann Ltd. Retrieved from http://www.perseus.tufts.edu/hopper/text?doc=Perseus%3Atext%3A1999.01.0174%3Atext%3DPhaedrus%3Apage%3D275

[2] Quoted in http://stakeholders.ofcom.org.uk/market-data-research/market-data/communications-market-reports/cmr12/market-context/

[3] Ofcom (2012, July 18). *The communications market report 2012*. Retrieved from http://media.ofcom.org.uk/files/2012/07/CMR_analyst_briefing_180712.pdf

[4] Ofcom, 2012 (see n. 3).

[5] Seltzer, L.J., Prososki, A.R., Ziegler, T.E., & Pollak, S.D. (2012). Instant messages vs. speech: Hormones and why we still need to hear each other. *Evolution and Human Behavior, 33*, 42–45. doi:10.1016/j.evolhumbehav.2011.05.004

[6] Lord, L. (2013, 14 January). Generation Y, dating and technology: Digital natives struggle to connect offline. Retrieved from http://www.huffingtonpost.ca/2013/01/14/generation-y-online-dating-technology-relationships_n_2457722.html

[7] Turkle, S. (2012). *Alone together: Why we expect more from technology and less from each other*. New York: Basic Books, p. 1.

[8] Howard-Jones, P. (2011). *The impact of digital technologies on human wellbeing: Evidence from the sciences of mind and brain*. Retrieved from http://www.nominettrust.org.uk/sites/default/files/NT%20SoA%20-%20The%20impact%20of%20digital%20technologies%20on%20human%20wellbeing.pdf, p. 17.

[9] Burke, M., Kraut, R., & Marlow, C. (2011). Social capital on Facebook: Differentiating uses and users. *Proceedings of the SIGCHI Conference on*

Human Factors in Computing Systems, 573–580. doi:10.1145/1978942.1979023

10 Bessière, K., Kiesler, S., Kraut, R., & Boneva, B.S. (2008). Effects of Internet use and social resources on changes in depression. *Information, Communication, and Society, 11*(1), 47–70. doi:10.1080/13691180701858851

11 Valkenburg, P.M., & Peter, J. (2007). Preadolescents' and adolescents' online communication and their closeness to friends. *Developmental Psychology, 43*(2), 267–277. doi:10.1037/0012-1649.43.2.267

12 Grieve, R., Indian, M., Witteveen, K., Tolan, G.A., & Marrington, J. (2013). Face-to-face or Facebook: Can social connectedness be derived online? *Computers in Human Behavior, 29*(3), 604–609. doi:10.1016/j.chb.2012.11.017

13 Pollet, T.V., Roberts, S.G.B., & Dunbar, R.I.M. (2011). Use of social network sites and instant messaging does not lead to increased offline social network size, or to emotionally closer relationships with offline network members. *Cyberpsychology, Behavior, and Social Networking, 14*(4), 253–258. doi:10.1089/cyber.2010.0161

14 Di Pellegrino, G., Fadiga, L., Fogassi, L., Gallese, V., & Rizzolatti, G. (1992). Understanding motor events: A neurophysiological study. *Experimental Brain Research, 91*, 176–180. Retrieved from http://www.fulminiesaette.it/_uploads/foto/legame/DiPellegrinoEBR92.pdf

15 Sagi, A., & Hoffman, M.L. (1976). Empathic distress in the newborn. *Developmental Psychology, 12*(2), 175–176. doi:10.1037/0012-1649.12.2.175

16 Knafo, A., Zahn-Waxler, C., Van Hulle, C., Robinson, J.L., & Rhee, S.H. (2008). The developmental origins of a disposition toward empathy: Genetic and environmental contributions. *Emotion, 8*(6), 737–752. doi:10.1037/a001417

17 Ioannidou, F., & Konstantikaki, V. (2008). Empathy and emotional intelligence: What is it really about? *International Journal of Caring Science, 1*(3), 118–123. Retrieved from http://www.caringsciences.org/volume001/issue3/Vol1_Issue3_03_Ioannidou_Abstract.pdf, p. 118.

18 Konrath, S.H., O'Brien, E.H., & Hsing, C. (2011). Changes in dispositional empathy in American college students over time: A meta-analysis. *Personality and Social Psychology Review, 15*(2), 180–198. doi:10.1177/1088868310377395

19 McPherson, M., Smith-Lovin, L., & Brashears, M.E. (2006). Social isolation in America: Changes in core discussion networks over two decades. *American Sociological Review, 71*(3), 353–375. doi:10.1177/000312240607100301

20 Rosen, L.D. (2012). *iDisorder: Understanding our obsession with technology and overcoming its hold on us*. New York: Palgrave Macmillan.

[21] Engelberg, E., & Sjöberg, L. (2004). Internet use, social skills, and adjustment. *CyberPsychology & Behavior, 7*(1), 41–47. doi:10.1089/109493104322820101

[22] He, J.B., Liu, C.J., Guo, Y.Y., & Zhao, L. (2011). Deficits in early stage face perception in excessive Internet users. *Cyberpsychology, Behavior, and Social Networking, 14*(5), 303–308. doi:10.1089/cyber.2009.0333

[23] McDowell, M.J. (2004). Autism, early narcissistic injury and self-organization: A role for the image of the mother's eyes? *Journal of Analytical Psychology, 49*(4), 495–520. doi:10.1111/j.0021-8774.2004.00481.x

[24] Waldman, M., Nicholson, S., & Adilov, N. (2006). *Does television cause autism?* Working Paper No. 12632. Cambridge, MA: National Bureau of Economic Research. Waldman, M., Nicholson, S., & Adilov, N. (2012). *Positive and negative mental health consequences of early childhood television watching*. Working Paper No. 17786. Cambridge, MA: National Bureau of Economic Research.

[25] Hertz-Picciotto, I., & Delwiche, L. (2009). The rise in autism and the role of age at diagnosis. *Epidemiology, 20*(1), 84–90. doi:10.1097/EDE.0b013e3181902d15

[26] Amodio, D.M., & Frith, C.D. (2006). Meeting of minds: The medial frontal cortex and social cognition. *Nature Reviews Neuroscience, 7*, 268–277. doi:10.1038/nrn1884

[27] Finkenauer, C., Pollman, M.M.H., Begeer, S., & Kerkhof, P. (2012). Examining the link between autistic traits and compulsive Internet use in a non-clinical sample. *Journal of Autism and Developmental Disorders, 42*, 2252–2256. doi:10.1007/s10803-012-1465-4

[28] About ECHOES (n.d.). Retrieved from http://echoes2.org/?q=node/2

[29] Clayton, R. B., Nagurney, A., & Smith, J. R. (2013). Cheating, breakup, and divorce: Is Facebook use to blame? *Cyberpsychology, Behavior, and Social Networking, 16/10*(717–720), 2152–2723. doi:10.1089/cyber.2012.0424

[30] Anderson, B., Fagan, P., Woodnutt, T., & Chamorro-Prezumic, T. (2012). Facebook psychology: Popular questions answered by research. *Psychology of Popular Media Culture, 1*(1), 23–37. doi:10.1037/a0026452

[31] Marshall, T.C. (2012). Facebook surveillance of former romantic partners: Associations with post-breakup recovery and personal growth. *Cyberpsychology, Behavior, and Social Networking, 15*(10), 521-526. doi:10.1089/cyber.2012.0125

[32] Marshall, 2012 (see n. 31), p. 521.

[33] Stern, L.A., & Taylor, K. (2007). Social networking on Facebook. *Journal of the Communication, Speech & Theatre Association of North Dakota, 20*,

9-20. Retrieved from http://www.cstand.org/userfiles/file/journal/2007.pdf#page=9

34 Tokunaga, R.S. (2011). Social networking site or social surveillance site? Understanding the use of interpersonal electronic surveillance in romantic relationships. *Computers in Human Behavior,* 27(2), 705-713. doi:10.1016/j.chb.2010.08.014

35 Muise, A., Christofides, E., & Desmarais, S. (2009). More information than you ever wanted: Does Facebook bring out the green-eyed monster of jealousy? *CyberPsychology & Behavior, 12*(4), 441-444. doi:10.1089/cpb.2008.0263. Muscanell, N.L., Guadagno, R.E., Rice, L., & Murphy S. (2013). Don't it make my brown eyes green? An analysis of Facebook use and romantic jealousy. *Cyberpsychology, Behavior and Social Networking, 16*(4), 237-242. doi:10.1089/cyber.2012.0411

36 Facebook fuelling divorce, research claims (2009, December 21). Retrieved from http://www.telegraph.co.uk/technology/facebook/6857918/Facebook-fuelling-divorce-research-claims.html

37 Facebook fuelling divorce, research claims, 2009 (see n. 36).

Chapter 12 SOCIAL NETWORKING AND SOCIETY

1 Maag, C. (2012, November). A hoax turned fatal draws anger but no charges. Retrieved from: http://www.nytimes.com/2007/11/28/us/28hoax.html?_r=0

2 LeBlanc, J.C. (2012, October). Cyberbullying and suicide: A retrospective analysis of 22 cases. *AAP Experience National Conference & Exhibition Council on School Health*. Retrieved from https://aap.confex.com/aap/2012/webprogram/Paper18782.html

3 Tokunaga, R.S. (2010). Following you home from school: A critical review and synthesis of research on cyberbullying victimization. *Computers in Human Behavior, 26*(3), 277-287. doi:10.1016/j.chb.2009.11.014

4 Lehart, L., Madden. M., Smith, A., Purcell, K., Zickuhr, & K., Rainie, L. (2011). *Teens, kindness and cruelty on social network sites*. Retrieved from http://pewinternet.org/Reports/2011/Teens-and-social-media.aspx, pp. 26-27.

5 de Balzac, H. (2010). *Father Goriot*. (E. Marriage, Trans). The Project Gutenberg Ebook. Retrieved from http://www.gutenberg.org/files/1237/1237-h/1237-h.htm (Original work published 1835.)

6 Volk, A.A., Camilleri, J.A., Dane, A.V., & Marini, Z.A. (2012). Is adolescent bullying an evolutionary adaptation? *Aggressive Behavior, 38*(3), 222-238. doi:10.1002/ab.21418

[7] Olweus, D. (2012). Cyberbullying: An overrated phenomenon? *European Journal of Developmental Psychology, 9*(5), 520–538. doi:10.1080/17405629.2012.682358, p. 529.

[8] Bonanno, R.A., & Hymel, S. (2013). Cyber bullying and internalizing difficulties: Above and beyond the impact of traditional forms of bullying. *Journal of Youth and Adolescence, 42*(5), 685–697. doi:10.1007/s10964-013-9937-1

[9] Pornari, C. D., & Wood, J. (2010). Peer and cyber aggression in secondary school students: The role of moral disengagement, hostile attribution bias, and outcome expectancies. *Aggressive Behavior, 36*(2), 81–94. doi:10.1002/ab.20336

[10] Bandura, A. (1986). *Social foundation of thought and action: A social cognitive theory*. Englewood Cliffs, NJ: Prentice Hall.

[11] Pornari & Wood, 2010 (see n. 9).

[12] Perren, S., & Gutzwiller-Helfenfinger, E. (2012). Cyberbullying and traditional bullying in adolescence: Differential roles of moral disengagement, moral emotions, and moral values. *European Journal of Developmental Psychology, 9*(2), 195–209. doi:10.1080/17405629.2011.643168

[13] Robson, C., & Witenberg, R.T. (2013). The influence of moral disengagement, morally based self-esteem, age, and gender on traditional and cyber bullying. *Journal of School Violence, 12*, 211–231. doi:10.1080/15388220.2012.762921

[14] Hardaker, C. (2010). Trolling in asynchronous computer-mediated communication: From user discussions to academic definitions. *Journal of Politeness Research: Language, Behaviour, Culture*, 6(2), 215–242. doi: 10.1515/jplr.2010.011

[15] Carey, T. (2011, September 24). 'Help me, mummy. It's hot here in hell': A special investigation into the distress of grieving families caused by the sick Internet craze 'trolling'. Retrieved from http://www.dailymail.co.uk/news/article-2041193/Internet-trolling-Investigation-distress-grieving-families-caused-trolls.html

[16] Quoted in Paton, G. (2010, October). Facebook 'encourages children to spread gossip and insults'. Retrieved from http://www.telegraph.co.uk/education/educationnews/8067093/Facebook-encourages-children-to-spread-gossip-and-insults.html

[17] Jackson, L.A., & Wang, J.L. (2013). Cultural differences in social networking site use: A comparative study of China and the United States. *Computers in Human Behavior, 29*(3), 910–921. doi:10.1016/j.chb.2012.11.024

[18] Anderson, B., Fagan, P., Woodnutt, T., & Chamorro-Prezumic, T. (2012). Facebook psychology: Popular questions answered by research. *Psychology of Popular Media Culture, 1*(1), 23–37. doi:10.1037/a0026452

19 Huang, C. (2011, June 6). Facebook and Twitter key to Arab Spring uprisings: Report. Retrieved from http://www.thenational.ae/news/uae-news/facebook-and-twitter-key-to-arab-spring-uprisings-report

20 Waldorf, L. (2012). White noise: Hearing the disaster. *Journal of Human Rights Practice, 4*(3), 469–474. doi:10.1093/jhuman/hus025

21 Flores, A., & James, C. (2013). Morality and ethics behind the screen: Young people's perspectives on digital life. *New Media & Society, 15*, 834–852. doi:10.1177/1461444812462842

22 Donne, J. (1839). Devotions upon emergent occasions. In H. Alfred (Ed.), The works of John Donne (pp. 574- 575). Retrieved from http://www.luminarium.org/sevenlit/donne/meditation17.php

Chapter 13 THE *SOMETHING* ABOUT VIDEO GAMES

1 Entertainment Software Association (2013). *Essential facts about the computer and video game industry*. Retrieved from http://www.theesa.com/facts/pdfs/esa_ef_2013.pdf

2 Entertainment Software Association, 2013 (see n. 1).

3 Lazzaro, N. (2004). *Why we play games: Four keys to more emotion without story*. Retrieved from http://www.xeodesign.com/xeodesign_whyweplaygames.pdf

4 D'Angelo, W. (2012, April 23). Top 10 in sales – first person shooters [Weblog post]. Retrieved from http://www.vgchartz.com/article/250080/top-10-in-sales-first-person-shooters/

5 Demetrovics, Z., Urbán, R., Nagygyörgy, K., Farkas, J., Zilahy, D., Mervó, B., . . . & Harmath, E. (2011). Why do you play? The development of the motives for online gaming questionnaire (MOGQ). *Behaviour Research Methods, 43*(3), 814–825. doi:10.3758/s13428-011-0091-y. Yee, N. (2006). Motivations for play in online games. *CyberPsychology & Behavior, 9*(6), 772–775. doi:10.1089/cpb.2006.9.772

6 Kuss, D. J., & Griffiths, M. D. (2012). Internet gaming addiction: A systematic review of empirical research. *International Journal of Mental Health and Addiction, 10*(2), 278–296. doi:10.1007/s11469-011-9138-5

7 Hopson, J. (2001, April 27). Behavioural game design. Retrieved from http://www.gamasutra.com/view/feature/3085/behavioral_game_design.php

8 Yee, N. (2002). Facets: 5 motivation factors for why people play MMORPG's. Retrieved from http://www.nickyee.com/facets/home.html

9 The reason that Internet addiction studies are included is because cyberpsychologists are currently unclear as to whether video game addiction is the same thing as Internet addiction. Ten years ago, when lots of these

studies were being done, the two were conflated, as researchers assumed Internet addiction was the same thing as video game addiction, or that video game addiction was a manifestation of Internet addiction. Thus, researchers looked at Internet addiction in samples of excessive video gamers. We would be unable to gain a complete picture of the current literature without also including Internet addiction.

10 Kuss & Griffiths (2012). Hur, M.H. (2012). Current trends of internet addiction disorder research: A review of 2000-2008 Korean academic journal articles. *Asia Pacific Journal of Social Work and Development, 22*(3), 187-201. doi:10.1080/02185385.2012.691718

11 Back in 1998, and therefore predating widespread video gaming on the Internet, Dr Kimberly Young modified pre-existing criteria used to diagnose pathological gambling in order to suggest that pathological Internet use shared similar features: preoccupation, tolerance, withdrawal, failure to control, longer use than intended, functional impairment, lying and escape (Young, K.S. (1998). Internet addiction: The emergence of a new clinical disorder. *CyberPsychology & Behavior, 1*(3), 237-244. doi:10.1089/cpb.1998.1.237). As the director of the Centre for Internet Addiction Recovery, Dr Young takes the view that 'Internet addicts suffer from emotional problems such as depression and anxiety-related disorders and often use the fantasy world of the Internet to psychologically escape unpleasant feelings or stressful situations' (Young, K. (2012, March 15). FAQs. Retrieved from http://netaddiction.com/faqs/). Consequences include regular loss of sleep, changes to diet, relationship difficulties, damage to real-world social life, loss of income or employment, poorer academic performance, irritability or anxiety when not using the Internet and an inability to cut back or stop Internet use. As if that weren't enough, excessive use has been linked to higher levels of hostility, stress, loneliness, depression and increased suicidal thoughts (Ko, C.H., Yen, J.Y., Yen, C.F., Chen, C.S., & Chen, C.C. (2012). The association between Internet addiction and psychiatric disorder: A review of the literature. *European Psychiatry, 27*(1), 1-8. doi:10.1016/j.eurpsy.2010.04.011). Another lobbyist is David Greenfield (no relation), who heads up the Center for Internet Behaviour in Connecticut and is the author of *Virtual Addiction* (Greenfield, D.N. (1999). *Virtual Addiction: Help for netheads, cyberfreaks, and those who love them*. Oakland, CA: New Harbinger). Greenfield believes that some services available over the Internet offer an unprecedented and alluring cocktail of stimulating content, ease of access, convenience, low cost, visual stimulation, autonomy and anonymity, all of which contribute to a highly psychoactive experience. Defining 'psychoactive' as mood altering,

and potentially behaviourally impacting, Greenfield claims that online sex, gaming, gambling and shopping can all produce a mood-altering effect, suggesting that a wide variety of Internet activities could all be lumped together as 'addictive'.

12 Signs of gaming addiction in adults. (n.d.). Retrieved from http://www.video-game-addiction.org/internet-addictions-adults.html

13 Starcevic, V. (2013). Is Internet addiction a useful concept? *Australian and New Zealand Journal of Psychiatry, 47*(1), 16–19. doi:10.1177/0004867412461693

14 In the United States, a review of excessive Internet use in youths showed prevalence ranged between 0 and 26.3% (Moreno M.A., Jelenchick, L., Cox, E., Young, H., & Christakis, D.A. (2011). Problematic Internet use among US youth: A systematic review. *Archives of Pediatrics & Adolescent Medicine, 165*(9), 797–805. doi:10.1001/archpediatrics.2011.58). Meanwhile, in Hong Kong, Daniel Shek, a psychology professor at the Polytechnic University and an expert on 'healthy parenting', came up with an estimated prevalence of Internet addiction of 20% in Chinese adolescents (Shek, D.T., Tang, V.M., & Lo, C.Y. (2008). Internet addiction in Chinese adolescents in Hong Kong: Assessment, profiles, and psychosocial correlates. *Scientific World Journal, 8*, 776–787. doi:10.1100/tsw.2008.104). In contrast, in a European study Konstantinos Siomos, a child and adolescent psychiatrist and chair of the Hellenic Society for the Study of Internet Addiction Disorder, surveyed over 2,000 Greek teenagers, again sampled using a diagnostic questionnaire of Internet addiction. Siomos found that the prevalence of Internet addiction was 8.2% (Siomos, K.E., Dafouli, E.D., Braimiotis, D.A., Mouzas, O.D., & Angelopoulos, N.V. (2008). Internet addiction among Greek adolescent students. *CyberPsychology & Behavior, 11*(6), 653–657. doi:10.1089/cpb.2008.0088). A review of the publications produced until the end of 2009 showed, from different studies mainly conducted in the Far East, highly varied prevalence rates of Internet addiction (Ko et al., 2012: see n. 11).

15 Gentile, D. (2009). Pathological video-game use among youth ages 8 to 18: A national study. *Psychological Science, 20*(5), 594–602. doi:10.1111/j.1467-9280.2009.02340.x

16 Kuss & Griffiths, 2012 (see n. 6).

17 Gentile, D.A., Choo, H., Liau, A., Sim, T., Li, D., Fung, D., & Khoo, A. (2011). Pathological video game use among youths: A two-year longitudinal study. *Pediatrics, 127*(2), 319–329. doi:10.1542/peds.2010-1353

18 Weinstein, A., & Lejoyeux, M. (2010). Internet addiction or excessive Internet use. *American Journal of Drug and Alcohol Abuse, 36*(5), 277–283. doi:10.3109/00952990.2010.491880

[19] Weinstein, A.M. (2010). Computer and video game addiction: A comparison between game users and non-game users. *American Journal of Drug and Alcohol Abuse, 36*(5), 268–276. doi:10.3109/00952990.2010.491879

[20] The ventral striatum is the lower part and the dorsal striatum the upper part of a large area, the striatum, which occupies a large central part of the brain in all mammals. In higher animals the striatum is subdivided into the upper part, called the putamen, and the lower, the caudate nucleus. Within the ventral striatum/caudate nucleus, another area, the nucleus accumbens, is a dopamine-rich region closely linked to drug addiction. The striatum is also directly and reciprocally connected to the substantia nigra, the primary site of degeneration in Parkinson's disease, a movement disorder. There is no single 'function' for the striatum which has diffuse and complex anatomical connections and which has been related to a variety of processes ranging from reward to movement.

[21] Kühn, S., Romanowski, A., Schilling, C., Lorenz, R., Mörsen, C., Seiferth, N., . . . & Gallinat, J. (2011). The neural basis of video gaming. *Translational Psychiatry, 1*(11), e53. doi:10.1038/tp.2011.53

[22] Linnet, J., Peterson, E., Doudet, D.J., Gjedde, A., & Moller, A. (2010). Dopamine release in ventral striatum of pathological gamblers losing money. *Acta Psychiatrica Scandinavica, 112*(4), 326–333. doi:10.1111/j.1600-0447.2010.01591.x

[23] Kühn et al., 2011 (see n. 21).

[24] Erickson, K.I., Boot, W.R., Basak, C., Neider, M.B., Prakash, R.S., Voss, M.W., . . . & Kramer, A.F. (2010). Striatal volume predicts level of video game skill acquisition. *Cerebral Cortex, 20*(11), 2522–2530. doi:10.1093/cercor/bhp293

[25] Drevets, W.C., Price, J.C., Kupfer, D.J., Kinahan, P.E., Lopresti, B., Holt, D., & Mathis, C. (1999). PET measures of amphetamine-induced dopamine release in ventral versus dorsal striatum. *Neuropsychopharmacology, 21*(6), 694–709. doi:10.1016/S0893-133X(99)00079-2

[26] Robbins, T. W., & Everitt, B. J. (1992). Functions of dopamine in the dorsal and ventral striatum. *Seminars in Neuroscience, 4*(2), 119–127. Retrieved from http://www.sciencedirect.com/science/article/pii/104457659290010Y. MacDonald, P.A., MacDonald, A.A., Seergobin, K.N., Tamjeedi, R., Ganjavi, H., Provost, J.S., & Monchi, O. (2011). The effect of dopamine therapy on ventral and dorsal striatum-mediated cognition in Parkinson's disease: Support from functional MRI. *Brain, 134*(5), 1447–1463. doi:10.1093/brain/awr075

[27] Koepp, M.J., Gunn, R.N., Lawrence, A.D., Cunningham, V.J., Dagher, A., Jones, T., . . . & Grasby, P.M. (1998). Evidence for striatal dopamine release during a video game. *Nature, 393*(6682), 266–267. doi:10.1038/30498

28 Metcalf, O., & Pammer, K. (2014). Sub-types of gaming addiction: Physiological arousal deficits in addicted gamers differ based on preferred genre. *European Addiction Research, 20*(1), 23–32. doi:10.1159/000349907
29 Han, D.H., Lee, Y.S., Yang, K.C., Kim, E.Y., Lyoo, I.K., & Renshaw, P.F. (2007). Dopamine genes and reward dependence in adolescents with excessive Internet video game play. *Journal of Addiction Medicine, 1*(3), 133–138. doi:10.1097/ADM.0b013e31811f465f
30 Lush, T. (2011, August 29). At war with *World of Warcraft*: An addict tells his story. Retrieved from http://www.theguardian.com/technology/2011/aug/29/world-of-warcraft-video-game-addict
31 King, D.L., Delfabbro, P.H., & Griffiths, M.D. (2011). The role of structural characteristics in problematic video game play: An empirical study. *International Journal of Mental Health and Addiction, 9*(3), 320–333. doi:10.1007/s11469-010-9289-y
32 Lazzaro, 2004 (see n. 3).
33 Trepte, S., & Reinecke, L. (2010). Avatar creation and video game enjoyment: Effects of life-satisfaction, game competitiveness, and identification with the avatar. *Journal of Media Psychology: Theories, Methods, and Applications,* 22(4), 171–184. doi:10.1027/1864-1105/a000022
34 Bavelier, D., Green, C.S., & Dye, M.W. (2010). Children, wired: For better and for worse. *Neuron, 67*(5), 692–701. doi:10.1016/j.neuron.2010.08.035, p. 698.
35 Nunneley, S. (2013, April 30). Guardian analysis of top 50 games sold in 2012 found 'more than half contain violent content labels' [Weblog post]. Retrieved from http://www.vg247.com/2013/04/30/guardian-analysis-of-top-50-games-sold-in-2012-found-more-than-half-contain-violent-content-labels/

Chapter 14 VIDEO GAMES AND ATTENTION

1 Dowd, M. (2011, December 6). Silence is golden. Retrieved from http://www.nytimes.com/2011/12/07/opinion/dowd-silence-is-golden.html?_r=0
2 Christakis, D.A., Zimmerman, F.J., DiGiuseppe, D.L., & McCarty, C.A. (2004). Early television exposure and subsequent attentional problems in children. *Pediatrics, 113*, 708–713. Retrieved from http://pediatrics.aappublications.org/content/113/4/708.short
3 Some experts think that video gaming is indeed more detrimental than TV. In his recent review, psychologist Paul Howard-Jones points to the difference between the two media in terms of the degree of personal involvement and interactivity. He concludes: 'In terms of content . . . it seems the internet

leisure activities popular with children, such as games, might not teach the types of attentional capabilities required for "paying attention" in the classroom and other contexts. Given the additional interactivity and the levels of psychological and cognitive engagement they can provide, a case can be made that some internet activities (such as games) might pose a greater threat to some attentional abilities other than television' (Howard-Jones, P. (2011). *The impact of digital technologies on human wellbeing: Evidence from the sciences of mind and brain*. Retrieved from http://www.nominettrust.org.uk/sites/default/files/NT%20SoA%20-%20The%20impact%20of%20digital%20technologies%20on%20human%20wellbeing.pdf).

4 Swing, E.L., Gentile, D.A., Anderson, C.A., & Walsh, D.A. (2010). Television and video game exposure and the development of attention problems. *Pediatrics, 126*(2), 214–221. doi:10.1542/peds.2009-1508

5 Swing et al., 2010 (see n. 4).

6 Gentile, D.A., Swing, E.L., Lim, C.G., & Khoo, A. (2012). Video game playing, attention problems, and impulsiveness: Evidence of bidirectional causality. *Psychology of Popular Media Culture, 1*(1), 62. doi:10.1037/a0026969

7 McKinley, R.A., McIntire, L.K., & Funke, M.A. (2011). Operator selection for unmanned aerial systems: Comparing video game players and pilots. *Aviation, Space and Environmental Medicine, 82*(6), 635–642. doi:10.3357/ASEM.2958.2011

8 Appelbaum, L.G., Cain, M.S., Darling, E.F., & Mitroff, S.R. (2013). Action video game playing is associated with improved visual sensitivity, but not alterations in visual sensory memory. *Attention, Perception, & Psychophysics,* 75(6), 1161–1167.

9 Quoted in Video gamers really do see more. (2013, June 11). *Duke Today*. Retrieved from http://today.duke.edu/2013/06/vidvision

10 Boot, W.R., Blakely, D.P., & Simons, D.J. (2011). Do action video games improve perception and cognition? *Frontiers in Psychology*, 2, 1–6. doi:10.3389/fpsyg.2011.00226

11 Bavelier, D., Green, C.S., Pouget, A., & Schrater, P. (2012). Brain plasticity through the life span: Learning to learn and action video games. *Annual Review of Neuroscience, 35*, 391–416. doi:10.1146/annurev-neuro-060909-152832. Castel, A.D., Pratt, J., & Drummond, E. (2005). The effects of action video game experience on the time course of inhibition of return and the efficiency of visual search. *Acta Psychologica, 119*(2), 217–230. doi:10.1016/j.actpsy.2005.02.004. Donohue, S.E., Woldorff, M.G., & Mitroff, S.R. (2010). Video game players show more precise multisensory temporal processing abilities. *Attention, Perception & Psychophysics,* 72(4), 1120–1129. doi:10.3758/APP.72.4.1120. Dye,

M.W.G., Green, C.S., & Bavelier, D. (2009). Increasing speed of processing with action video games. *Current Directions in Psychological Science, 18*(6), 321–326. doi:10.1111/j.1467-8721.2009.01660.x. Feng, J., Spence, I., & Pratt, J. (2007). Playing an action video game reduces gender differences in spatial cognition. *Psychological Science, 18*(10), 850–855. doi:10.1111/j.1467-9280.2007.01990.x. Green, C.S., & Bavelier, D. (2003). Action video game modifies visual selective attention. *Nature, 423*(6939), 534–537. Retrieved from http://www.nature.com/nature/journal/v423/n6939/abs/nature01647.html. Green, C.S., & Bavelier, D. (2007). Action-video-game experience alters the spatial resolution of vision. *Psychological Science, 18*(1), 88–94. doi:10.1111/j.1467-9280.2007.01853.x. Green, C.S., & Bavelier, D. (2012). Learning, attentional control, and action video games. *Current Biology,* 22(6), R197–R206. doi:10.1016/j.cub.2012.02.012. Green, C.S., Pouget, A., & Bavelier, D. (2010). Improved probabilistic inference as a general learning mechanism with action video games. *Current Biology,* 20, 1573–1579. doi:10.1016/j.cub.2010.07.040. Hubert-Wallander, B., Green, C.S., & Bavelier, D. (2011). Stretching the limits of visual attention: The case of action video games. *Wiley Interdisciplinary Reviews: Cognitive Science,* 2(2), 222–230. doi:10.1002/wcs.116. Subrahmanyam, K., & Greenfield, P.M. (1994). Effect of video game practice on spatial skills in girls and boys. *Journal of Applied Developmental Psychology, 15*(1), 13–32. doi:10.1016/0193-3973(94)90004-3

12 Green & Bavelier, 2003 (see n. 11), p. 536. The subjects were between 18 and 23 years old and divided into two separate groups. The video gamers were already familiar with playing action video games such as *Grand Theft Auto*, for a minimum of one hour a day, at least four days a week during the previous six months. The second group, the non-players, had had little or no video game usage in the previous six months.

13 See citations in n. 11.

14 Rosser, J.C.J., Lynch, P.J., Cuddihy, L., Gentile, D.A., & Klonsky, J., Merrell, R., & Curet, M. (2007). The impact of video games on training surgeons in the 21st century. *Archives of Surgery, 142*(2), 181–186. Retrieved from http://cat.inist.fr/?aModele=afficheN&cpsidt=18510967

15 What is Big Brain Academy? (n.d.). Retrieved from http://www.bigbrainacademy.com/ds/what/index.html

16 Boot, Blakely, & Simons, 2011 (see n. 10).

17 Han, D.H., Renshaw, P.F., Sim, M.E., Kim, J.I., Arenella, L.S., & Lyoo, I. K. (2008). The effect of Internet video game play on clinical and extrapyramidal symptoms in patients with schizophrenia. *Schizophrenia Research, 103*(1–3), 338–340. doi:10.1016/j.schres.2008.01.026

18 Bavelier, D., Green, C.S., Han, D.H., Renshaw, P.F., Merzenich, M.M., & Gentile, D.A. (2011). Brains on video games. *Nature Reviews Neuroscience, 12*(12), 763–768. doi:10.1038/nrn3135

19 Walshe, D.G., Lewis, E.J., Kim, S.I., O'Sullivan, K., & Wiederhold, B.K. (2003). Exploring the use of computer games and virtual reality in exposure therapy for fear of driving following a motor vehicle accident. *CyberPsychology & Behavior, 6*(3), 329–334. doi:10.1089/109493103322011641

20 Fernández-Aranda, F., Jiménez-Murcia, S., Santamaría, J.J., Gunnard, K., Soto, A., Kalapanidas, E., . . . & Penelo, E. (2012). Video games as a complementary therapy tool in mental disorders: PlayMancer, a European multicentre study. *Journal of Mental Health, 21*(4), 364–374. doi:10.3109/09638237.2012.664302

21 Gambotto-Burke, A. (2011, August 13). Hi-tech stimuli help to dull the pain. Retrieved from http://www.theaustralian.com.au/news/health-science/hi-tech-stimuli-help-to-dull-the-pain/story-e6frg8y6-1226113730661

22 Coyne, S.M., Padilla-Walker, L.M., Stockdale, L., & Day, R.D. (2011). Game on . . . girls: Associations between co-playing video games and adolescent behavioral and family outcomes. *Journal of Adolescent Health, 49*(2), 160–165. doi:10.1016/j.jadohealth.2010.11.249

23 Bessière, K., Seay, A. F., & Kiesler, S. (2007). The ideal elf: Identity exploration in *World of Warcraft*. *CyberPsychology & Behavior, 10*(4), 530–535. doi:10.1089/cpb.2007.9994

24 Xanthopoulou, D., & Papagiannidis, S. (2012). Play online, work better? Examining the spillover of active learning and transformational leadership. *Technological Forecasting and Social Change, 79*(7), 1328–1339. doi:10.1016/j.techfore.2012.03.006

25 Bailey, K., West, R., & Anderson, C.A. (2010). A negative association between video game experience and proactive cognitive control. *Psychophysiology, 47*(1), 34–42. doi:10.1111/j.1469-8986.2009.00925.x

26 Braver, T.S., Gray, J.R., & Burgess, G.C. (2007). Explaining the many varieties of working memory variation: Dual mechanisms of cognitive control. In A. Conway, C. Jarrold, M. J. Kane, A. Miyake & J. N. Towse (Eds.), *Variation in working memory* (pp. 76–106). Oxford: Oxford University Press.

27 Bailey, West, & Anderson, 2010 (see n. 25).

28 Ventura, M., Shute, V., & Zhao, W. (2013). The relationship between video game use and a performance-based measure of persistence. *Computers & Education, 60*(1), 52–58. doi:10.1016/j.compedu.2012.07.003

29 ADHD and ADD (attention deficit disorder) are general terms frequently used to describe individuals who have attention deficit hyperactivity disorder or, as the abbreviated name suggests, attention problems without

the hyperactive and impulsive behaviours. The terms ADHD and ADD are often used interchangeably both for those who do, and for those who do not, have symptoms of hyperactivity and impulsiveness, and for our purposes we can consider the two together under the same umbrella terminology relating to attentional problems.

30 Howard-Jones, 2011 (see n. 3), p. 52.

31 Parkes, A., Sweeting, H., Wight, D., Henderson, M. (2013). Do television and electronic games predict children's psychosocial adjustment? Longitudinal research using the UK Millennium Cohort Study. *Archives of Disease in Childhood, 98*(5), 341–348. doi:10.1136/archdischild-2011-301508

32 Researchers use terms such as 'excessive', 'obsessive', 'compulsive', 'pathological', 'harmful' and 'addictive' when referring to Internet use that results in harmful consequences to a user and an inability to control Internet use, as 'Internet addiction' is not a formally recognised disorder. These terms are used throughout to refer to the same behaviour – an inability to cut back or control Internet use, despite significant negative consequences.

33 Collins, E., Freeman, J., & Chamarro-Premuzic, T. (2012). Personality traits associated with problematic and non-problematic massively multiplayer online role playing game use. *Personality and Individual Differences, 52*(2), 133–138. doi:10.1016/j.paid.2011.09.015

34 Ha, J.H., Yoo, H.J., Cho, I.H., Chin, B., Shin, D., & Kim, J.H. (2006). Psychiatric comorbidity assessed in Korean children and adolescents who screen positive for Internet addiction. *Journal of Clinical Psychiatry, 67*(5), 821–826. doi:10.4088/JCP.v67n0517

35 Yen, J.Y., Ko, C.H., Yen, C.F., Wu, H.Y., & Yang, M.J. (2007). The comorbid psychiatric symptoms of Internet addiction: Attention deficit and hyperactivity disorder (ADHD), depression, social phobia, and hostility. *Journal of Adolescent Health, 41*, 93–98. doi:10.1016/j.jadohealth.2007.02.002

36 Swing et al., 2010 (see n. 4).

37 Chan, P.A., & Rabinowitz, T. (2006). A cross-sectional analysis of video games and attention deficit hyperactivity disorder symptoms in adolescents. *Annals of General Psychiatry, 5*(16), 5–16. doi:10.1186/1744-859X-5-16, p. 4.

38 Bioulac, S., Arfi, L., & Bouvard, M.P. (2008). Attention deficit/hyperactivity disorder and video games: A comparative study of hyperactive and control children. *European Psychiatry, 23*(2), 134–141. doi:10.1016/j.eurpsy.2007.11.002

39 Doward, J, & Craig, E. (2012, May 6). Ritalin use for ADHD children soars

fourfold. Retrieved from http://www.theguardian.com/society/2012/may/06/ritalin-adhd-shocks-child-psychologists

40 Zuvekas, S.H., & Vitiello, B. (2012). Stimulant medication use in children: A 12-year perspective. *American Journal of Psychiatry, 169*(2), 160–166. doi:10.1176/appi.ajp.2011.11030387

41 Hollingworth, S.A., Nissen, L. M., Stathis, S.S., Siskind, D.J., Varghese, J.M., & Scott, J.G. (2011). Australian national trends in stimulant dispensing: 2002–2009. *Australian and New Zealand Journal of Psychiatry, 45*(4), 332–336. doi:10.3109/00048674.2010.543413

42 A major thought to flag here, however, is that whatever findings may transpire on one group of subjects, we must always be aware of possible cultural factors making an all-important difference. For example, a Korean scientist, Seok Young Moon, all too aware of the issue, concluded: 'While investigating whether teachers' and parents' perspectives on ADHD are influenced by culture, I found that cultural influence plays an important role: In Korea, according to Confucianism, parents and teachers tend to focus more on children's academic achievement and take children's distractive behaviours as a negative reflection on themselves and their authority. Korean teachers and parents try to take personal responsibility for children's distractive behaviours, and have negative attitudes toward medication because the medication does not help to increase academic improvement. U.S. parents and teachers, influenced by western culture's focus on independence, tend not to take personal responsibility for the children's behaviours but to focus more on children's current problems and treatment. U.S. parents and teachers did not mind a third party's engagement in dealing with children with ADHD and their behaviours. U.S. parents were more positive about medical treatments because medication helps to reduce children's distractive behaviours' (Moon, S.Y. (n.d.). Cultural perspectives on attention deficit hyperactivity disorder: A comparison between Korea and the US. *Journal of International Business and Cultural Studies,* 1–11. Retrieved from http://ww.aabri.com/manuscripts/11898.pdf).

43 Turner, D.C., Robbins, T.W., Clark, L., Aron, A.R., Dowson, J., & Sahakian, B.J. (2003). Cognitive enhancing effects of modafinil in healthy volunteers. *Psychopharmacology, 165*(3), 260–269. doi:10.1007/s00213-002-1250-8

44 Han, D.H., Lee, Y.S., Na, C., Ahn, J.Y., Chung, U.S., Daniels, M.A., . . . & Renshaw, P.F. (2009). The effect of methylphenidate on Internet video game play in children with attention-deficit/hyperactivity disorder. *Comprehensive Psychiatry, 50*(3), 251–256. doi:10.1016/j.comppsych.2008.08.011, p. 251.

45 Howard-Jones, 2011 (see n. 3).

Chapter 15 VIDEO GAMES, AGGRESSION AND RECKLESSNESS

1 Fifty-six children aged 10 to 13 years named other children who displayed certain forms of physical and verbal aggressive behaviour that day, as well as evaluating the intentions of these aggressive behaviours, if any (Polman, H., De Castro, B.O., & van Aken, M.A. (2008). Experimental study of the differential effects of playing versus watching violent video games on children's aggressive behavior. *Aggressive Behavior, 34*(3), 256–264. doi:10.1002/ab.20245).

2 Griffiths, M. (1999). Violent video games and aggression: A review of the literature. *Aggression and Violent Behavior, 4*(2), 203–212. doi:10.1016/S1359-1789(97)00055-4. Dill, K.E., & Dill, J.C. (1999). Video game violence: A review of the empirical literature. *Aggression and Violent Behavior, 3*(4), 407–428. doi:10.1016/S1359-1789(97)00001-3. Anderson, C.A., & Dill, K.E. (2000). Video games and aggressive thoughts, feelings, and behavior in the laboratory and in life. *Journal of Personality and Social Psychology, 78*(4), 772–790. doi:10.1037/0022-3514.78.4.772

3 Konijn, E.A., Nije Bijvank, M., & Bushman, B.J. (2007). I wish I were a warrior: The role of wishful identification in the effects of violent video games on aggression in adolescent boys. *Developmental Psychology, 43*(4), 1038–1044. doi:10.1037/0012-1649.43.4.1038

4 Weaver, A.J., & Lewis, N. (2012). Mirrored morality: An exploration of moral choice in video games. *Cyberpsychology, Behavior, and Social Networking, 15*(11), 610–614. doi:10.1089/cyber.2012.0235

5 Weaver & Lewis, 2012 (see n. 4).

6 Anderson, C.A. (2003). Violent video games: Myths, facts, and unanswered questions. Retrieved from http://www.apa.org/science/about/psa/2003/10/anderson.aspx

7 Bavelier, D., Green, C.S., Han, D.H., Renshaw, P.F., Merzenich, M. M., & Gentile, D. A. (2011). Brains on video games. *Nature Reviews Neuroscience, 12*(12), 763–768. doi:10.1038/nrn3135, p.765.

8 These effects were also more marked for men than for women: given the far higher levels of testosterone in the male body, a tendency for aggression will be much more easily realised (Hasan, Y., Bègue, L., & Bushman, B.J. (2012). Viewing the world through 'blood-red tinted glasses': The hostile expectation bias mediates the link between violent video game exposure and aggression. *Journal of Experimental Social Psychology, 48*(4), 953–956. doi:10.1016/j.jesp.2011.12.019).

9 Ferguson, C.J. (2009). Violent video games: Dogma, fear, and pseudoscience. *Skeptical Inquirer, 33*, 38–43. Retrieved from http://www.tamiu.edu/~cferguson/skeptinq.pdf

[10] Olson, C.K. (2010). Children's motivations for video game play in the context of normal development. *Review of General Psychology, 14*(2), 180–187. doi:10.1037/a0018984

[11] Anderson, C.A., Sakamoto, A., Gentile, D.A., Ihori, N., Shibuya, A., Yukawa, S., . . . & Kobayashi, K. (2008). Longitudinal effects of violent video games on aggression in Japan and the United States. *Pediatrics, 122*(5), e1067–e1072. doi:10.1542/peds.2008-1425

[12] Möller, I., & Krahé, B. (2009). Exposure to violent video games and aggression in German adolescents: A longitudinal analysis. *Aggressive Behavior, 35*(1), 75–89. doi:10.1002/ab.20290

[13] Wallenius, M., & Punamäki, R.L. (2008). Digital game violence and direct aggression in adolescence: A longitudinal study of the roles of sex, age, and parent–child communication. *Journal of Applied Developmental Psychology, 29*(4), 286–294. doi:10.1016/j.appdev.2008.04.010

[14] Anderson, C.A., Shibuya, A., Ihori, N., Swing, E.L., Bushman, B.J., Sakamoto, A., . . . & Saleem, M. (2010). Violent video game effects on aggression, empathy, and prosocial behavior in eastern and western countries: A meta-analytic review. *Psychological Bulletin, 136*(2), 151. doi:10.1037/a0018251

[15] Ferguson, C.J., & Kilburn, J. (2010). Much ado about nothing: The misestimation and overinterpretation of violent video game effects in Eastern and Western nations: Comment on Anderson et al. (2010). *Psychological Bulletin, 136*(2), 174–178. doi:10.1037/a0018566

[16] Bushman, B.J., Rothstein, H. R., & Anderson, C.A. (2010). Much ado about something: Violent video game effects and a school of red herring: Reply to Ferguson and Kilburn (2010). *Psychological Bulletin, 136*(2), 182–187. doi:10.1037/a0018718

[17] Ferguson, 2009 (see n. 9). Gunter, W.D., & Daly, K. (2012). Causal or spurious: Using propensity score matching to detangle the relationship between violent video games and violent behavior. *Computers in Human Behavior, 28*(4), 1348–1355. doi:10.1016/j.chb.2012.02.020

[18] Carnagey, N.L., Anderson, C.A., & Bushman, B.J. (2007). The effect of video game violence on physiological desensitization to real-life violence. *Journal of Experimental Social Psychology, 43*(3), 489–496. doi:10.1016/j.jesp.2006.05.003

[19] Carnagey, Anderson, & Bushman, 2007 (see n. 18).

[20] Bushman, B.J., & Anderson, C.A. (2009). Comfortably numb desensitizing effects of violent media on helping others. *Psychological Science, 20*(3), 273–277. doi:10.1111/j.1467-9280.2009.02287.x

[21] Mathiak, K., & Weber, R. (2006). Toward brain correlates of natural

behavior: fMRI during violent video games. *Human Brain Mapping, 27*(12), 948–956. doi:10.1002/hbm.20234

22 Weber, R., Ritterfeld, U., & Mathiak, K. (2006). Does playing violent video games induce aggression? Empirical evidence of a functional magnetic resonance imaging study. *Media Psychology*, 8(1), 39–60. doi:10.1207/S1532785XMEP0801_44

23 Llinás, R.R., & Paré, D. (1991). Of dreaming and wakefulness. *Neuroscience, 44*(3), 521–535. doi.org/10.1016/0306-4522(91)90075-Y

24 Nunneley, S. (2013, April 30). Guardian analysis of top 50 games sold in 2012 found 'more than half contain violent content labels' [Weblog post]. Retrieved from http://www.vg247.com/2013/04/30/guardian-analysis-of-top-50-games-sold-in-2012-found-more-than-half-contain-violent-content-labels/

25 Harlow, J.M. (1993). Recovery from the passage of an iron bar through the head. *History of Psychiatry, 4*(14), 274–281. Retrieved from http://hpy.sagepub.com/content/4/14/274.short, p. 1673.

26 Tataranni, P.A., & DelParigi, A. (2003). Functional neuroimaging: A new generation of human brain studies in obesity research. *Obesity Reviews, 4*(4), 229–238. doi:0.1046/j.1467-789X.2003.00111.x

27 Tanabe, J., Thompson, L., Claus, E., Dalwani, M., Hutchison, K., & Banich, M.T. (2007). Prefrontal cortex activity is reduced in gambling and nongambling substance users during decision-making. *Human Brain Mapping, 28*(12), 1276–1286. doi:10.1002/hbm.20344

28 Callicott, J.H., Bertolino, A., Mattay, V.S., Langheim, F.J., Duyn, J., Coppola, R., . . . & Weinberger, D.R. (2000). Physiological dysfunction of the dorsolateral prefrontal cortex in schizophrenia revisited. *Cerebral Cortex, 10*(11), 1078–1092. doi:10.1093/cercor/10.11.1078

29 Welsh, M. C., & Pennington, B. F. (1988). Assessing frontal lobe functioning in children: Views from developmental psychology. *Developmental Neuropsychology, 4*(3), 199–230. doi:10.1080/87565648809540405

30 Davis,. C., Levitan, R.D., Muglia, P., Bewell, C., & Kennedy, J.L. (2004). Decision-making deficits and overeating: A risk model for obesity. *Obesity Research, 12*(6), 929–935. doi:10.1038/oby.2004.113. Pignatti, R., Bertella, L., Albani, G., Mauro, A., Molinari, E., & Semenza, C. (2006). Decision-making in obesity: A study using the Gambling Task. *Eating and Weight Disorders: EWD, 11*(3), 126–132. Retrieved from http://www.ncbi.nlm.nih.gov/pubmed/17075239

31 Oltmanns, T.F. (1978). Selective attention in schizophrenic and manic psychoses: The effect of distraction on information processing. *Journal of Abnormal Psychology, 87*(2), 212–225. Retrieved from http://www.

ncbi.nlm.nih.gov/pubmed/649860. Parsons, B., Gandhi, S., Aurbach, E. L., Williams, N., Williams, M., Wassef, A., & Eagleman, D. M. (2012). Lengthened temporal integration in schizophrenia. *Neuropsychologia, 51*(2), 372–376. doi:10.1016/j.neuropsychologia.2012.11.008

32 Kasanin, J.S. (Ed.) (1944). *Language and thought in schizophrenia*. Berkeley, CA: University of California Press. In the case of schizophrenics, where there is an imbalance of modulating, fountaining chemicals such as dopamine, it might be that excessive release of these powerful agents can suppress the connectivity, particularly in the prefrontal cortex (Ferron, A., Thierry, A.M., Le Douarin, C., & Glowinski, J. (1984) Inhibitory influence of the mesocortical dopaminerglc system on spontaneous activity or excitatory response induced from the thalamic mediodorsal nucleus in the rat medial prefrontal cortex. *Brain Research, 302*, 257–265. doi:10.1016/0006-8993(84)90238-5. Gao, W.J., Wang, Y., & Goldman-Rakic, P.S. (2003). Dopamine modulation of perisomatic and peridendritic inhibition in prefrontal cortex. *Journal of Neuroscience, 23*(5), 1622–1630. Retrieved from http://neurobio.drexel.edu/GaoWeb/papers/J.%20Neurosci.%202003.pdf), reducing the robustness of cognitive processes and thus enhancing disproportionately the impact of the incoming senses (Greenfield, S.A. (2001). *The private life of the brain: Emotions, consciousness, and the secret of the self*. New York: Wiley).

33 Tsujimoto, S. (2008). The prefrontal cortex: Functional neural development during early childhood. *The Neuroscientist, 14*, 345–358. doi:10.1177/1073858408316002

34 Shimamura, A.P. (1995). Memory and the prefrontal cortex. *Annals of the New York Academy of Sciences, 769*(1), 151–160. doi:10.1111/j.1749-6632.1995.tb38136.x

35 Ferron et al., 1984 (see n. 32).

36 Lazzaro, N. (2004). *Why we play games: Four keys to more emotion without story*. Retrieved from http://www.xeodesign.com/xeodesign_whyweplaygames.pdf

37 Fischer, P., Greitemeyer, T., Morton, T., Kastenmüller, A., Postmes, T., Frey, D., . . . & Odenwälder, J. (2009). The racing-game effect: Why do video racing games increase risk-taking inclinations? *Personality and Social Psychology Bulletin, 35*(10), 1395–1409. doi:10.1177/0146167209339628

38 Hull, J.G., Draghici, A.M., & Sargent, J.D. (2012). A longitudinal study of risk-glorifying video games and reckless driving. *Psychology of Popular Media Culture, 1*(4), 244. doi:10.1037/a0029510

39 Koepp, M.J., Gunn, R.N., Lawrence, A.D., Cunningham, V.J., Dagher, A., Jones, T., . . . & Grasby, P.M. (1998). Evidence for striatal dopamine release during a video game. *Nature, 393*(6682), 266–267. doi:10.1038/30498

40 Kelly, C.R., Grinband, J., Hirsch, J. (2007). Repeated exposure to media violence is associated with diminished response in an inhibitory frontolimbic network. *PLOS ONE*, 2(12), e1268. doi:10.1371/journal.pone.0001268

41 Yuan, K., Qin, W., Wang, G., Zeng, F., Zhao, L., Yang, X., . . . & Tian, J. (2011). Microstructure abnormalities in adolescents with Internet addiction disorder. *PLOS ONE*, *6*(6), e20708. doi:10.1371/journal.pone.0001268

42 A subsequent study looking specifically at gaming addiction showed abnormalities in cortical thickness. Specifically, increased cortical thickness was found in a range of regions, which correlated with the duration of the gaming addiction (Yuan, K., Cheng, P., Dong, T., Bi, Y., Xing, L., Yu, D., . . . & Tian, J. (2013). Cortical thickness abnormalities in late adolescence with online gaming addiction. *PLOS ONE*, *8*(1), e53055. doi:10.1371/journal.pone.0053055).

43 Kim, Y.R., Son, J.W., Lee, S.I., Shin, C.J., Kim, S.K., Ju, G., . . . & Ha, T.H. (2012). Abnormal brain activation of adolescent Internet addict in a ball-throwing animation task: Possible neural correlates of disembodiment revealed by fMRI. *Progress in Neuro-Psychopharmacology and Biological Psychiatry*, *39*(1), 88–95. doi:10.1016/j.pnpbp.2012.05.013

44 Kim et al., 2012 (see n. 43).

Chapter 16 THE *SOMETHING* ABOUT SURFING

1 Polly, J. (2008, March 22). Surfing the Internet. Retrieved from http://www.netmom.com/about-net-mom/26-surfing-the-internet.html

2 But a brief cautionary note: such a utopian state of affairs must be offset against the consideration that the Internet is only as useful as the information it disseminates. For example, Steve Bratt, now CEO of the World Wide Web Foundation, gave an insightful explanation for the 3.3 billion-person gap between mobile phone users and Internet users. The problem is that, for a person in a developing country, the current Internet is far less useful for everyday life than it might seem: 'Maybe they can look at scores from the playoffs, but if they want to find a local doctor, if they want to understand which crops to plant or how much money they can get for their crops, if they want to be able to teach their kids a language other than English or French or Chinese, there's just nothing for them there' (Kessler, S. (2011, February 4). Why the web is useless in developing countries – and how to fix it [Weblog post]. Retrieved from http://mashable.com/2011/02/04/web-developing-world/).

3 Bohannon, J. (2011, December). *Without Google and Wikipedia I am stupid.* Speech given at Online Educa Berlin, Berlin, Germany.

4 Sparrow, B., Liu, J., & Wegner, D.M. (2011). Google effects on memory: Cognitive consequences of having information at our fingertips. *Science, 333*(6043), 776–778. doi:10.1126/science.1207745

5 Squire, L. R., & Zola, S. M. (1996). Structure and function of declarative and nondeclarative memory systems. *Proceedings of the National Academy of Sciences, 93*(24), 13515–13522. Retrieved from http://www.ncbi.nlm.nih.gov/pmc/articles/PMC33639/

6 Sparrow, Liu, & Wegner, 2011 (see n. 4), p. 776.

7 Small, G.W., Moody, T.D., Siddarth, P., & Bookheimer, S.Y. (2009). Your brain on Google: Patterns of cerebral activation during Internet searching. *American Journal of Geriatric Psychiatry, 17*, 116–126. doi:10.1097/JGP.0b013e3181953a02

8 Eliot, T.S. (1942). Little Gidding. Retrieved from http://www.columbia.edu/itc/history/winter/w3206/edit/tseliotlittlegidding.html

9 Thurber, J. (1939, February 18). Fables for our time – III. *The New Yorker.* Retrieved from http://www.newyorker.com/archive/1939/02/18/1939_02_18_019_TNY_CARDS_000176433, p.19.

10 Desjarlais, M. (2013). Internet exploration behaviours and recovery from unsuccessful actions differ between learners with high and low levels of attention. *Computers in Human Behavior, 29*(3), 694–705. doi:10.1016/j.chb.2012.12.006

11 Nicholas, D., Rowlands, I., Clark, D., & Williams, P. (2011). Google Generation II: Web behaviour experiments with the BBC. *Aslib Proceedings, 63*(1), 28–45. doi:10.1108/00012531111103768, p. 44.

12 In 2011, 86% of the UK Internet population visited a video site at least once. (Experian Hitwise (2011). *Online video: Bringing social media to life*. Retrieved from file:///C:/Users/owner/Downloads/Experian%20Hitwise%20-%20Online%20Video%20Bringing%20Social%20Media%20to%20Life.pdf). In the United States, in August 2012, 188 million people viewed an online video with an average of 22 hours' worth of online video viewing per person that month (comScore (2012, September 19). Online video content reaches all-time high of 188 million viewers [Weblog post]. Retrieved from https://www.comscore.com/esl/Insights/Press_Releases/2012/9/comScore_Releases_August_2012_US_Online_Video_Rankings). The majority of online content viewed is through YouTube, which dominates visits to online video sites. In the past few years, YouTube and other sites for sharing video files over the Internet have soared from obscurity to a pivotal position in the media landscape. Networks fear that the availability of their clips so freely and flexibly will depress television viewing, but unauthorized clips are also free advertising for television shows and, as YouTube has grown quickly,

major networks have responded by making their content available on their own sites.

13 Waldfogel, J. (2009). Lost on the web: Does web distribution stimulate or depress television viewing? *Information Economics and Policy, 21*(2), 158–168. doi:10.1016/j.infoecopol.2008.11.002

14 Watson, R. (2011, January 28). Out and about [Weblog post]. Retrieved from http://toptrends.nowandnext.com/2011/01/28/out-and-about

Chapter 17 THE SCREEN IS THE MESSAGE

1 McLuhan, M. (1994). *Understanding media: The extensions of man*. Cambridge, MA: MIT Press, p. 9.

2 Sellen, A. J., & Harper, R. H. (2003). *The myth of the paperless office*. Cambridge, MA: MIT Press.

3 The study investigated whether there is any difference in comprehension in 15–16-year-olds between reading on a computer screen and in print, and found that students who read in print scored significantly higher on reading comprehension tests than those who read on a screen. A crucial issue was how readily you could get an overview of what was in front of you: readers of the paper text would have immediate access to the text in its entirety. This access, moreover, is built on both visual and tactile cues: the reader can see as well as feel the spatial extension and physical dimensions of the text, as the material substrate of paper provides physical, tactile, spatio-temporally fixed cues to the length of the text that they are about to read. By contrast, those reading on the screen are restricted to seeing and sensing only one page of the text at any given time. Hence, their overview of the organization, structure and flow of the text might be hampered (Mangen, A., Walgermo, B.R., & Brønnick, K. (2013). Reading linear texts on paper versus computer screen: Effects on reading comprehension. *International Journal of Educational Research, 58*, 61–68. doi:10.1016/j.ijer.2012.12.002).

4 Another study of fifth grade students found that they were more efficient reading from a traditional text than scrolling through a computer screen. The researchers suggested that 'difficulties in reading from computers may be due to disrupted mental maps of the text, which may be reflected in poorer understanding and ultimately poorer recall of presented material' (Kerr, M.A., & Symons, S.E. (2006). Computerized presentation of text: Effects on children's reading of informational material. *Reading and Writing, 19*(1), 1–19. doi:10.1007/s11145-003-8128-y).

5 Cataldo, M.G., & Oakhill, J. (2000). Why are poor comprehenders inefficient searchers? An investigation into the effects of text representation and spatial

memory on the ability to locate information in text. *Journal of Educational Psychology, 92*(4), 791–799. doi:10.1037/0022-0663.92.4.791

The permanence of words printed on paper helps the reader by providing unequivocal and fixed spatial cues for text memory and recall. In order to respond appropriately to multiple-choice questions, the subjects in Mangen's study were required to locate, access and retrieve essential pieces of information either on paper or on screen. Comprehension became harder when the information required to complete such a task, like answering questions in a reading comprehension assessment, was not immediately visible, for instance when the reader had to integrate information occurring at locations in a text which were spatially far apart. Such integration requires that the reader has constructed a solid mental representation of the structure of the text. Even with relatively short distances, it is not unreasonable to assume that the fact the reader cannot touch the digital text in the way they touch the pages of a book with their fingers may have challenged their mental reconstruction of the physical layout of the text. In turn, this physical distancing may have impeded their overview as well as ability to access, locate and retrieve required pieces of textual information.

6 For example, e-book technologies based on electronic ink, such as Kindle and Kobo readers, merely reflect light and are hence more reader-friendly with respect to visual ergonomics, while LCD computer screens cause visual fatigue because they emit light. Various studies have gone on to show that certain features of the LCD screen, such as refresh rate, contrast levels and fluctuating light, interfere with cognitive processing and hence potentially impair long-term memory, as well as *computer vision syndrome*, a temporary condition resulting from focusing the eyes on a computer display for protracted, uninterrupted periods of time. Symptoms of this syndrome include headaches, blurred vision, neck pain, redness in the eyes, fatigue, eye strain, dry eyes, irritated eyes, double vision, polyopia and difficulty refocusing the eyes (Blehm, C., Vishnu, S., Khattak, A., Mitra, S., & Yee, R.M. (2005). Computer vision syndrome: A review. *Survey of Opthalmology, 50*(3), 253–262. doi:10.1016/j.survophthal.2005.02.008).

7 Jeong, H. (2012). A comparison of the influence of electronic books and paper books on reading comprehension, eye fatigue, and perception. *Electronic Library, 30*(3), 390–408. doi:10.1108/02640471211241663

8 Carr, N. (2011). *The shallows: What the Internet is doing to our brains*. New York: Norton, p. 118.

9 Rideout, V.J., Foehr, U.G., & Roberts, D.F. (2010). *Generation M^2: Media in the lives of 8- to 18-year-olds*. Retrieved from http://kaiserfamilyfoundation.

wordpress.com/uncategorized/report/generation-m2-media-in-the-lives-of-8-to-18-year-olds/

10 Kessler, S. (2011). 38% of college students can't go 10 minutes without tech. [Weblog post]. Retrieved from http://mashable.com/2011/05/31/college-tech-device-stats/

11 Ophir, E., Nass, C., & Wagner, A.D. (2009). Cognitive control in media multitaskers. *Proceedings of the National Academy of Sciences, 106*(37), 15583–15587. doi:10.1073/pnas.0903620106

12 Gorlick, A. (2009, August 24). Media multitaskers pay mental price, Stanford study shows. Retrieved from http://news.stanford.edu/news/2009/august24/multitask-research-study-082409.html

13 Daniel, D.B., & Woody, W.D. (2013). E-textbooks at what cost? Performance and use of electronic v. print texts. *Computers & Education, 62*, 18–23. doi:10.1016/j.compedu.2012.10.016

14 Kraushaar, J.M., & Novak, D.C. (2010). Examining the effects of student multitasking with laptops during the lecture. *Journal of Information Systems Education, 21*, 241–251. Retrieved from http://jise.org/Contents/Contents-21-2.htm

15 Sana, F., Weston, T., & Cepeda, N.J. (2013). Laptop multitasking hinders classroom learning for both users and nearby peers. *Computers & Education, 62*, 24–31. doi:10.1016/j.compedu.2012.10.003

16 Rosen, L.D., Carrier, L.M., & Cheever, N.A. (2013). Facebook and texting made me do it: Media-induced task-switching while studying. *Computers in Human Behavior, 29*(3), 948–958. doi:10.1016/j.chb.2012.12.001

17 Junco, R., & Cotten, S.R. (2011). Perceived academic effects of instant messaging use. *Computers & Education, 56*(2), 370–378. doi:10.1016/j.compedu.2010.08.020

18 Rosen, Carrier, & Cheever, 2013 (see n. 16). Kirschner, P.A., & Karpinski, A.C. (2010). Facebook and academic performance. *Computers in Human Behavior, 26*(6), 1237–1245. doi:10.1016/j.chb.2010.03.024

19 Kirschner & Karpinski, 2010 (see n. 18).

20 Bowman, L.L., Levine, L.E., Waite, B.M., & Gendron, M. (2010). Can students really multitask? An experimental study of instant messaging while reading. *Computers & Education, 54*(4), 927–931. doi:10.1016/j.compedu.2009.09.024

21 A similar kind of study recruited participants who completed a reading comprehension task either uninterrupted or while concurrently holding an instant messaging conversation. Multi-taskers took significantly longer to complete the task, indicating that concurrent instant messaging use impaired efficiency. However, while there were no differences between groups in reading comprehension scores, the more time participants

reported spending on instant messaging the lower their reading comprehension scores. Additionally, the more time participants reported spending on instant messaging the lower their self-reported GPA (Fox, A.B., Rosen, J., & Crawford, M. (2009). Distractions, distractions: does instant messaging affect college students' performance on a concurrent reading comprehension task? *CyberPsychology & Behaviour, 12*(1), 51–53. doi:10.1089/cpb.2008.0107).

22 DeStefano, D., & LeFevre, J.A. (2007). Cognitive load in hypertext reading: A review. *Computers in Human Behavior, 23*, 1616–1641. doi:10.1016/j.chb.2005.08.012

23 Ackerman, R., & Goldsmith, M. (2011). Metacognitive regulation of text learning: On screen versus on paper learning. *Journal of Experimental Psychology: Applied, 17*(1), 18–32. doi:10.1037/a0022086, p. 29.

24 Liu, Z. (2005). Reading behavior in the digital environment: Changes in reading behavior over the past ten years. *Journal of Documentation, 61*(6), 700–712. doi:10.1016/j.chb.2005.08.012

25 Kretzschmar, F., Pleimling, D., Hosemann, J., Füssel, S., Bornkessel-Schlesewsky, I., & Schlesewsky, M. (2013). Subjective impressions do not mirror online reading effort: concurrent EEG-eyetracking evidence from the reading of books and digital media. *PLOS ONE, 8*(2), e56178. doi:10.1371/journal.pone.0056178

26 Daniel & Woody, 2013 (see n. 13).

27 Morse, D., Tardival, G.M., & Spicer, J. (1996). *A comparison of the effectiveness of a dichotomous key and a multi-access key to woodlice*. Technical Report 14-96. Retrieved from kar.kent.ac.uk/21343/1/WoodliceMorse.pdf

28 Farrell, N. (2013, January 7). Ebook craze is slowing [Weblog post]. Retrieved from http://news.techeye.net/internet/ebook-craze-is-slowing

29 Indvik, L. (2012, June 18). Ebook sales surpass hardcover for the first time in U.S. [Weblog post]. Retrieved from http://mashable.com/2012/06/17/ebook-hardcover-sales/

30 Flood, A. (2013, February 22). Decline in independent bookshops continues with 73 closures in 2012. Retrieved from http://www.theguardian.com/books/2013/feb/22/independent-bookshops-73-closures-2012

31 Smith, G.E., Housen, P., Yaffe, K., Ruff, R., Kennison, R.F., Mahncke, H.W., & Zelinski, E.M. (2009). A cognitive training program designed based on principles of brain plasticity: Results from the improvement in memory with plasticity-based adaptive cognitive training study. *Journal of the American Geriatrics Society, 57*, 594–603. doi:10.1111/j.1532-5415.2008.02167.x. Thorell, L.B., Lindqvist, S., Nutley, S.B., Bohlin, G. & Klingberg, T. (2009). Training and transfer effects of executive functions

in preschool children. *Developmental Science, 12*, 106–113. doi:10.1111/j.1467-7687.2008.00745.x

32 Owen, A.M., Hampshire, A., Grahn, J.A., Stenton, R., Dajani, S., Burns, A.S. . . . & Ballard, C.G. (2010). Putting brain training to the test. *Nature, 465*(7299), 775–778. doi:10.1038/nature09042

33 Lee, K.M., Jeong, E.J., Park, N., & Ryu, S. (2011). Effects of interactivity in educational games: A mediating role of social presence on learning outcomes. *International Journal of Human-Computer Interaction, 27*(7), 620–633. doi:10.1080/10447318.2011.555302

34 Tanenhaus, J. (n.d.). Computers and special needs: Enhancing self esteem and language. Retrieved from www.kidneeds.com/diagnostic_categories/articles/computers.pdf

35 Kagohara D.M., van der Meer, L., Ramdoss, D., O'Reilly, M.F., Lancioni, G.E., Davis, T.N., . . . & Sigafoos, J. (2013). Using iPods and iPads in teaching programs for individuals with developmental disabilities: A systematic review. *Research in Developmental Disabilities, 34*(1), 147–156. doi:10.1016/j.ridd.2012.07.027

36 Li, Q., & Ma, X. (2010). A meta-analysis of the effects of computer technology on school students' mathematics learning. *Educational Psychology Review*, 22, 215–243. doi:10.1007/s10648-010-9125-8

37 Cheung, A.C.K., & Slavin, R.E. (2012). How features of educational technology applications affect student reading outcomes: A meta-analysis. *Educational Research Review*, 7(3), 198–215. doi:10.1016/j.edurev.2012.05.002

38 Gosper, M., Green, D., McNeil, M., Phillips, R., Preston, G. & Woo, K. (2008). *The impact of web-based lecture technologies on current and future practices in learning and teaching*. Retrieved from http://mq.edu.au/ltc/altc/wblt/docs/report/ce6-22_final2.pdf

39 Massingham, P., & Herrington, T. (2006). Does attendance matter? An examination of student attitudes, participation, performance and attendance. *Journal of University Teaching and Learning Practice, 3*(2), 82–103. Retrieved from http://ro.uow.edu.au/jutlp/vol3/iss2/3

40 Brown, B.W., & Liedholm, C.E. (2002). Can web courses replace the classroom in principles of microeconomics? *American Economic Review Papers and Proceedings*, 92(2), 444–448. Retrieved from http://www.jstor.org/stable/3083447

41 Figlio, D.N., Rush, M., & Yin, L. (2010). *Is it live or is it Internet? Experimental estimates of the effects of online instruction on student learning*. NBER Working Paper No. w16089. Retrieved from http://www.nber.org/papers/w16089.pdf

42 Korat, O., & Shamir, A. (2007). Electronic books versus adult readers:

Effects on children's emergent literacy as a function of social class. *Journal of Computer Assisted Learning, 23*(3), 248–259. doi:10.1111/j.1365-2729.2006.00213.x

43 Li & Ma, 2010 (see n. 36).

44 Lai, E. (2012, October 16). Chart: Top 100 iPad rollouts by enterprises & schools [Weblog post]. Retrieved from http://www.forbes.com/sites/sap/2012/08/31/top-50-ipad-rollouts-by-enterprises-schools/

45 Ramachandran, V. (2013, June 20). Apple scores $30m iPad deal with L.A. schools [Weblog post]. Retrieved from http://mashable.com/2013/06/19/la-ipad-tablets-in-schools/

46 Hu, W. (2011, January 4). Math that moves: Schools embrace the iPad. Retrieved from http://www.nytimes.com/2011/01/05/education/05tablets.html?pagewanted=all&_r=0

47 Harris, S. (2012, May 29). The iPad generation: Pupils as young as four taught lessons with a touchscreen. Retrieved from http://www.dailymail.co.uk/news/article-2151403/The-iPad-generation-Pupils-young-taught-lessons-touchscreen.html

48 Paton, G. (2012, November 12). Teachers' obsession with technology sees gadgets worth millions sit in cupboards. Retrieved from http://www.telegraph.co.uk/news/9681828/Teachers-obsession-with-technology-sees-gadgets-worth-millions-sit-in-cupboards.html

49 Furió, D., González-Gancedo, S., Juan, M., Seguí, I., & Rando, N. (2013). Evaluation of learning outcomes using an educational iPhone game vs. traditional game. *Computers & Education, 64*, 1–23. doi:10.1016/j.compedu.2012.12.001

50 Sung, E., & Mayer, R.E. (2013). Online multimedia learning with mobile devices and desktop computers: An experimental test of Clark's methods-not-media hypothesis. *Computers in Human Behavior, 29*(3), 639–647. doi:10.1016/j.chb.2012.10.022

51 Richtel, M. (2011, October 22). A Silicon Valley school that doesn't compute. Retrieved from http://www.nytimes.com/2011/10/23/technology/at-waldorf-school-in-silicon-valley-technology-can-wait.html?pagewanted=all

52 Richtel, 2011 (see n. 51).

53 Clark, C., & Hawkins, L. (2010). Young people's reading: The importance of the home environment and family support. Retrieved from http://www.literacytrust.org.uk/assets/0000/4954/Young_People_s_Reading_2010.pdf

54 Topping, K. (2013). What kids are reading: The book-reading habits of students in British schools 2013. Retrieved from http://www.readforpleasure.co.uk/documents/2013wkar_fullreport_lowres.pdf

Chapter 18 THINKING DIFFERENTLY

1 For example, a basic feature of screen-based interaction is the directory tree. This unprecedented constraining of options has become so much a normal part of our lives that we no longer question it, even when we are not sitting directly in front of a screen. Everyone knows the frustration of calling an organisation and having our query not dealt with by a real human being, but by an automated answering system that inevitably gives us a fixed menu of options with different numbers to press. These directory trees could become the pattern of daily life as we try to gather information, offering us menus with a fixed number of possibilities, where, in order to get to an option that is not immediately presented, we have to plod up and down through various branch lines of categories and sub-categories. Given that the human brain becomes good, and is good only, at what it rehearses, perhaps all that up and down toing and froing will leave a significant mark on our erstwhile flexible brain processes and, in particular, how we approach problems. Such a rigid and systematic strategy may, on the one hand, impart a certain rigour and logic to our debating ability but, on the other hand, turn out to be highly restrictive.

2 There are many different kinds of IQ tests using a wide variety of methods. Some are visual, some verbal; some use abstract reasoning problems, and still others concentrate on arithmetic, spatial imagery, reading, vocabulary, memory or general knowledge. Modern comprehensive IQ tests no longer give a single score. Although they still provide an overall rating, they also give values for different abilities, identifying particular strengths and weaknesses of an individual's brain power.

3 Kurzweil, R. (2005). *The singularity is near: When humans transcend biology*. New York: Penguin.

4 Benyamin, B., Pourcain, B., Davis, O.S., Davies, G., Hansell, N.K., Brion, M.J., . . . & Visscher, P.M. (2013). Childhood intelligence is heritable, highly polygenic and associated with FNBP1L. *Molecular Psychiatry, 19*(2), 253–258. doi:10.1038/mp.2012.184

5 This figure fits well with the calculation of Roger Gosden in his book *Designing Babies*, where he gives an estimate of 0.3 for inheritability of IQ, where a score of 0 indicates a trait attributable entirely to environmental factors and 1 a trait attributable just to genes. However, the crucial issue is that even the inherited component of IQ is the result of many different and diverse genes. If a major gene *for* IQ were suddenly to be discovered, it would only account for some 5% at most and therefore boost an IQ score of 100 to a paltry 101.5 (Gosden, R.G. (1999). *Designing babies: The brave new world of reproductive technology*. New York: Freeman).

[6] Flynn, J.R. (2006). The Flynn effect: Rethinking intelligence and what affects it. In *Introduction to the Psychology of Individual Differences*. Porto Alegre, Brazil: ArtMed.

[7] Johnson, S. (2006). *Everything bad is good for you: How today's popular culture is actually making us smarter*. New York: Penguin.

[8] Pernille Olesen and his colleagues at the Karolinska Institute in Sweden investigated the changes in brain activity induced by working memory training. Experiments were carried out in which healthy adult human subjects practised working memory tasks for five weeks. Brain activity was measured with functional magnetic resonance imaging (fMRI) before, during and after training. After training, brain activity that was related to working memory had indeed increased in key parts of the outer layer of the brain, the cortex (Olesen, P.J., Westerberg, H., & Klingberg, T. (2003). Increased prefrontal and parietal activity after training of working memory. *Nature Neuroscience, 7*(1), 75–79. doi:10.1038/nn1165).

[9] Johnson, 2006 (see n. 7), p. 39.

[10] Paton, G. (2010, October 16). Facebook 'encourages children to spread gossip and insults'. Retrieved from http://www.telegraph.co.uk/education/educationnews/8067093/Facebook-encourages-children-to-spread-gossip-and-insults.html

[11] Dickens, C. (2007). *Hard times*. New York: Pocket Books, p. 1.

[12] This notion of real understanding as opposed to information processing fits in well with the distinction of 'crystallised' as opposed to 'fluid' intelligence, the terms first developed by Raymond Cattell (see Chapter 7) (Cattell, R.B. (Ed.) (1987). *Intelligence: Its structure, growth and action*. Amsterdam: Elsevier).

[13] Flynn, 2006 (see n. 6).

[14] Flynn, J.R. (1987). Massive IQ gains in 14 nations: What IQ tests really measure. *Psychological Bulletin, 101*, 171–191. Retrieved from http://www.iapsych.com/iqmr/fe/LinkedDocuments/flynn1987.pdf. Flynn, J.R. (1994). *IQ gains over time*. In R.J. Sternberg (Ed.), *Encyclopedia of human intelligence* (pp. 617–623). New York: Macmillan. Geake, J.G. (2008). The neurobiology of giftedness. Retrieved from http://hkage.org.hk/b5/events/080714%20APCG/01-%20Keynotes%20%26%20Invited%20Addresses/1.6%20Geake_The%20Neurobiology%20of%20Giftedness.pdf

[15] Flynn, 1994 (see n. 14).

[16] Flynn, 1994 (see n. 14).

[17] Song, M., Zhou, Y., Li, J., Liu, Y., Tian, L., Yu, C., & Jiang, T. (2008). Brain spontaneous functional connectivity and intelligence. *Neuroimage, 41*(3), 1168–1176. doi:10.1016/j.neuroimage.2008.02.036

18 Janowsky, J.S., Shimamura, A.P., & Squire, L.R. (1989). Source memory impairment in patients with frontal lobe lesions. *Neuropsychologia, 27*(8), 1043–1056. doi:10.1016/0028-3932(89)90184-X

19 Gabriel, S., & Young, A.F. (2011). Becoming a vampire without being bitten: The narrative collective-assimilation hypothesis. *Psychological Science*, 22(8), 990–994. doi:10.1177/0956797611415541, p. 993.

20 Quoted in Flood, A. (2011, September 7). Reading fiction 'improves empathy' study finds. *Guardian*. Retrieved from http://www.theguardian.com/books/2011/sep/07/reading-fiction-empathy-study

21 Macintyre, B. (2009, November 5). The Internet is killing storytelling. Retrieved from http://www.thetimes.co.uk/tto/opinion/columnists/benmacintyre/article2044914.ece

22 Scohnfeld. E. (2009, March 7). Eric Schmidt tells Charlie Rose Google is 'unlikely' to buy Twitter and wants to turn phones into TVs [Weblog post]. Retrieved from http://techcrunch.com/2009/03/07/eric-schmidt-tells-charlie-rose-google-is-unlikely-to-buy-twitter-and-wants-to-turn-phones-into-tvs/

23 Sass, L. (2001). Schizophrenia, modernism, and the 'creative imagination': On creativity and psychopathology. *Creativity Research, 13*(1), 55–74. doi:10.1207/S15326934CRJ1301_7

24 Burnet's clonal selection hypothesis explains how the immune system combats infection by selecting certain types of B and T lymphocytes for the destruction of specific antigens invading the body.

25 van Rheenen, E. (2014, January 2). 12 predictions Isaac Asimov made about 2014 in 1964. Retrieved from http://mentalfloss.com/article/54343/12-predictions-isaac-asimov-made-about-2014-1964

Chapter 19 MIND CHANGE BEYOND THE SCREEN

1 Office for National Statistics (2012). *What are the chances of surviving to age 100?* Retrieved from http://www.ons.gov.uk/ons/dcp171776_260525.pdf

2 While there may not be single genes for complex mental traits, there are specific genes and genetic profiles for certain diseases such as cystic fibrosis and the degenerative neurological disorder, Huntington's disease. As we saw in Chapter 5, genes don't work in isolation but need the context of the brain and body and the environment to manifest, but the fact remains that a faulty gene will occasionally lead directly, or most often indirectly, to some kind of correspondingly faulty outcome. So, although genes are usually not the whole story, the detection of a malfunctioning gene can have significant

health benefits. The genetically based technologies therefore hold out the very real promise of bespoke medication, fitted to an individual's particular genetic profile so that side effects can be minimised (pharmacogenomics). Even better, an individual's particular risk factors for certain diseases can be predicted by screening their genome for preventive measures (lifestyle, diet or treatment), which can then start as soon as possible (What is pharmacogenomics? (2013, August 12). Retrieved from http://ghr.nlm.nih.gov/handbook/genomicresearch/pharmacogenomics).

3 *Regenerative medicine* is a therapy that offers another exciting and realistic alternative, as well as providing a very valuable tool to gain a better understanding of the diseases themselves. The rationale is completely different from conventional treatments. The idea is not to treat the symptoms but to harness biological mechanisms that convert basic all-purpose stem cells which are injected into the region of the body where the specialised types of cells are deficient. Stem cells, derived from the microscopic ball of some 200 that make up the early stage embryo, are extraordinary because they have the capacity to produce every single type of cell in the body, whether of the heart, bone or even brain. This regenerative strategy does not try to compensate for the aberrant effects of a disease as a result of cell death, but from the get-go it actually provides substitutes, generating new cells and supporting ailing cells with the natural chemicals produced by the newcomers. In this way, stem cell therapy brings us that bit closer to a real cure for a whole range of diseases, such as the degenerative movement disorder Parkinson's disease, but not for Alzheimer's disease, where the sites of damage are too widespread (Pera, R.A.R., & Gleeson, J.G. (2008). Stem cells and regeneration [Special review issue]. *Human Molecular Genetics, 17*(R1), R1–R2. doi:10.1093/hmg/ddn186).

4 Knapp, M., & Prince, M. (2007). *Dementia UK*. Retrieved from http://www.alzheimers.org.uk/site/scripts/download.php?fileID=1

5 Prince, M., Bryce, R., Albanese, E., Wimo, A., Ribeiro, W., & Ferri, C. P. (2013). The global prevalence of dementia: A systematic review and metaanalysis. *Alzheimer's & Dementia, 9*(1), 63–75. Retrieved from http://www.sciencedirect.com/science/article/pii/S1552526012025319

6 Hurd, M.D., Martorell, P., Delavande, A., Mullen, K.J., & Langa, K.M. (2013). Monetary costs of dementia in the United States. *New England Journal of Medicine, 368*(14), 1326–1334. doi:10.1056/NEJMsa1204629

7 Atkins, S. (2013). *First steps in living with dementia*. Oxford: Lion Hudson.

8 Currently, the diagnosis of Alzheimer's disease is based provisionally on symptoms, and ultimately on post-mortem histological verification. By the time the patient presents with the characteristic cognitive impairments,

extensive atrophy of the affected brain regions has typically already been underway for some ten or even twenty years. Arguably, there has been no dramatically different new drug introduced to combat Alzheimer's disease specifically, or neurodegenerative disorders more generally since 1996, when approval from the United States Food and Drug Administration (USFDA) was granted for donepezil under the brand *Aricept*. The reason is that there is as yet no accepted or proven basic mechanism that could consequently be targeted pharmaceutically. One well-established idea is that the key problem is a deficit of a certain chemical messenger, the transmitter acetylcholine, as a result of the death of specific neurons where it is operational (Bartus, R.T., Dean, R.L., Pontecorvo, M.J., & Flicker, C. (1985). The cholinergic hypothesis: A historical overview, current perspective, and future directions. *Annals of the New York Academy of Sciences*, *444*(1), 332–358. doi:10.1111/j.1749-6632.1985.tb37600.x. Terry, A.V., & Buccafusco, J.J. (2003). The cholinergic hypothesis of age and Alzheimer's disease-related cognitive deficits: Recent challenges and their implications for novel drug development. *Journal of Pharmacology and Experimental Therapeutics*, *306*(3), 821–827). Hence the treatment of choice at the moment is Aricept (or an equivalent such as galantamine, sold, for example, as Reminyl), a drug which temporarily boosts levels of the dwindling transmitter acetylcholine by protecting it from normal enzymatic degradation. However, this theory fails to account for a well-known discrepancy: not all areas of the brain affected by Alzheimer's use acetylcholine, nor are all acetylcholine-using areas of the brain affected by the disease. Not surprisingly, therefore, Aricept does not prevent the continuing death of cells, since it merely tackles just one biochemical symptom.

The other main contender for accounting for the process of neurodegeneration is the *amyloid hypothesis*, where neuronal death is attributed to disruption of the cell structure by toxic deposits of a substance named after the Greek for starch, *amyloid*, which is characteristic of the post-mortem Alzheimer brain (Hardy, J., & Allsop, D. (1991). Amyloid deposition as the central event in the aetiology of Alzheimer's disease. *Trends in Pharmacological Sciences*, *12*, 383–388. doi:10.1016/0165-6147(91)90609-V. Hardy, J.A., & Higgins, G.A. (1992). Alzheimer's disease: The amyloid cascade hypothesis. *Science*, 256(5054), 184–185. doi:10.1126/science.1566067. Pákáski, M., & Kálmán, J. (2008). Interactions between the amyloid and cholinergic mechanisms in Alzheimer's disease. *Neurochemistry International*, *53*(5), 103–111. doi:10.1016/j.neuint.2008.06.005). However, the amyloid hypothesis does not explain the fact that only certain cells are vulnerable in neurodegenerative diseases, the absence of amyloid deposits in some otherwise faithful animal models of dementia, or indeed the occurrence post-mortem of amyloid in the healthy non-Alzheimer brain. Again, it is small wonder that, despite the popularity of amyloid formation as a pharmaceutical target since the 1990s, no treatment based on this theory has yet proved effective in the clinic.

9 Of course many neuroscientists, including my own group, have their own ideas as to what this crucial, pivotal neurodegenerative process may be. For a technical review of our group research on dementia, see Greenfield, S. (2013). Discovering and targeting the basic mechanism of neurodegeneration: The role of peptides from the C-terminus of acetylcholinesterase. *Chemico-biological Interactions, 203(3),* 543–546. doi:10.1016/j.cbi.2013.03.015

10 Baker, R. (1999). *Sex in the future: Ancient urges meet future technology.* London: Macmillan.

11 Rosegrant, S. (n.d.). The new retirement: No retirement? [Weblog post]. Retrieved from http://home.isr.umich.edu/sampler/the-new-retirement/

12 Forecasts from *The Futurist* magazine. (n.d.). Retrieved from http://www.wfs.org/Forecasts_From_The_Futurist_Magazine

13 Glass (n.d.). Retrieved from http://www.google.com/glass/start/

14 The actual term 'augmented reality' is believed to have been coined by Professor Tom Caudell, working for Boeing, and first used in 1990. Since then a variety of applications of increasing sophistication have been developed, culminating in Google Glass (Sung, D. (2011, March 1). The history of augmented reality [Weblog post]. Retrieved from http://www.pocket-lint.com/news/108888-the-history-of-augmented-reality).

15 Graham, M., Zook, M., & Boulton, A. (2012). Augmented reality in urban places: Contested content and the duplicity of code. *Transactions of the Institute of British Geographers*, *38*(3), 464–479. doi:10.1111/j.1475-5661.2012.00539.x

16 ABI Research (2013, February 21). Wearable computing devices, like Apple's iWatch, will exceed 485 million annual shipments by 2018. Retrieved from https://www.abiresearch.com/press/wearable-computing-devices-like-apples-iwatch-will

17 Lookout (2012). *Mobile mindset study.* Retrieved from https://www.lookout.com/resources/reports/mobile-mindset

18 Securenvoy (2012, February 16). 66% of the population suffer from nomophobia: The feat of being without their phone [Weblog post]. Retrieved from http://www.securenvoy.com/blog/2012/02/16/66-of-the-population-suffer-from-nomophobia-the-fear-of-being-without-their-phone/

19 Keen, A. (2013, February 26). Why life through Google Glass should be for our eyes only [Weblog post]. Retrieved from http://edition.cnn.com/2013/02/25/tech/innovation/google-glass-privacy-andrew-keen

20 Haworth, A. (2013, October 20). Why have young people in Japan stopped having sex? Retrieved from http://www.theguardian.com/world/2013/oct/20/young-people-japan-stopped-having-sex. Low birthrate could slash South Korea's youth population in half by 2060: Report. (2013, January 8). Retrieved from http://www.japantimes.co.jp/news/2013/01/08/asia-pacific/low-birthrate-could-slash-south-koreas-youth-population-in-half-by-2060-report/
21 Haworth, 2013 (see n. 20).
22 Haworth, 2013 (see n. 20).
23 Trends in obesity prevalence (n.d.). Retrieved from http://www.noo.org.uk/NOO_about_obesity/trends

Chapter 20 MAKING CONNECTIONS

1 Wang, Y. (2013, March 25). More people have cell phones than toilets U.N. study shows. Retrieved from http://newsfeed.time.com/2013/03/25/more-people-have-cell-phones-than-toilets-u-n-study-shows/#ixzz2cEZUrSIF
2 Frequently asked questions (2007, April 10). Retrieved from http://www-03.ibm.com/ibm/history/documents/pdf/faq.pdf
3 Haldane, J.B.S. (1923). *Daedalus: Or, science and the future*. London: Kegan Paul. Retrieved from http://vserver1.cscs.lsa.umich.edu/~crshalizi/Daedalus.html
4 Haldane, 1923 (see n. 3).
5 Quoted in Apt46 (2011, May 18). Socrates was against writing [Weblog post]. Retrieved from http://apt46.net/2011/05/18/socrates-was-against-writing/
6 Muir, E. (1952). The horses. Retrieved from http://www.poemhunter.com/best-poems/edwin-muir/the-horses/
7 Bettelheim, B. (1959). Joey: A 'mechanical boy'. Retrieved from http://www.weber.edu/wsuimages/psychology/FacultySites/Horvat/Joey.PDF
8 Oxford dictionaries word of the year (2013, November 19). Retrieved from http://blog.oxforddictionaries.com/press-releases/oxford-dictionaries-word-of-the-year-2013/
9 James, O. (2008). *Affluenza*. London: Vermilion.
10 Russell, B. (1924). Icarus or the future of science. Retrieved from http://www.marxists.org/reference/subject/philosophy/works/en/russell2.htm
11 Criado-Perez, C. (2013, August 7). Diary: Internet trolls, Twitter rape threats and putting Jane Austen on our banknotes. Retrieved from http://www.newstatesman.com/2013/08/internet-trolls-twitter-rape-threats-and-putting-jane-austen-our-banknotes

12 Zimmer, B. (2012, April 26). What is YOLO? Only teenagers know for sure. Retrieved from http://www.bostonglobe.com/ideas/2012/08/25/what-yolo-only-teenagers-know-for-sure/Idso04FecrYzLa4KOOYpXO/story.html

13 I've previously dubbed the three basic tendencies for self-expression: *someone* (the drive for status), where you are individual but not fulfilled; *anyone* (the appeal of the collective identity as previously exemplified in various political movements such as fascism and communism); *nobody* (the need for abnegating the sense of self and living in/for the moment). See Greenfield, S. (2008). *I.D.: The quest for meaning in the 21st century*. London: Hodder & Stoughton.

14 Examples of such software might include:

Other people's minds. The aim here would be to combat problems in empathy. The experience would start with a conventional visual sequence of fast-moving events, driven by the user. The speed of the images would be slowed incrementally, with longer periods introduced for speech, then conversation. Note that it would be valuable for such software to use voices with different inflections, recreating the experience of prosody. Questions would be inserted intermittently, querying the various outcomes that might potentially result from what the different people in the ongoing scene might do, and progressing according to what these suggest. Previous performance would set the skill level for empathy.

What does it all mean? Building up over time, this would become an individual's conceptual framework. The user enters random ideas – brainstorming or, indeed, as if blogging, interesting facts learned, even titles of books read. An individual framework would be developed that then feeds into other responses/activities; e.g. the notion 'the government is betraying us' might be cross-referenced with other examples within the existing personal framework, then to a wider, more objective database. Evaluations would show progress based on the understanding of abstract ideas, but from an individual perspective.

Consequences. The idea here would be to reinforce the message that, after all, actions really do have consequences. It would consist of a suite of games in which permanent change results from action: for example, if someone is shot dead, they remain dead thereafter. For every action, such as being shot, the programme would cut to real-life footage that includes a brief report from someone on what it actually feels like to be shot or bereaved, for example.

Imagine. The idea here would be to tackle the constraints imposed by anything from PowerPoint to word processing to company answerphone messages, all suggesting that life has only a fixed number of options. So, no menus! The starting point is a word/idea/action of the user's own that freely links to anything else and is prompted by previous entries across the whole range of other programmes. Icons/pictures of the entry are slowly replaced by words/voice. Over time, the entries build up into an increasingly complex, evolving conceptual framework.

My life story. The aim is to reclaim a sense of privacy. It would be a Facebook-type activity, *but* for the user only, and locked into real time. Since this 'diary' will be impossible to share with anyone else, the user will develop a sense of privacy and an enduring sense of self with a clear narrative that the user learns does not require feedback or comments from others. It may be best appreciated as a smartphone app, in which the user could can confide wherever and whenever they wished.

Who am I? This would be an attempt to bolster up a sense of identity. Here there would be feedback to the user based on the user's inputs over time. As performance on the whole range of activities accumulates, an analysis of the responses builds up of the types of personality traits emerging and/or changing.

FURTHER READING

Atkins, S. (2013). *First steps to living with dementia.* Oxford: Lion.

Baker, R. (1999). *Sex in the future: Ancient urges meet future technology.* London: Macmillan.

Begley, S. (2008). *The plastic mind.* London: Constable & Robinson.

Bowlby J. (1969). *Attachment and loss*, Vol. 1: *Loss.* New York: Basic Books.

Carr, N. (2011). *The shallows: What the Internet is doing to our brains.* New York: Norton.

Flynn, J.R. (2006). The Flynn Effect: Rethinking intelligence and what affects it. In *Introduction to the Psychology of Individual Differences.* Porto Alegre, Brazil: ArtMed.

Frost, J.L. (2010). *A history of children's play and play environments: Toward a contemporary child-saving movement.* New York: Routledge.

Gentile, D.A. (Ed.) (2003). *Media violence and children: A complete guide for parents and professionals*. Westport, CT: Praeger.

Gosden, R.G. (1999). *Designing babies: The brave new world of reproductive technology*. New York: Freeman.

Greenfield, S. (2011). *You and me: The neuroscience of identity*. London: Notting Hill.

Greenfield, S.A. (2001). *The private life of the brain: Emotions, consciousness, and the secret of the self*. New York: Wiley.

Greenfield, S.A. (2007). *I.D.: The quest for meaning in the 21st Century*. London: Hodder.

Harkaway, N. (2012). *The blind giant: Being human in a digital world*. London: Vintage.

Johnson, S. (2006). *Everything bad is good for you: How today's popular culture is actually making us smarter*. New York: Penguin.

Keen, A. (2007). *The cult of the amateur*. London: Nicholas Brealey.

Kurzweil, R. (2005). *The singularity is near: When humans transcend biology*. New York: Penguin.

McLuhan, M. (1994). *Understanding media: The extensions of man*. Cambridge, MA: MIT Press.

Palmer, S. (2007). *Toxic childhood: How the modern world is damaging our children and what we can do about it*. London: Orion.

Pickren, W., & Rutherford, A. (2010). *A history of modern psychology in context*. Hoboken, NJ: Wiley.

Purves, D., Augustine, G.J., Fitzpatrick, D., Hall, W.C., LaMantia, A.S., & White, L.E. (Eds.) (2012). *Neuroscience* (5th ed.). Sunderland, MA: Sinauer.

Rosen, L.D. (2012). *iDisorder: Understanding our obsession with technology and overcoming its hold on us*. New York: Macmillan.

Sellen, A. J., & Harper, R. H. (2003). *The myth of the paperless office*. Cambridge, MA: MIT Press.

Turkle, S. (2011). *Alone together: Why we expect more from technology and less from each other*. New York: Basic Books.

Watson, R. (2010). *Future files: A brief history of the next 50 years*. London: Nicholas Brealey.

ACKNOWLEDGEMENTS

I would like to thank, more than anyone, Dr Olivia Metcalf: as soon as I sent her the first draft of *Mind Change* with the tentative request that she might be able to help me with the references, she committed immediately to be 'in this for the long haul': this was just as well since the volume of reports and papers to sift through turned out to be far greater than either of us had anticipated. It is no exaggeration to say that Olivia has completely raised the game of the book. Through the endless email iterations between Oxford and Melbourne she has been more conscientious, constructively critical and enthusiastic than I could ever have dreamed. However, the book itself would not even have been started were it not for Will Murphy at Random House New York, who had the original idea and approached me with an invitation. I'm enormously grateful to him, his colleague Mika Kasuga, and more immediately to Judith Kendra at Random House UK for all the detailed help and advice they have given over the last two years. I'd also like to thank my good friend Professor Clive Coen for proof-reading the final draft of the MS. Finally, it would be impossible for me to write any book at all without the unflagging support and fantastic friendship of my agent, Caroline Michel. *Mind Change* is dedicated to Professor John Stein FRCP, for his backing me unstintingly both professionally and personally for over 35 years. John is the best example possible of the definition of a mentor: 'someone who believes in you more than you believe in yourself'.

INDEX